COVID-19 in Dental Practice

S. R. Prabhu • Amrita Pattanaik
Shankargouda Patil
Lakshman Samaranayake • S. M. Balaji
Editors

COVID-19 in Dental Practice

A Reference Manual for Oral Healthcare Professionals

Springer

Editors
S. R. Prabhu
School of Dentistry
University of Queensland
Brisbane, QLD, Australia

Amrita Pattanaik
National Institute of Mental Health and Neuro Sciences (NIMHANS)
Bengaluru, India

Shankargouda Patil
College of Dental Medicine
Roseman University of Health Sciences
South Jordan, UT, USA

Lakshman Samaranayake
University of Hong Kong
Faculty of Dentistry
Hong Kong, Hong Kong

S. M. Balaji
Balaji Dental & Craniofacial Hospital and Research Institute
Chennai, Tamil Nadu, India

ISBN 978-3-032-25999-8 ISBN 978-3-032-26000-0 (eBook)
https://doi.org/10.1007/978-3-032-26000-0

This Springer imprint is published by the registered company Springer Nature Switzerland AG
The registered company address is: Gewerbestrasse 11, 6330 Cham, Switzerland

- *Religious diversity* is associated with fewer cases and substantially fewer deaths, potentially reflecting stronger community networks and cooperative norms.
- *Female leadership* is associated with reductions in both morbidity and mortality, with a more pronounced effect on mortality. While the magnitudes are modest, these findings suggest that communication style, trust-building, and inclusive governance may influence public behaviour and policy effectiveness during crises.
- *Technology use* presents a nuanced pattern, increasing infections but slightly reducing mortality, consistent with greater mobility alongside improved detection, tracing, and health communication.

Taken together, the comparison of Figs. 3.2 and 3.3 reveals that COVID-19 outcomes were shaped less by short-term policy choices alone and more by long-standing national characteristics that governed exposure, vulnerability, and system response. Factors that increased infections often also increased deaths, but health system capacity, governance quality, and prior epidemic experience were especially important in breaking the link between widespread transmission and fatal outcomes. This integrated perspective reinforces the central message of the chapter: pandemic resilience is deeply structural, rooted in demographic composition, institutional strength, and social capacity that predate the crisis itself.

While this section has focused on the framework and findings of Chang et al. [1], these patterns are not unique to a single study. A growing body of cross-country research has examined similar questions using alternative data, methodologies, and outcome measures, including excess mortality, vaccination uptake, and non-pharmaceutical interventions. The following section situates the Chang et al. [1] results within this broader literature, highlighting areas of convergence, extension, and nuance that further illuminate why countries experienced such divergent pandemic trajectories.

3.2.6 Evidence from Other Cross-Country Studies

Beyond the framework developed by Chang et al. [1], a rapidly expanding cross-country literature has examined why national experiences of the COVID-19 pandemic diverged so sharply. Collectively, these studies reinforce the central role of structural conditions while also highlighting how policy choices, behavioural responses, and institutional quality interact with those foundations.

A prominent strand of this literature emphasises measurement and governance. Using data from seventy-two countries, Nojković et al. [2] compare official COVID-19 mortality, excess mortality, and the gap between the two. Their analysis shows that lower excess mortality was achieved in countries with stricter epidemiological measures, higher vaccination rates, stronger health systems, younger populations, and more democratic institutions. Importantly, they demonstrate that official death statistics were more susceptible to manipulation in autocratic regimes, leading them to conclude that excess mortality provides a more reliable indicator of pandemic performance.

Other studies explicitly distinguish between intrinsic national characteristics and actionable policy levers. Sun et al. [3] apply a gradient boosting approach to excess deaths across eighty countries, separating structural features such as demography and baseline health from policy-related factors including vaccination uptake, public trust, and health interventions. Their findings show that actionable public health measures substantially improve explanatory and predictive power beyond intrinsic characteristics alone, with vaccination rates and confidence in official guidance emerging as critical determinants.

Environmental exposure and cultural norms have also been shown to shape outcomes. Ozkan et al. [4], analysing data from 110 countries, find that higher climate risk, weaker readiness to adapt to climate change, and greater individualism are all associated with higher COVID-19 mortality. These results suggest that environmental vulnerability and social norms can amplify the effects of public health shocks.

Machine learning approaches further underscore the dynamic nature of pandemic determinants. Zhou et al. [5] use an interpretable extreme gradient boosting framework to study COVID-19 case fatality rates across 156 countries over multiple pandemic phases. Their analysis reveals that the importance of determinants shifted over time: health conditions and universal health coverage dominated early in the pandemic, while vaccination rates became the primary driver during the Omicron period. Simulations indicate that a 5% increase in vaccination coverage reduced case fatality rates by more than 30% in countries with low baseline vaccination coverage, highlighting the gains from equitable vaccine access.

Socioeconomic inequality has likewise featured prominently. Davies [6] shows that during the first wave of the pandemic, higher income inequality, measured by the Gini coefficient, was strongly associated with higher COVID-19 mortality. This finding reinforces the view that pandemics exploit existing social and economic fault lines rather than affecting populations uniformly.

Trust and governance are other central themes. Farzanegan and Hofmann [7] document that higher political trust correlates with fewer COVID-19 cases and deaths across more than 70 countries and that effective risk communication critically depends on underlying levels of trust. Complementing this, da Silva et al. [8] analyse data from 213 countries and find that governance indicators, including control of corruption, government effectiveness, regulatory quality, and rule of law, are inversely related to excess mortality. Countries with stronger governance also launched vaccination programmes earlier and achieved higher coverage.

A separate body of research examines specific policy interventions. Using time-series data from Our World in Data, Agyapon-Ntra and McSharry [9] compare the effectiveness of non-pharmaceutical measures across countries. They find that mask mandates are the most cost-effective, significantly reducing transmission more than school closures or mobility restrictions. Gathering bans are also effective, while international travel controls and public information campaigns have limited impact. Compliance is higher in countries with greater literacy and income support.

Finally, long-standing environmental and health risks have been shown to worsen pandemic outcomes. Bretschger et al. [10] demonstrate that air pollution and obesity significantly increased infection and death rates across OECD and

Dedicated to the victims of COVID-19 and to the healthcare professionals who served them with courage and compassion.

Foreword

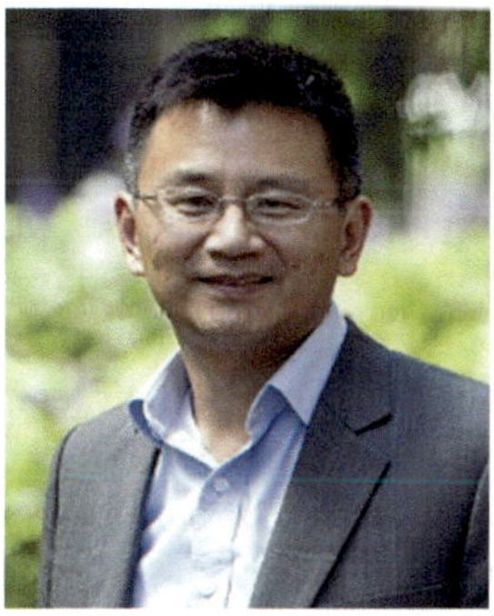

The COVID-19 pandemic may have been unexpected to most people, but not for healthcare professionals working in public health and infectious diseases. Strangely, many infectious disease threats, even those that have caused large numbers of deaths, have not made their mark on history in the way that other major events of the twentieth century have. There is much more written about the Great War than the 1918 influenza pandemic that probably caused a greater loss of life. The 1957, 1968, and 2009 influenza pandemics are now only historical footnotes. Prior to the COVID-19 pandemic, two other coronaviruses had been shown to have significant outbreak potential: SARS coronavirus in 2002–4 and MERS coronavirus, which has been an ongoing threat since 2013.

Since the first early reports of illness associated with a new respiratory virus emerged in late 2019, COVID-19 quickly caused major disruptions to the lives of billions of people over the first months of 2020. In the first years of the pandemic, there was substantial direct mortality from severe COVID-19. While official government accounts reported around six million deaths, more careful studies estimating 'excess' mortality by comparing death rates to the pre-pandemic baseline have suggested there were 15–18 million attributed deaths to COVID-19 in 2020 and 2021. This difference between official and estimated deaths not only reflects undiagnosed cases but also disruptions to health services, economic activity, and many other aspects of life. Few of these impacts were positive, and many had indirect adverse effects on health and well-being.

It is not only important to document the impact of COVID-19 on health but also our approaches to the various dilemmas that it posed—how we described its clinical features, how to prevent transmission, how to mitigate its impact, particularly on those with the least capacity to safely isolate, how to maintain essential services and the functioning of society. We also need to remember the post-pandemic sequelae—its impacts on preventative health, on education and the mental health of children, trust in government and science, the rise in political polarisation, disinformation, and misinformation.

Five years on, COVID-19 is a different disease now. This is largely due to the dominance of the Omicron variant of SARS-CoV-2, which is associated with milder disease, widespread population immunity from vaccination and natural infection, and, to a lesser degree, the availability of antiviral treatments and improved medical care.

In this context, this book, *COVID-19 in Dental Practice*, has been written. It provides dental practitioners with an accessible, evidence-based understanding of COVID-19, its evolution, clinical and oral features, patterns of transmission in dental settings, and the implications for safe, day-to-day practice.

We have learned a lot about how COVID-19 behaves, how it affects oral health, and how best to protect dental professionals, their teams, and their patients. In some respects, this is a historical document, but COVID-19 continues to circulate and will remain with us. This book brings together current science, practical guidance, and the lessons learned across different phases of the pandemic. By doing so, the book aims to help dental professionals respond confidently not only to COVID-19 but, more importantly, to future respiratory infectious threats.

Professor of Infectious Diseases Allen C. Cheng
Monash University
Melbourne, VIC, Australia
February 2026

Personal Reflections

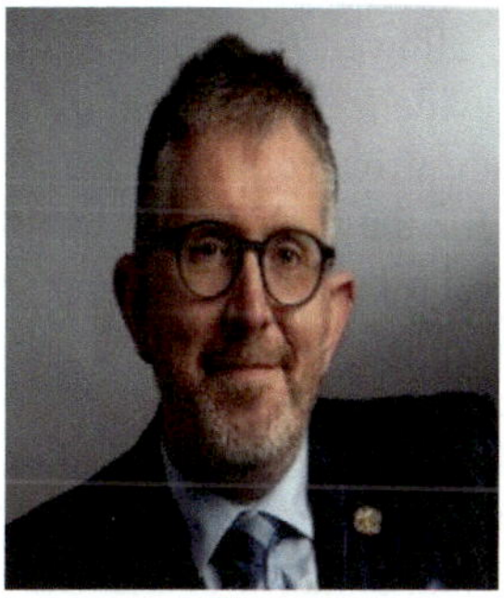

In November 2019, the world became interested in the novel SARS-CoV-2 virus, which became known as COVID-19, as it emerged in Wuhan, China. The virus initially gripped the Far East and then spread to Europe and North America, with different countries adopting individual approaches to virus control and minimising population-level infection risks whilst ensuring that those infected received treatment.

Nobody knew what was to unfold as the virus spread around the globe. Whilst countries took different approaches to border control, virus-spread precautions, lockdowns, and restrictions on daily life, the COVID-19 SARS-2 virus continued to rampage worldwide. The dental profession was resilient, and whilst the dental team worked through the various stages of the pandemic to ensure patients were not disenfranchised and did what was possible within national restrictions, this was a period of considerable uncertainty.

As with many people in dentistry and other professions during the first wave, I focused my attention as a clinical academic and dental leader on ensuring the safety of our students and patients, and on prioritising dental treatment for those with the greatest need. Little did I know that in doing so, I was to fall ill with the SARS-CoV-2 virus and come close to death. I spiralled into critical illness and multi-organ failure and required over seven weeks of extracorporeal membrane oxygenation in the intensive care unit, followed by months of rehabilitation. Whilst I was fortunate to survive, over seven million people succumbed to the SARS-CoV-2 virus and the consequences of critical illness throughout the world.

Dentistry was one of many professions worldwide that consistently delivered clinical care throughout the various phases of the pandemic. The aspects of close patient contact, aerosol-generating procedures, and face-to-face care delivery all required continual re-thinking throughout the pandemic. Practices, clinics, and offices were forced to close and reopen as required, operate under new and ever-evolving safety protocols, and rapidly redefine what 'safe practice' truly meant as new information and virus waves evolved. What emerged was not only a crisis but a catalyst for change and innovation.

COVID-19 transformed every aspect of the healthcare sector. Improved infection control protocols, ventilation in clinics and waiting areas, teledentistry, and adaptable clinical pathways suddenly became essential for protecting patients and dental teams. While we now have greater respect for this microscopic pathogen and respiratory viruses in general due to the pandemic, the lessons learned from COVID-19 should not be forgotten despite the publication of this book.

The COVID-19 pandemic allowed the dental profession to highlight the long-standing strengths, including evidence-based dental care, attention to detail throughout the patient journey and team-driven clinical care. The pandemic also highlighted other aspects of importance for the profession: well-being and wellness, sustainability, knowledge of population health measures, and the ethics of adaptability during a public health crisis.

COVID-19 in Dental Practice is a testament to the considerable work of the dental profession in addressing the challenges presented by a global public health emergency, along with the innovative and inventive methods in which the dental industry adapted to the different phases and stages of the COVID-19 pandemic. This book also serves as a historical record and a guide for any future public health scenario. The book captures the science of COVID-19 in dentistry and the lived experience of the profession during a period of ongoing disruption and change. This book details the problems and solutions, and, most importantly, the knowledge our profession has developed that will continue to shape dental education, dental health policy, and patient safety.

Most importantly, *COVID-19 in Dental Practice* celebrates the dental team who, from behind the masks, ensured the delivery of clinical care. The COVID-19 pandemic demonstrated that dentistry is not just about technical delivery, but an ever-adapting community of highly committed professionals united by a commitment to population health, scientific care, and compassion.

As you read *COVID-19 in Dental Practice*, I hope you will deepen your understanding of the pandemic's impact on dental care worldwide, with renewed clarity. COVID-19 posed numerous challenges for dentistry but also offered opportunities for change and growth. This book is an excellent resource that recounts the profession's journey through the pandemic and provides a solid foundation for the future.

Consultant and Professor in Orthodontics Grant McIntyre
University of Dundee
Dundee, UK
Vice-President (Dental) and Dean of The Faculty of Dental Surgery
The Royal College of Surgeons of Edinburgh
Edinburgh, UK
January 2026

Preface

The COVID-19 pandemic changed our lives in unexpected ways. For those of us in dentistry, it redefined not just how we worked but also how we approached safety, teamwork, and our responsibility to patients. During the early stages of the pandemic, dental professionals were not well-informed about COVID-19, despite being exposed to patients infected with the virus. Nevertheless, amidst this uncertainty, we observed colleagues adapt with courage, compassion, and remarkable resilience. This book is written in honour of that spirit.

Although the initial crisis has passed, the threat of new variants and future outbreaks remains. The lessons we have learned, often under significant pressure, are too valuable to ignore. *COVID-19 in Dental Practice: A Reference Manual for Oral Healthcare Professionals* was developed to safeguard these lessons and to assist the profession in remaining prepared, confident, and well-informed.

The book is divided into four clear sections: the global impact of the pandemic; the biology and behaviour of the virus; its systemic clinical features; and the oral health considerations that are still evolving. Together, they offer a practical, evidence-based guide for clinicians navigating a post-pandemic world.

More than 30 experts worldwide have contributed their knowledge and experience to this project. Their insights have helped develop a resource that we hope will support dental professionals for many years. Our hope is that this book serves not only as a reference but also as a reminder of our collective resilience and the important role dentistry plays within the broader field of health.

Acknowledgements Our sincere gratitude goes to Professor Allen Chen for his thoughtful and generous Foreword, which frames this volume with a deep understanding of the profession's responsibilities during and beyond the pandemic.

We are also grateful to Professor Grant McIntyre for sharing his personal reflections on experiencing COVID-19 firsthand. His account brings a human dimension to this book and reminds us of the profound impact the pandemic has had on colleagues across healthcare.

Our warm thanks extend to all chapter contributors, whose expertise and commitment have shaped this book into a comprehensive and practical resource for dental practitioners. Their collective effort has strengthened the profession's understanding of COVID-19 and its implications for safe, evidence-based dental care.

We also wish to acknowledge the exceptional support of the Springer production team, whose professionalism, attention to detail, and steady guidance have been invaluable in bringing this book to completion.

Brisbane, QLD, Australia S. R. Prabhu
Bengaluru, Karnataka, India Amrita Pattanaik
South Jordan, UT, USA Shankargouda Patil
Hong Kong, Hong Kong Lakshman Samaranayake
Chennai, Tamil Nadu, India S. M. Balaji

Contents

Editors and Contributors

Editors

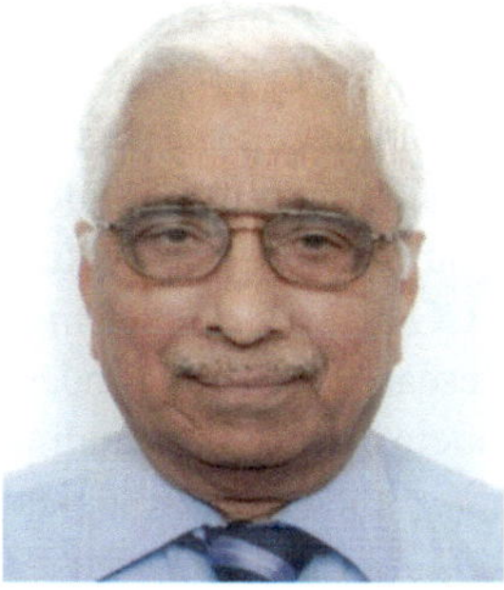

S. R. Prabhu BDS; MDS (Oral Path); FFDRCSI (Oral Med); FDSRCS(Edin); FDSRCPS(Glasgow); FDSRCS(Eng.); FFGDP RCS(UK); MOMed RCS(Edin); FICD is an Honorary academic at the School of Dentistry in Brisbane and a globally recognised expert in oral and maxillofacial pathology and oral medicine. With academic and leadership roles in India, Kenya, Sudan, Trinidad and Tobago, Malaysia, Saudi Arabia, the UAE, and Australia, he has helped shape dental education internationally. He is a Fellow of all four Royal Colleges of Surgeons in the UK and Ireland, a former international advisor for the Caribbean and UAE regions, and an examiner for the membership examinations of the Royal College of Surgeons of Edinburgh. In collaboration with Professor Jeff Hill of the University of Alabama at Birmingham School of Dentistry, he has conducted HIV/AIDS education workshops for oral healthcare professionals across Asia and the Caribbean. He has published numerous articles in peer-reviewed journals and edited several books on various topics related to oral diseases, published by renowned international academic publishers. He currently serves on the editorial board of the *International Dental Journal* (IDJ), published by the FDI World Dental Federation, Geneva.

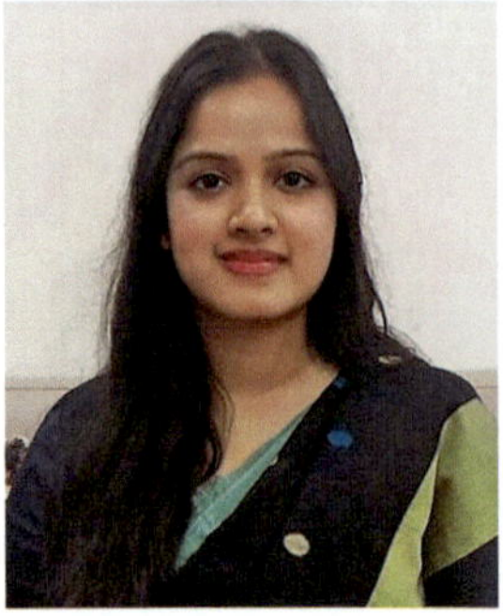

Amrita Pattanaik MBBS, MD is a medical scientist at the Department of Neurovirology, National Institute of Mental and Neurosciences, Bengaluru. She holds a post-graduate degree in Clinical Microbiology and brings a wealth of expertise in virology and neuro-infections. With several years of experience as a virologist in premier institutes, including the Manipal Institute of Virology in Manipal, India, she has served as the medical officer in charge of multiple pivotal laboratories, among them the WHO Southeast Asia Japanese Encephalitis Laboratory, COVID-19 diagnostic facilities, and the National Referral Laboratory for HIV diagnosis. In addition to overseeing viral diagnostic testing, she has actively contributed to research on rabies and COVID-19. She is currently involved in projects that include exploring the clinical and molecular aspects of viral brain infections, evaluating antecedent viral infections in Guillain-Barré Syndrome, and investigating viral immunology in paediatric COVID-19 cases, which is Indian Council of Medical Research (ICMR) funded. Her work is committed to advancing the understanding of viral diseases, especially their neurological implications.

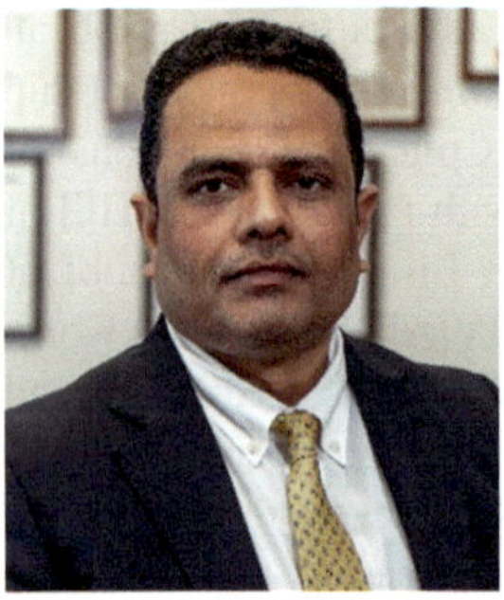

Shankargouda Patil BDS, MDS, PhD, FRCPath, FDS RCPS (Glasg), FICD and FPFA is a Professor at the College of Dental Medicine, Roseman University of Health Sciences, Utah, USA, and serves as Vice President of both the Utah Section of the American Association of Dental, Oral, and Craniofacial Research (AADOCR) and the Roseman University Faculty Senate. A distinguished academician and researcher, he brings deep expertise in oral pathology and medical biotechnology.

He earned his PhD in Medical Biotechnology from the University of Siena, Italy; his MDS in Oral Pathology from Sree Balaji Dental College, Chennai; and his BDS from PMNM Dental College, Bagalkot. He is a Fellow of the Royal College of Pathology (London), the Royal College of Physicians and Surgeons (Glasgow), the International College of Dentists, and the Pierre Fauchard Academy, and is a Full Member of Sigma Xi.

With over 300 peer-reviewed publications, 3 textbook chapters, an h-index of 54, and more than 18,000 citations, he is recognised internationally for his scholarly impact. As a contributor to the Global Burden of Disease (GBD) network, his work appears in *The Lancet* and other leading journals. He is included in Marquis Who's Who in America and Stanford University.

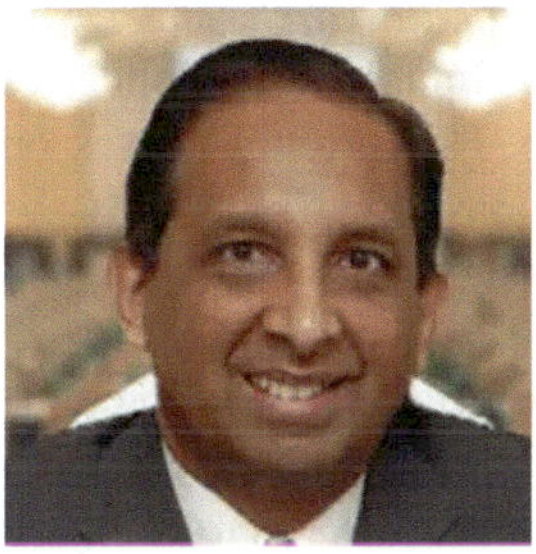

Lakshman Samaranayake DSc, DDS (Glas), FRCPath, FDSRCS(Edin), FRACDS, FDS RCPS (Glas), FHKCPath, FCDSHK. Professor Emeritus, Faculty of Dentistry, University of Hong Kong, Hong Kong is a distinguished figure in clinical microbiology, and he is celebrated for his contributions to research, publication, and executive-level administration. After graduating in Sri Lanka, he honed his expertise in clinical microbiology and later served as a Consultant Microbiologist in the UK. Throughout his career, he has worked at various prestigious institutions worldwide, including universities in the UK, Canada, Hong Kong, Australia, and the UAE, and has accumulated an impressive publication record of over 450 articles, which have been cited more than 35,000 times (h-index 103). He holds the esteemed position of Editor-in-Chief of the *International Dental Journal*. He is recognised for his authorship of seminal works such as Samaranayake's *Essential Microbiology for Dentistry* (6th Ed). Additionally, he has taken on exceptional leadership roles as the Executive Dean of dental schools in both Hong Kong and Australia, affiliated with the Universities of Hong Kong and Queensland, respectively, where he facilitated the establishment of the No. 1 dental school in the world at the University of Hong Kong, according to the QS World University Rankings from 2014 to 2016. Highly sought after as a speaker and workshop moderator, Prof. Samaranayake has shared his insights and expertise with professionals across more than 40 countries. His outstanding contributions to surgical sciences have been acknowledged through prestigious accolades, including the King James IV Professorship of the Royal College of Surgeons (Edinburgh) and the Distinguished Scientist Award from the International Association for Dental Research (IADR). Furthermore, he holds multiple visiting, adjunct, and honorary professorial appointments at universities in India, Indonesia, Oman, the UAE, Sri Lanka, and Thailand.

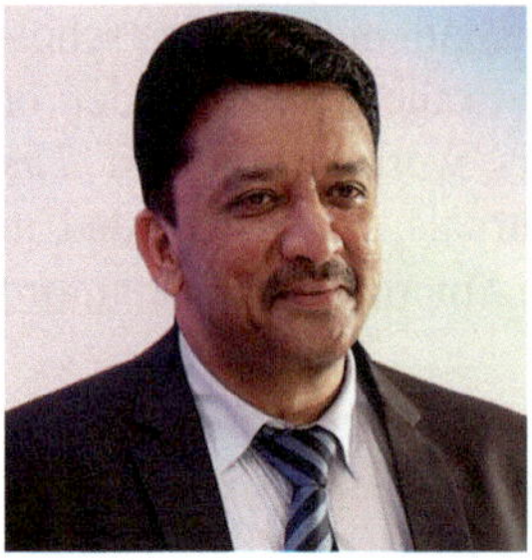

S. M. Balaji MDS, MFDS RCPS (Glasg), FDS RCPS (Glasg), PhD, DSc (Hon) is an eminent Oral and Cranio-Maxillofacial Surgeon from Chennai, India, and Director and Consultant of Balaji Dental and Craniofacial Hospital, a globally recognised centre for cranio-maxillofacial surgery. He is the Editor-in-Chief of the *Annals of Maxillofacial Surgery*, Executive Editor of the *Indian Journal of Dental Research*, and Dean/Executive Vice-President of the International College of Continuing Dental Education. He currently serves on the FDI Council and is President-Elect of the International College of Dentists (India, Sri Lanka, and Nepal Section).

A prolific academician, Prof. Balaji has authored the bestselling *Textbook of Oral and Maxillofacial Surgery* (Elsevier) and *Clinical Cranio-Maxillofacial Surgery* and has published over 140 scientific papers with significant global citations. He has delivered prestigious orations, including the Dr M. S. Ginwalla and Dr R. Ahmed Orations, and has received numerous honours, such as the Dr B. C. Roy National Award and the Prof. David Precious Award for cleft research.

With more than three decades of pioneering contributions and innovations in maxillofacial surgery, Prof. Balaji continues to represent India at leading international forums and serves as Honorary Consultant to hospitals across Seychelles, Maldives, Mauritius, and Swaziland.

Contributors

Mohammad Abusamak Faculty of Dentistry, Dalhousie University, Halifax, Nova Scotia, Canada

Shilpi Ajwani Sydney Dental Hospital and Oral Health Services, Sydney Local Health District, NSW Health, Sydney, NSW, Australia

M. A. Ashwini Department of Neurovirology, National Institute of Mental Health and Neurosciences, Bengaluru, Karnataka, India

Jane C. Atkinson (Retired) National Institutes of Health, Bethesda, MD, USA

Devi Atukorallaya Department of Oral Biology, Dr. Gerald Niznick College of Dentistry, Rady Faculty of Health Sciences, University of Manitoba, Winnipeg, MB, Canada

S. M. Balaji Balaji Dental, Craniofacial Hospital & Research Institute, Chennai, Tamil Nadu, India

Suresha Bandara Infectious Diseases Practitioner, Detroit, MI, USA

Shilpa Bhandi College of Dental Medicine, Roseman University of Health Sciences, South Jordan, UT, USA

Meghashyam Bhat Department of Public Health Dentistry, Sharavathi Dental College and Hospital, Shivamogga, Karnataka, India
School of Dentistry, Adelaide University, Adelaide, SA, Australia

Sreevidya Bhat Department of Public Health Dentistry, Srinivas Institute of Dental Sciences, Surathkal, Mangaluru, India

Arjun Bhugra Transplant Virology, Department of Microbiology and Virology, Queen Elizabeth The Queen Mother Hospital, East Kent Hospitals University NHS Foundation Trust, Margate, UK

Sophie Chen Department of Oral Biology, Dr. Gerald Niznick College of Dentistry, Rady Faculty of Health Sciences, University of Manitoba, Winnipeg, MB, Canada

Manohar Lal Choudhary Indian Council of Medical Research (ICMR)-National Institute of Virology (NIV), Pune, Maharashtra, India

Avinash Choudekar Virology Laboratory, Department of Microbiology, All India Institute of Medical Sciences, New Delhi, Delhi, India

Ananda P. Dasanayake Department of Epidemiology, New York University College of Dentistry, New York, NY, USA

Pedro Miguel dos Santos Abrantes Department of Medical Biosciences, Faculty of Natural Sciences, University of the Western Cape, Bellville, South Africa

Dennis Fernando Medmark, Chantilly, VA, USA

Pronami Gogoi ICMR-National Institute of Virology, Pune, Maharashtra, India

Matt Hopcraft Melbourne Dental School, University of Melbourne, Melbourne, VIC, Australia

Nuwan Indika Business Analytics, College of Business, Loyola University New Orleans, New Orleans, LA, USA

Rasika Manori Jayasinghe Department of Prosthetic Dentistry, Faculty of Dental Sciences, University of Peradeniya, Peradeniya, Sri Lanka
Department of Prosthetic Dentistry, Mahsa International college (Penang), Butter worth, Malaysia

Ruwan Duminda Jayasinghe Department of Oral Medicine and Periodontology, Faculty of Dental Sciences, University of Peradeniya, Peradeniya, Sri Lanka

Joseph Katz Department of Oral Diagnostic Sciences, University of Florida College of Dentistry, Gainesville, FL, USA

Himanshu Kaushal Indian Council of Medical Research (ICMR)-National Institute of Virology (NIV), Pune, Maharashtra, India
Academy of Scientific and Innovative Research (AcSIR), Ghaziabad, India

Wajihul Hasan Khan Virology Laboratory, Department of Microbiology, All India Institute of Medical Sciences, New Delhi, Delhi, India

Hasna H. Kunhipurayil College of Dental Medicine, Qatar University Health, Qatar University, Doha, Qatar

Frank W. Licari College of Dental Medicine, Roseman University of Health Sciences, South Jordan, UT, USA

Lonika Lodha Department of Neurovirology, National Institute of Mental Health and Neurosciences (NIMHANS), Bengaluru, Karnataka, India

Basavaraj Mathapati Indian Council of Medical Research (ICMR)-National Institute of Virology (NIV), Pune, Maharashtra, India

Vesna Miletic Faculty of Medicine and Health, Sydney Dental School, The University of Sydney, Surry Hills, Sydney, NSW, Australia

Souvik Mitra ICMR-National Institute of Virology, Pune, Maharashtra, India

Shivdas Rajaram Naik Kasturba Medical College, Manipal, Karnataka, India

Priyasi Mittal ICMR-National Institute of Virology, Pune, India

Shankargouda Patil College of Dental Medicine, Department of Oral and Maxillofacial Pathology, College of Dental Medicine, Roseman University of Health Sciences, South Jordan, UT, USA

Amrita Pattanaik National Institute of Mental Health and Neuro Sciences (NIMHANS), Bengaluru, India

S. R. Prabhu School of Dentistry, University of Queensland, Brisbane, QLD, Australia

Vijayalakshmi Reddy Department of Neurovirology, NIMHANS, Bengaluru, Karnataka, India

T. S. Roberts Faculty of Dentistry, Maxillofacial Pathology, University of the Western Cape, Cape Town, South Africa

Lakshman Samaranayake Faculty of Dentistry, University of Hong Kong, Hong Kong, Hong Kong

Salima Shebbo College of Dental Medicine, Qatar University Health, Qatar University, Doha, Qatar

Faleh Ahmad Tamimi Faculty of Dental Medicine and Oral Health Sciences, McGill University, Montreal, QC, Canada

Kelvin J.K. Tan UQ Business School, The University of Queensland, Brisbane, QLD, Australia

Neeky Yassari Dental Student, New York University College of Dentistry, New York, NY, USA

Sue-Ching Yeoh Sydney Dental School, Faculty of Medicine and Health, The University of Sydney, Sydney, Australia

COVID-19 Abbreviations

Ab-test	Antibody Test (serology)
Ag-test	Antigen Test
AI	Artificial Immunity (immunity from vaccination)
ARDS	Acute Respiratory Distress Syndrome
Asx	Asymptomatic
AZ	AstraZeneca vaccine (ChAdOx1-S)
Booster	Additional vaccine dose to increase immunity
CFR	Case Fatality Rate
COVID-19	Coronavirus Disease 2019
Ct value	Cycle Threshold (PCR measure of viral load)
CT	Community Transmission
CT	Contact Tracing
CTP	Contact Tracing Program
Fomite	Contaminated object/surface
FTC	Flatten the Curve
HCP	Healthcare Personnel
HCW	Healthcare Worker
HI	Herd Immunity
ICU	Intensive Care Unit
IFR	Infection Fatality Rate
L&D	Lockdown and Distancing
MIS-C	Multisystem Inflammatory Syndrome in Children
mRNA	Messenger RNA (technology used in Pfizer/Moderna vaccines)
NPIs	Non-Pharmaceutical Interventions (masking, distancing)
PCR	Polymerase Chain Reaction (gold-standard diagnostic test)
PHEIC	Public Health Emergency of International Concern
PHSM	Public Health and Social Measures
PPE	Personal Protective Equipment
R_0 (R-naught)	Basic Reproduction Number
RAT	Rapid Antigen Test (also called rapid test)
Rt	Effective Reproduction Number

RT-PCR	Reverse Transcriptase PCR
SARS-CoV-2	Severe Acute Respiratory Syndrome Coronavirus 2
Symp	Symptomatic
VOC	Variant of Concern
VOI	Variant of Interest

Part I

COVID-19: Know the Basics

Coronavirus-19 Disease (COVID-19): Origin, Controversies, Pandemic Politics and Myths

1

S. R. Prabhu

1.1 Introduction

1.1.1 The Origin and Impact of COVID-19

COVID-19 refers to coronavirus disease 2019. The "19" in COVID-19 indicates the year 2019, when the disease was first identified. The full name is coronavirus disease 2019. According to established guidelines for naming new infectious diseases, it was officially named by the World Health Organisation (WHO) on 11 February 2020 [1]. Previously, the disease was referred to by various provisional names, including "2019-nCoV" or "Wuhan coronavirus." The WHO chose "COVID-19" to avoid stigmatising any geographical location, animal, or group of people, which aligns with their naming policy for new diseases [1].

In December 2019, a series of pneumonia cases of unknown origin were reported in Wuhan, China, linked to a seafood market. This outbreak marked the start of a global public health crisis. By 7 January 2020, the causative agent was identified as a novel coronavirus, later named Severe Acute Respiratory Syndrome Coronavirus 2 (SARS-CoV-2) [1]. Researchers focused on bats and other wildlife known to carry coronaviruses. However, theories about an accidental release from a research laboratory in Wuhan have also gained attention, although no conclusive evidence has confirmed this scenario [2]. As infections spread internationally, the World Health Organisation (WHO) officially declared COVID-19 a pandemic on 11 March 2020 [1].

SARS-CoV-2 belongs to the broader coronavirus family, which includes the pathogens responsible for severe acute respiratory syndrome (SARS) and Middle East Respiratory Syndrome (MERS). Although initially believed to spread mainly through respiratory droplets, later research confirmed the virus's potential for

S. R. Prabhu (✉)
School of Dentistry, University of Queensland, Brisbane, QLD, Australia
e-mail: r.prabhu@uq.edu.au

S. R. Prabhu et al. (eds.), *COVID-19 in Dental Practice*,
https://doi.org/10.1007/978-3-032-26000-0_1

airborne transmission, especially in enclosed or poorly ventilated environments [3]. In response to the unprecedented rate of transmission and death, the global scientific community mobilised to develop effective vaccines. By the end of 2020, messenger RNA (mRNA) vaccines, notably BNT162b2 developed by Pfizer-Biontech, showed substantial effectiveness in preventing severe symptoms of the disease [4].

The pandemic's effects extended far beyond public health. Economic activity sharply declined as governments worldwide implemented lockdowns, closed borders, and imposed restrictions on movement. The International Monetary Fund (2020) called this period "The Great Lockdown," emphasising the scale of economic upheaval. Educational systems were similarly affected, prompting a swift shift to digital and remote learning methods [5].

Cultural and social norms shifted in response to the crisis. Terms such as "social distancing" entered the global vocabulary, while face coverings became both a protective measure and a symbol of collective responsibility. Empirical evidence indicates notable behavioural changes; for instance, a study by the Pew Research Center found a significant increase in mask usage among the US population during the early phase of the pandemic [6]. Furthermore, the pandemic exposed deep-rooted inequalities in healthcare access, prompting renewed calls for systemic reform and more equitable public health policies.

1.2 Controversies About the Origin of COVID-19

The origin of COVID-19 remains one of the most fiercely debated scientific and political issues of our time. The controversy revolves around two main theories: one proposes that the virus emerged naturally through spillover from animals to humans, while the other suggests it may have originated from a laboratory-related incident. Despite extensive investigations, conclusive evidence supporting either theory remains unavailable, fuelling ongoing debate among scientists, policymakers and the public.

The natural origin theory proposes that the virus originated from animals, likely bats, and was transmitted to humans, possibly via an intermediate host. This aligns with the emergence of other coronaviruses, such as SARS and MERS. However, despite thorough investigations, no definitive animal host has been identified, which leaves some uncertainty. Conversely, the lab-leak theory suggests that the virus may have accidentally escaped from a laboratory, such as the Wuhan Institute of Virology in China, which was studying bat coronaviruses [7]. This idea was initially dismissed as a conspiracy theory but has gained support following calls from US intelligence agencies and scientists for further investigation. What makes this debate particularly tense is its geopolitical aspect, along with accusations of cover-ups, misinformation and political interference, especially between the USA and China. It's not just about the origins of the virus; it's about trust, transparency, and how we prepare for future pandemics.

1.3 Pandemic Politics

The COVID-19 pandemic was not only a public health emergency but also a political flashpoint. In Australia, the government responded swiftly with strict border controls and centralised quarantine systems [8]. Although this helped delay widespread transmission, extended lockdowns, especially in Victoria, tested public patience and economic resilience [8]. In India, the second wave in early 2021 was disastrous. With over 400,000 new infections daily at its peak, hospitals were overwhelmed, oxygen shortages were common, and mass cremations painted a bleak picture [9]. In the USA, leadership changes, the politicisation of public health measures and inconsistent messaging undermined early efforts. Meanwhile, the development of mRNA vaccines was a scientific breakthrough. Vaccine hesitancy and disinformation prolonged waves of illness and death [10]. Brazil's story was marked by deep division. Federal authorities minimised the virus and discouraged mask-wearing and vaccinations, even as cases and death rates increased [11]. Despite this, the country's universal public health system provided a vital lifeline.

1.4 Myths and Misinformation

The pandemic was accompanied by myths and misinformation that hampered containment efforts.

- Myth: COVID-19 is just like the seasonal flu.
- *Reality*: COVID-19 and the seasonal flu share similarities as respiratory illnesses, but they differ significantly in terms of severity, transmission, and long-term impact.
- COVID-19 has a much higher mortality rate and long-term complications.
- *Myth: Vaccines alter human DNA.*
- *Reality: mRNA vaccines do not enter the cell nucleus and cannot modify DNA.*
- *Myth: The virus was deliberately engineered.*
- *Reality: No credible scientific evidence supports this claim.*

These myths, widely circulated on social media, have significantly influenced vaccine acceptance and adherence to public health guidelines.

1.5 Lessons Learned and Reflections

Countries that acted early and communicated consistently fared better. Those who took swift action by closing borders, enforcing quarantines, and increasing testing managed to delay or lessen the initial impact.

The COVID-19 pandemic revealed and intensified existing inequalities. Access to healthcare, vaccines, and reliable information varied greatly across and within countries. The rapid development of vaccines is a significant scientific achievement. However, scientific institutions must also ensure transparency and accountability to sustain public trust. Long-term investment in resilient health systems is now clearly essential. COVID-19 highlighted the high costs of underfunded health systems and emphasised the importance of pandemic preparedness. Investing in public health is not optional; it is vital. As the world transitions into a post-pandemic era, the enduring effects of COVID-19 persist. Long COVID continues to affect millions. Mental health issues have risen, and economies are still in recovery. Nevertheless, there is hope in the lessons learned and the international solidarity demonstrated during crises. A pandemic is not merely a biological event; it serves as a mirror reflecting our systems, values and preparedness. As we move forward, these lessons should not be disregarded; they act as guides for future readiness.

References

1. World Health Organisation. WHO Director-General's opening remarks at the media briefing on COVID-19. 2020, March 11. https://www.who.int/director-general/speeches/detail/who-director-general-s-opening-remarks-at-the-media-briefing-on-covid-19%2D%2D-11-march-2020.
2. World Health Organisation. Origins of the SARS-CoV-2 virus: joint WHO–China study. Geneva: WHO; 2021.
3. Centers for Disease Control and Prevention. Scientific brief: SARS-CoV-2 transmission. 2021. https://www.cdc.gov/coronavirus/2019-ncov/science/science-briefs/sars-cov-2-transmission.html.
4. Polack FP, Thomas SJ, Kitchin N, Absalon J, Gurtman A, Lockhart S, et al. Safety and efficacy of the BNT162b2 mRNA COVID-19 vaccine. N Engl J Med. 2020;383(27):2603–15. https://doi.org/10.1056/NEJMoa2034577.
5. UNESCO. COVID-19 educational disruption and response. 2020. https://en.unesco.org/covid19/educationresponse.
6. Pew Research Centre. More Americans say they are regularly wearing masks in stores and other businesses. 2020. https://www.pewresearch.org/fact-tank/2020/06/23/more-americans-say-they-are-regularly-wearing-masks-in-stores-and-other-businesses/.
7. Alwine J, Goodrum F, Banfield B, et al. The harms of promoting the lab leak hypothesis for SARS-CoV-2 origins without evidence. J Virol. 2024;98:e01240–24. https://doi.org/10.1128/jvi.01240-24.
8. Duckett S, Stobart A. Australia's COVID-19 response: the triumphs and the challenges. Aust Health Rev. 2022;46(3):234–42.
9. Ministry of Health and Family Welfare (India). COVID-19 dashboard [internet]. New Delhi: MoHFW; 2023. [cited 2025 Jun 21]. Available from: https://www.mohfw.gov.in/.
10. Nwachukwu G, Rihan A, Nwachukwu E, Uduma N, Elliott KS, Tiruneh YM. Understanding COVID-19 vaccine hesitancy in the United States: a systematic review. Vaccine. 2024;12:747. https://doi.org/10.3390/vaccines12070747.
11. Rocha R, Atun R, Massuda A. Brazil's COVID-19 crisis and the role of health systems. Lancet. 2022;399(10326):1930–41.

Global Burden of COVID-19 (2019–2024) 2

Meghashyam Bhat and Sreevidya Bhat

2.1 Introduction

In recent times, a global health emergency has posed unprecedented challenges, leading to widespread morbidity and mortality and affecting economies and healthcare systems worldwide. The pandemic was caused by coronavirus disease 2019 (COVID-19), a disease caused by an RNA virus known as severe acute respiratory syndrome coronavirus 2 (SARS-CoV-2). The disease primarily affects humans and animals, including bats, mice, and wild animals. In humans, the virus affects the gastrointestinal system, liver, central nervous system, and, mainly, the respiratory system. Those affected present with fever, dry cough, and breathlessness. Death may occur due to pneumonia and acute respiratory distress syndrome [1]. The virus was named SARS-CoV-2 by the WHO after examining the throat swab of a patient affected by the novel coronavirus [2]. SARS-CoV has been described for more than 75 years now [3]. The first person to be affected with COVID-19 was in Wuhan, Hubei Province, China, in December 2019, leading to a rapid global spread that has resulted in millions of infections and deaths worldwide. On 30 January 2020, following the Emergency Committee's recommendations, WHO declared the outbreak a public health emergency of international concern. The disease had spread to 20 countries by February 2020 [4].

The pandemic has caused a significant mortality burden worldwide, with estimates suggesting the impact could be even greater than reported figures indicate,

M. Bhat (✉)
Department of Public Health Dentistry, Sharavathi Dental College and Hospital, Shivamogga, Karnataka, India

School of Dentistry, Adelaide University, Adelaide, SA, Australia
e-mail: meghashyam.bhat@adelaide.edu.au

S. Bhat
Department of Public Health Dentistry, Srinivas Institute of Dental Sciences, Surathkal, Mangaluru, India

S. R. Prabhu et al. (eds.), *COVID-19 in Dental Practice*,
https://doi.org/10.1007/978-3-032-26000-0_2

especially in vulnerable populations. By May 2020, according to a WHO report, more than five million cases had been confirmed, and the death toll surpassed 300 across 213 countries, highlighting the urgent need for effective public health interventions to limit the spread of SARS-CoV-2 [5]. The COVID-19 outbreak resulted in widespread health crises and economic difficulties, requiring a comprehensive understanding of its effects on various populations and health systems globally. This chapter examines the global burden of COVID-19 and its implications for public health policy and resource allocation. Grasping these dynamics is essential for preparing for future pandemics and strengthening global health resilience.

2.2 Epidemiology

COVID-19 has exhibited different epidemiological patterns across various regions, influenced by factors such as population density, the country's healthcare infrastructure, and public health measures implemented to control the virus's spread. These disparities in epidemiological patterns have led to the adoption of tailored public health strategies to effectively address the unique challenges posed by COVID-19 in different settings.

Global prevalence: The COVID-19 prevalence rate differs greatly between countries, reflecting variations in socioeconomic factors, healthcare access, and public health measures. Recognising these disparities is crucial for effective policymaking and resource distribution. The estimates also provide insights into the pandemic's dynamics. According to a study by Luoca, the cumulative prevalence ranged from 31% (95% CI = 22–50) for Peru to 0.12% (0.074–0.26) for Japan. Other country estimates included 27% for Mexico, 22% for Brazil, 12% for the United States, 11% for the United Kingdom, 8.2% for France, 7.4% for Sweden, 4.2% for Canada, and 1.8% for Germany [6].

2.3 Incidence, Regional Variation, and Trend

The incidence of COVID-19 has varied significantly over time and across regions, influenced by public health measures and population mobility. Understanding the patterns of spread and trends is vital for developing effective strategies to manage future outbreaks. By May 2020, the disease was widespread in 213 countries, with over five million people infected and more than 300,000 deaths. The global case fatality rate (CFR) was 6.5% [7]. By January 2022, the global cumulative incidence had increased to 349.6 million confirmed cases and 5.6 million deaths [8]. At the end of 2024, the WHO reported that the worldwide cumulative incidence of confirmed cases had reached approximately 800 million, with total deaths exceeding 6.9 million, emphasising the ongoing challenges posed by COVID-19 [9]. The cumulative incidence was higher in the Americas and Oceania than in Asia and Africa (Fig. 2.1) [10]. The highest cumulative infection rate was in the European region (0.326), while Africa had the lowest (0.011). The CFR was highest in Africa

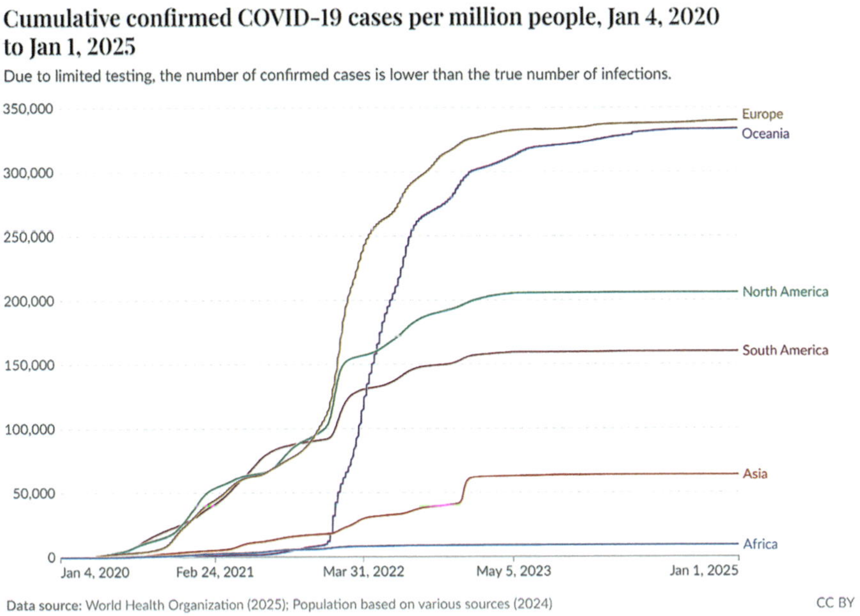

Fig. 2.1 Regional variation in cumulative COVID-19 incidence, with the highest levels observed in the Americas and Oceania

(0.020) and lowest in Oceania (0.002). The cumulative infection rate was greater (0.353) and the CFR lower (0.006) in upper-middle- and high-income countries compared to low-income countries, which had a lower cumulative infection rate (0.006) but a higher CFR (0.016) [11]. CFR varied across regions, with higher rates observed in low-income countries than in high-income countries, highlighting the need for targeted public health strategies to address these disparities. These differences emphasise the importance of understanding socioeconomic factors that contribute to variations in case fatality rates globally, especially in low-income regions.

In Italy, where nearly a quarter of the population is of older age (>65 years), the CFR was higher (6.5%). The median age of those who died was 78 years, and more than half of the deceased were aged 80 years or older [12]. Similar findings were observed in China, where the CFR was 8% among 70- to 79-year-olds, and 14.8% for those aged 80 years and older [13]. Those in critical condition and with comorbidities such as cardiovascular disease, diabetes, and chronic respiratory conditions exhibited higher CFR than those with no pre-existing conditions.

2.4 Mortality Burden of COVID-19

2.4.1 Global and Regional Mortality Rates

Approximately 95% of deaths related to COVID-19 occurred between 2020 and 2022 [9]. The age-standardised death rate for COVID-19 in 2021 was highest in sub-Saharan Africa (271.0 deaths per 100,000 population) and Latin America and the Caribbean (195.4 deaths per 100,000 population). In contrast, high-income super-regions such as Southeast Asia, East Asia, and Oceania experienced the lowest death rates (23.2 deaths per 100,000 population) [14].

Globally, the cumulative death rate for COVID-19 by January 2022 was 71.75 deaths per 100,000 people, with the highest rates seen in the Americas (14,039.95 deaths per 100,000 people) and Europe (12,512.57 deaths per 100,000 people). However, developing and underdeveloped countries experienced higher death rates despite lower incidence rates, highlighting the unequal impact of the pandemic [8]. A significant decline was observed from the latter half of 2022, likely due to increased immunity from infection and vaccination, as well as ongoing vigilance and improvements in healthcare systems (Fig. 2.2) [9, 10].

The impact of COVID-19 on children under 5 years old has been particularly concerning, as they are vulnerable to severe complications and mortality associated with the virus. The mortality risk for infants was higher than for older children or adults (20–45 years). The proportion of deaths in children was significantly lower (0.2%) compared to older people, >65 years (54%–85%), who faced the highest mortality risk. More than half of the deaths among children were of children younger than 5 years [15].

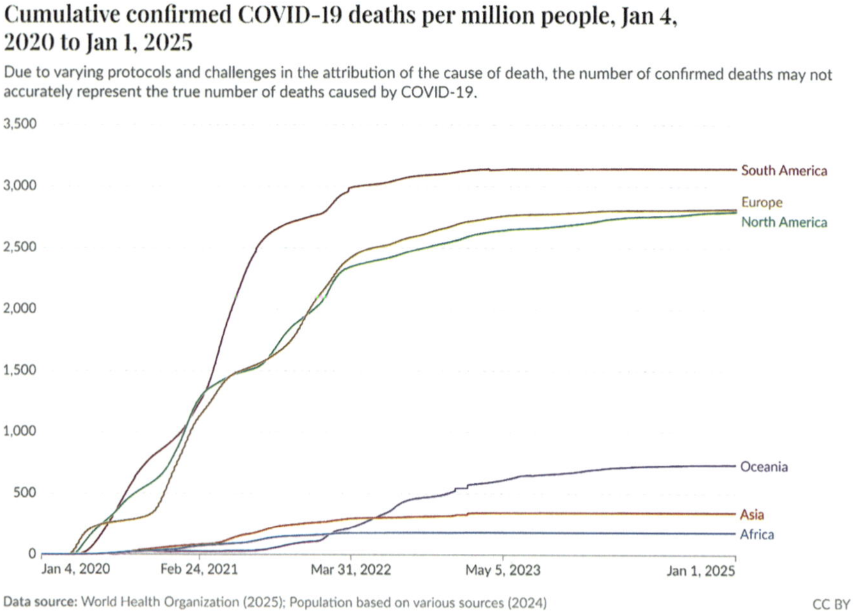

Fig. 2.2 Trends showing a marked reduction in COVID-19 transmission from late 2022, associated with increased immunity and improved healthcare capacity

2.4.2 Excess Mortality

Excess mortality, which captures both direct and indirect deaths caused by the pandemic, provides a more comprehensive measure of COVID-19's impact. According to the definition, excess mortality is "the difference in the total number of deaths during a crisis compared to those expected under normal conditions" [16]. An estimate based on available data indicates that, worldwide, there were 14.9 million excess deaths between January 2020 and December 2021, with significant regional variations. This figure is almost three times higher than the mortality rate reported during the same period. The Southeast Asia Region recorded the highest excess deaths (5.99 million), followed by the European Region (3.25 million) and the Region of the Americas (3.23 million) (Fig. 2.3) [10, 17]. The percentage of excess deaths attributable to COVID-19, compared to a scenario without the pandemic, was estimated at 7.97% in 2020 and 18.3% in 2021. The global response to COVID-19 required continuous adaptation of public health strategies, particularly as new variants emerge and vaccination coverage expands.

2.4.3 Loss of Life Expectancy and Years of Life Lost Due to COVID-19

COVID-19 has significantly impacted life expectancy, with estimates indicating millions of years of life lost (YLL) due to premature deaths, particularly among

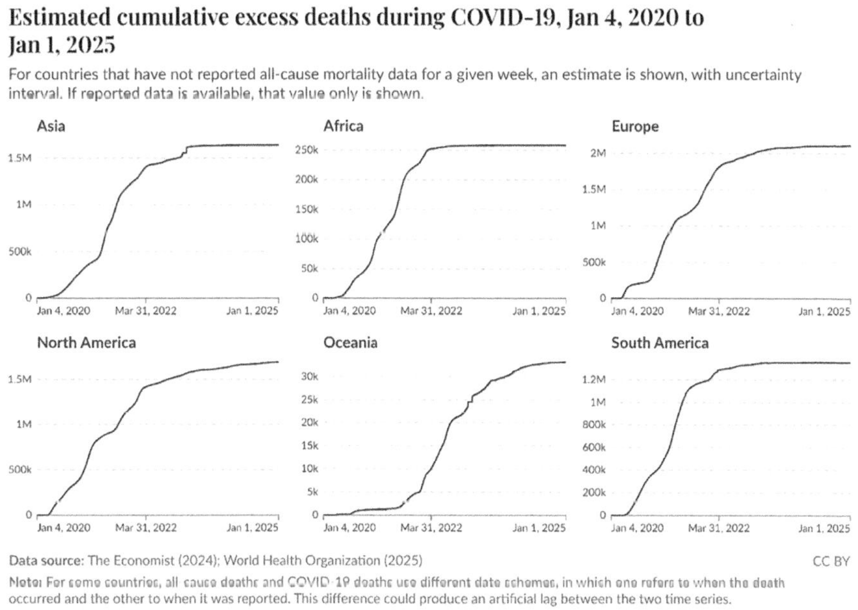

Fig. 2.3 Global distribution of excess deaths during the COVID-19 pandemic, with the Southeast Asia Region recording the highest mortality burden

vulnerable populations. A decade's efforts to improve life expectancy were disrupted in just 2 years of the COVID-19 pandemic. By 2021, global life expectancy had fallen by 1.8 years to 71.4 years, returning to levels last seen in 2012 and marking the first significant decline since 1950. The pandemic's impact varied across WHO regions and income groups. In the Regions of the Americas and Southeast Asia, life expectancy dropped by 3.0 years and healthy life expectancy at birth (HALE) by 2.5 years between 2019 and 2021. Meanwhile, in the Western Pacific Region, the loss of life expectancy and HALE was 0.1 years and 0.2 years, respectively [18]. According to the World Bank income groups, low-income countries experienced a smaller decline in LE (0.6 years) and HALE (0.6 years) compared to lower- and middle-income countries, which saw reductions of 2.4 and 2.0 years, respectively, and high-income countries, which experienced a decline of 2.5 years in life expectancy [18]. The reduction in life expectancy was estimated to be more pronounced among older adults, particularly those aged 65 and above, who faced the highest mortality risks during the pandemic. Men experienced a greater loss of life expectancy than women, owing to higher COVID-19 mortality rates, highlighting the need for targeted interventions to address these gender disparities in health outcomes. The average YLL due to COVID-19 between 2020 and 2021 is 16 years, with 45% attributable to deaths among individuals aged 55–75, 30% among those under 55, and 25% among those aged 75 and older [19].

YLLs due to COVID-19 were particularly high in older adults, who experienced the greatest burden of premature deaths. Globally, 85.6 million years of life were lost due to COVID-19 in the first two years of the pandemic, with significant disparities between countries [20].

2.4.4 Global Disability-Adjusted Life Years (DALYs) and Years of Life Lost (YLLs)

DALY, YLL, and Value of Statistical Life (VSL) provide measures of impact on health and economic loss worldwide. The estimated global DALYs, obtained through machine-learning analysis of data from January 2020 to April 2021, were 31,930 based on the global population [21]. In 2021, a study based on Global Burden of Disease data showed that COVID-19 caused 212.0 million DALYs globally, accounting for 9.0% of all-cause DALYs [22]. DALYs steadily increased from 2699 (thousand) during January to April 2020 to 13,683 during January to April 2021 [21]. The burden of DALYs was mainly due to YLL in low- and middle-income countries and due to YLD in high-income countries [22]. North America, Europe, and South America experienced significant increases in DALYs due to COVID-19. The five nations with the highest DALYs were the United States, Italy, Mexico, Brazil, and India, while Tanzania, Burundi, Laos, and Taiwan experienced lower DALYs [21].

Sociodemographic disparities were observed in DALYS related to COVID-19. The age-standardised DALYs were higher among males (3247 per 100,000 males) than females (1822 per 100,000 females). DALYs in people aged 50–69 years were lower (5834) compared to those aged 70 years and older (11,584) [23].

2.4.5 Regional and Socioeconomic Disparities

The burden of DALYs and YLLs varied considerably by region and socioeconomic status. Before the COVID-19 outbreak, the primary causes of DALYS were non-communicable diseases [21]. A few infectious diseases, such as HIV/AIDS, tuberculosis, and malaria, contributed to DALYs that were negatively correlated with the socioeconomic index (SDI). After the COVID-19 outbreak, the findings were conflicting, with DALYs showing a positive association with SDI. However, GBD 2021 data indicated that countries with lower SDI experienced higher age-standardised DALY rates for COVID-19, reflecting disparities in healthcare access and the pandemic's impact on vulnerable populations [22].

2.5 Economic Burden of COVID-19

2.5.1 Impact on National Economies

The pandemic had a significant impact on national economies, especially in low- and middle-income countries. In Latin America, for example, the direct medical costs of COVID-19 ranged from 258 million to 10,437 million, accounting for 2%–5% of national health expenditures [20]. Globally, the pandemic caused a decline in GDP growth, with low-income countries dedicating a larger share of their healthcare budgets to COVID-19 compared to high-income countries [24].

2.5.2 Value of Statistical Life (VSL)

The VSL indicator is measured using DALY and GDP to quantify healthy life years lost. It is a metric that translates health loss into economic loss. Globally, during the COVID-19 outbreak, the VSL increased from US$267 billion to US$996 billion between January and April [21].

2.5.3 Burden on Healthcare Systems and Policy Responses

The burden of COVID-19 on healthcare systems has been enormous. Hospitalisations increased as the number of cases rose, impacting healthcare resources beyond their capacity in many countries. Nearly 28.1 million COVID-19 hospitalisations were reported across 172 countries. These hospitalisations accounted for 5% of all confirmed cases. Average hospitalisations in 2020 were 155,000 per week, rising substantially to 526,000 per week in 2021, then decreasing to 140,000 per week in

2022, 40,000 in 2023, and 13,000 in 2024. Even the best healthcare systems were affected. The Italian health system, ranked as one of the best [25] worldwide, was also impacted by the pandemic. Regions with healthcare systems operating at standard levels faced shortages of beds, ICUs, ventilators, PPE, and healthcare workers [26, 27]. Moreover, insufficient supplies of healthcare resources, including personnel and medical supplies, worsened the challenges faced by health systems to critical levels. As a temporary measure for PPE shortages, healthcare personnel used plastic bags and cloth masks made at home, further increasing the risk of infection among healthcare professionals [28, 29] and patients without COVID-19. Countries such as China and the United States adopted additional interim arrangements by recognising alternative resources to manage the overwhelming demand for care [13, 30]. The pandemic has highlighted the urgent need for resilient healthcare systems that can adapt to sudden surges in patient volume and provide adequate protection for healthcare workers.

Healthcare workers are on the frontline of the response to COVID-19, often facing significant risks and challenges as they provide essential care to those infected. The infection rate among health careworkers globally was 11.0%. Contributing factors included household exposure, occupational exposure, inadequate infection prevention and control training, insufficient use of PPE, performing aerosol-generating procedures, inadequate hand hygiene, and working as a cleaner [31].

The socioeconomic impact of COVID-19 goes beyond immediate health effects, seriously disrupting education systems and labour markets around the world. Schools experienced extended closures, affecting millions of students and worsening existing educational inequalities, especially in low-income areas where access to remote learning resources was limited. According to the World Bank, about 1.6 billion learners were affected by school closures globally, with potential long-term impacts on human capital development [32]. Furthermore, the pandemic has caused significant job losses, notably in sectors such as hospitality and tourism, leading to increased poverty and economic instability, particularly in developing countries. As nations work towards recovery, tackling these complex challenges will be essential in rebuilding resilient education and economic systems that can endure future crises and support fair growth [17].

2.6 Impact of Vaccination

2.6.1 Global Impact of COVID-19 Vaccination

The introduction of COVID-19 vaccines was a vital part of the global plan to tackle the pandemic. By December 2021, COVID-19 vaccination efforts had prevented an estimated 14.4 million deaths worldwide, rising to 19.8 million when including excess deaths [33]. The vaccines also brought significant economic advantages, saving an estimated $155 billion through reduced infections and increased productivity [34].

2.6.2 Disparities in Vaccine Access

Despite the success of vaccination programmes, there were significant disparities in vaccine access between high-income and low-income countries. If low-income countries had achieved the 40% vaccination coverage target set by the WHO, an additional 111% of deaths could have been averted [35]. The lack of vaccine equity not only limited the impact of vaccination in low-income countries but also had broader economic implications, as the cost of not vaccinating these countries far outweighed the cost of manufacturing and distributing vaccines [36].

2.7 Long-Term Effects and Recovery

2.7.1 Post-COVID-19 Conditions

The long-term effects of COVID-19, often called post-COVID-19 conditions or long COVID, have increased the burden of the pandemic. These effects can include ongoing respiratory symptoms, neurological issues, and mental health problems, among others [37]. The occurrence and severity of long COVID differ by region and population, with higher rates seen in areas with fewer healthcare resources [38].

2.7.2 Recovery Time and Global Trends

The recovery time for COVID-19 varies greatly depending on the severity of the infection. Mild cases usually resolve within 2 weeks, while severe cases may take several weeks to months to recover from lung issues [39, 40]. Globally, the number of reported COVID-19 cases has decreased since mid-2022, but the virus still circulates, and recovery times remain a concern for individuals and healthcare systems [11].

2.8 Policy Implications and Future Directions

2.8.1 Strengthening Health Systems

The COVID-19 pandemic has highlighted the need for stronger healthcare systems, especially in low- and middle-income countries. Investments in healthcare infrastructure, including diagnostic capacity, treatment options, and vaccination programmes, are essential for reducing the impact of COVID-19 and preparing for future pandemics.

2.8.2 Addressing Disparities

The disparities in the burden of COVID-19 across regions and income groups highlight the need for targeted interventions and international cooperation. Policymakers must focus on vaccine equity, improve access to healthcare, and address the social and economic determinants of health to lessen the impact of COVID-19 and future pandemics [22].

2.8.3 Monitoring and Surveillance

Enhanced monitoring and surveillance systems are crucial for tracking the impact of COVID-19 and responding to future public health emergencies. Developing robust health information systems, particularly in low-income countries, will improve the accuracy of mortality and morbidity data and enable more effective policy responses [17, 20].

2.9 Conclusion

The global impact of COVID-19 has been significant, affecting mortality, morbidity, and economic outcomes. The pandemic has emphasised the importance of equitable healthcare access, strong health systems, and international cooperation to tackle public health emergencies. As the world advances, the lessons learned from the COVID-19 pandemic will be vital in preparing for future challenges and lessening the global burden of infectious diseases.

References

1. Weiss SR, Navas-Martin S. Coronavirus pathogenesis and the emerging pathogen severe acute respiratory syndrome coronavirus. Microbiol Mol Biol Rev. 2005;69(4):635–64.
2. Zhu N, Zhang D, Wang W, et al. A novel coronavirus from patients with pneumonia in China, 2019. N Engl J Med. 2020;382(8):727–33.
3. Wu D, Wu T, Liu Q, et al. The SARS-CoV-2 outbreak: what we know. Int J Infect Dis. 2020;94:44–8.
4. WHO. COVID-19 public health emergency of international concern (PHEIC) global research and innovation forum. 2020.
5. WHO, Coronavirus disease (COVID-19): situation report, 147, in Coronavirus disease (COVID-19): situation report, 147. 2020.
6. Louca S. COVID-19 prevalence in 161 countries and over time. medRXiv. 2020;
7. WHO, Coronavirus disease (COVID-19) Situation Report – 125, in Situation report, WHO, Editor. 2020.
8. Kim S, Yeniova A. Global, regional, and national incidence and mortality of COVID-19 in 237 countries and territories, January 2022: a systematic analysis for World Health Organization COVID-19 dashboard. Life Cycle. 2022:2.
9. WHO, COVID-19 Epidemiological Update – Special Edition 174, WHO, Editor. 2024.

10. Mathieu E, Ritchie H, Rodés-Guirao L, et al. COVID-19 Pandemic. 2020, OurWorldinData.org: Online Resource.
11. Du J, Lang H-m, Ma Y, et al. Global trends in COVID-19 incidence and case fatality rates (2019–2023): a retrospective analysis. Front Public Health. 2024;12:1355097.
12. Onder G, Rezza G, Brusaferro S. Case-fatality rate and characteristics of patients dying in relation to COVID-19 in Italy. JAMA J Am Med Assoc. 2020;323(18):1775–6.
13. Wu Z, McGoogan JM. Characteristics of and important lessons from the coronavirus disease 2019 (COVID-19) outbreak in China: summary of a report of 72 314 cases from the Chinese Center for Disease Control and Prevention. JAMA J Am Med Assoc. 2020;323(13):1239–42.
14. Naghavi M, Mohsen N, Kanyin Liane O, et al. Global burden of 288 causes of death and life expectancy decomposition in 204 countries and territories and 811 subnational locations, 1990–2021: a systematic analysis for the global burden of disease study 2021. Lancet. 2024;403(10440):2100–32.
15. WHO. Clinical characteristics and health outcomes for children hospitalized with COVID-19. World Health Organization; 2023.
16. Checchi F, Roberts L. HPN network paper 52: interpreting and using mortality data in humanitarian emergencies: a primer for non-epidemiologists. 2005.
17. Msemburi W, Karlinsky A, Knutson V, et al. The WHO estimates of excess mortality associated with the COVID-19 pandemic. Nature. 2023;613(7942):130–7.
18. WHO. World health statistics 2024: monitoring health for the SDGs, sustainable development goals. World Health Organization; 2024.
19. Pifarré i Arolas H, Acosta E, López-Casasnovas G, et al. Years of life lost to COVID-19 in 81 countries. Sci Rep. 2021;11(1):3504.
20. Espinosa O, Ramos J, Rojas-Botero ML, et al. Years of life lost to COVID-19 in 49 countries: a gender-and life cycle-based analysis of the first two years of the pandemic. PLoS Global Public Health. 2023;3(9):e0002172.
21. Fan CY, Fann JC, Yang MC, et al. Estimating global burden of COVID-19 with disability-adjusted life years and value of statistical life metrics. J Formos Med Assoc. 2021;120(Suppl 1):S106–s117.
22. Li X-C, Zhang Y-Y, Zhang Q-Y, et al. Global burden of viral infectious diseases of poverty based on global burden of diseases study 2021. Infect Dis Poverty. 2024;13(05):53–67.
23. Ferrari AJ, Santomauro DF, Aali A, et al. Global incidence, prevalence, years lived with disability (YLDs), disability-adjusted life-years (DALYs), and healthy life expectancy (HALE) for 371 diseases and injuries in 204 countries and territories and 811 subnational locations, 1990–2021: a systematic analysis for the Global Burden of Disease Study 2021. Lancet. 2024;403(10440):2133–61.
24. Micah AE, Bhangdia K, Cogswell IE, et al. Global investments in pandemic preparedness and COVID-19: development assistance and domestic spending on health between 1990 and 2026. Lancet Glob Health. 2023;11(3):e385–413.
25. Tandon A, Murray CJ, Lauer JA, et al. Measuring overall health system performance for 191 countries. Geneva: World Health Organization; 2000.
26. Armocida B, Formenti B, Ussai S, et al. The Italian health system and the COVID-19 challenge. Lancet Public Health. 2020;5(5):e253.
27. Odone A, Delmonte D, Scognamiglio T, et al. COVID-19 deaths in Lombardy, Italy: data in context. Lancet Public Health. 2020;5(6):e310.
28. Guerra FM, Bolotin S, Lim G, et al. The basic reproduction number (R0) of measles: a systematic review. Lancet Infect Dis. 2017;17(12):e420–8.
29. Wallinga J, Teunis P. Different epidemic curves for severe acute respiratory syndrome reveal similar impacts of control measures. Am J Epidemiol. 2004;160(6):509–16.
30. Marquez M, Moghe S. Inside a Brooklyn hospital that is overwhelmed with Covid-19 patients and deaths. CNN. 2020;90
31. Bansal A, Trieu M-C, Eriksson EM, et al. SARS-CoV-2 infection rates and associated risk factors in healthcare workers: systematic review and meta-analysis. Sci Rep. 2025;15(1):4705.

32. Azevedo JP, Hasan A, Goldemberg D, et al. Simulating the potential impacts of COVID-19 school closures on schooling and learning outcomes: a set of global estimates. World Bank Res Obs. 2021, 36(1):1–40.
33. Watson OJ, Barnsley G, Toor J, et al. Global impact of the first year of COVID-19 vaccination: a mathematical modelling study. Lancet Infect Dis. 2022;22(9):1293–302.
34. Yang J, Vaghela S, Yarnoff B, et al. Estimated global public health and economic impact of COVID-19 vaccines in the pre-omicron era using real-world empirical data. Expert Rev Vaccines. 2023;22(1):54–65.
35. Pai C, Finnane H. Inequalities in access to covid-19 vaccines and potential solutions for low- and middle-income countries. In Proceedings of the global public health conference. 2023.
36. Ferranna M. Causes and costs of global COVID-19 vaccine inequity. In: Seminars in immunopathology. Springer; 2024.
37. Zaman M, Sizemore RC. Long COVID: epidemiology, post-COVID-19 manifestations, possible mechanisms, treatment, and prevention strategies–a review. IMC J Med Sci. 2024;18:1.
38. Hou Y, Gu T, Ni Z, et al. Global prevalence of long COVID, its subtypes and risk factors: an updated systematic review and meta-analysis. medRxiv. 2025;
39. SeyedAlinaghi S, Abbasian L, Solduzian M, et al. Predictors of the prolonged recovery period in COVID-19 patients: a cross-sectional study. Eur J Med Res. 2021;26(1):41.
40. Schlemmer F, Valentin S, Boyer L, et al. Respiratory recovery trajectories after severe-to-critical COVID-19: a 1-year prospective multicentre study. Eur Respir J. 2023;61(4):2201532.

3 Global Determinants of COVID-19 Morbidity and Mortality

Kelvin J.K. Tan

3.1 Introduction

The COVID-19 pandemic triggered a global health crisis of unprecedented scale, yet its impacts were highly uneven across countries. Although all nations confronted the same virus, infection and death rates, reflected in morbidity and mortality outcomes, varied substantially across borders. By the end of 2025, cumulative global figures reported to the World Health Organisation indicate approximately 779 million confirmed cases and 7.1 million deaths worldwide. While some countries were able to contain transmission rapidly and limit fatalities, others experienced prolonged waves of infection accompanied by severe loss of life. These stark cross-country disparities, illustrated in Fig. 3.1, highlight the importance of understanding why some nations were affected more severely than others. The United States emerged as the hardest-hit country in terms of both confirmed cases and deaths. China and India followed as the countries with the highest numbers of confirmed cases, while Brazil and India recorded among the highest cumulative death tolls.

Early research mainly focused on government measures like lockdowns, mask mandates, and vaccination efforts. However, more recent studies have explored a deeper structural issue: whether some countries were inherently more vulnerable to the pandemic due to pre-existing factors.

This chapter places particular emphasis on the empirical analysis of Chang et al. [1], which provides one of the most comprehensive and influential cross-country examinations of this question. Using data from 91 nations, their study analyses 21 predetermined country-level factors spanning demographic composition, institutional arrangements, socioeconomic conditions, and healthcare capacity. We highlight this study as the central reference point for three reasons. First, its focus on pre-pandemic structural characteristics allows for a clean separation between underlying

K. J.K. Tan (✉)
UQ Business School, The University of Queensland, Brisbane, QLD, Australia
e-mail: k.tan@business.uq.edu.au

S. R. Prabhu et al. (eds.), *COVID-19 in Dental Practice*,
https://doi.org/10.1007/978-3-032-26000-0_3

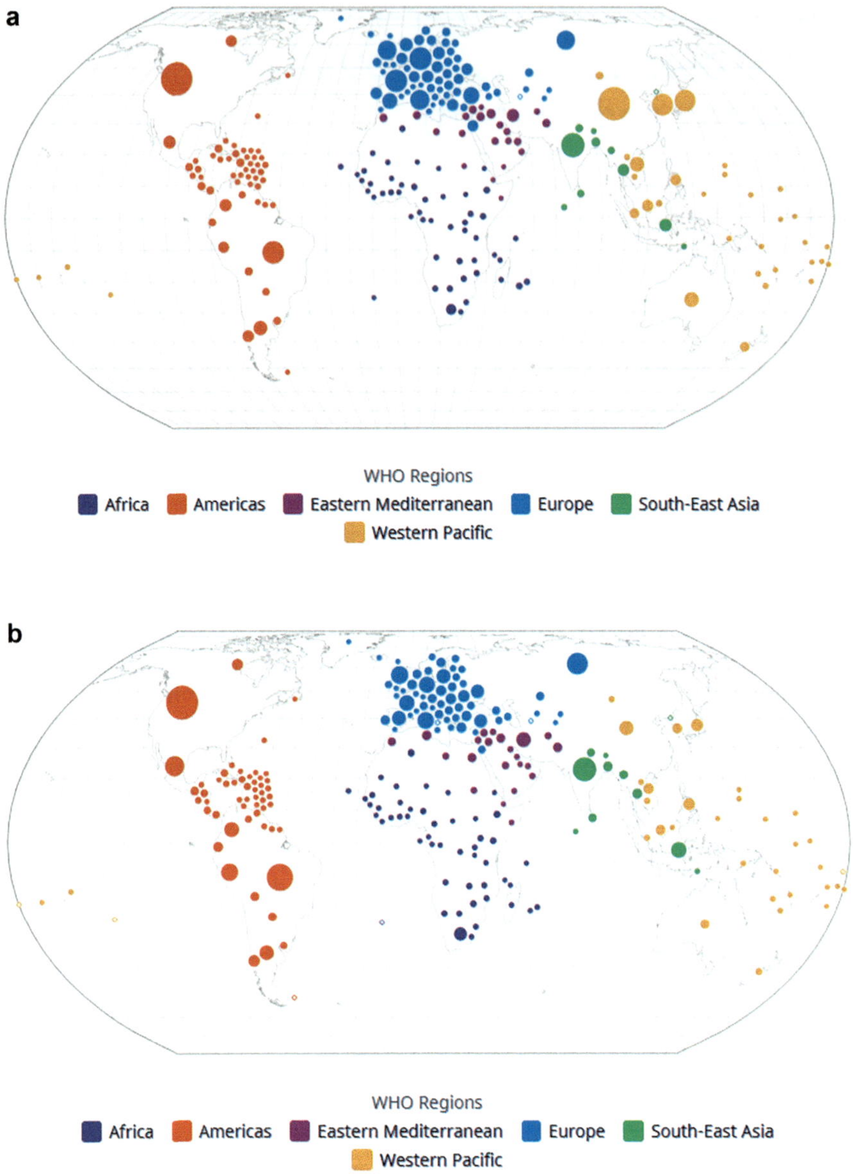
a
WHO Regions
Africa
Americas
Eastern Mediterranean
Europe
South-East Asia
Western Pacific
b
WHO Regions
Africa
Americas
Eastern Mediterranean
Europe
South-East Asia
Western Pacific

vulnerability and reactive policy measures. Second, the study has been highly influential within academia and is widely cited across economics, finance, public health, and policy research. Third, its impact extends well beyond scholarly audiences, attracting substantial attention from media outlets, policy discussions, blogs, and social media, with an Altimetric score of 424 as of December 2025. This combination of academic rigour and broad public engagement makes Chang et al. [1] a handy anchor for synthesising the literature on cross-country pandemic outcomes.

To disentangle structural vulnerabilities from reactive responses, Chang et al. [1] restrict their analysis to variables measured before the onset of the pandemic. These predetermined factors are organised into four domains: demographic and geographic characteristics, political and legal institutions, socioeconomic conditions, and healthcare-related factors. Pandemic outcomes are measured using the natural logarithm of one plus the number of confirmed COVID-19 cases and deaths per country per week, based on data from Johns Hopkins University's global COVID-19 database.

The empirical strategy follows the Fama-MacBeth two-step regression approach. In the first step, weekly cross-sectional regressions are estimated for each country. In the second step, the coefficients from these regressions are averaged over 2020, producing estimates that account for temporal variation while mitigating concerns about serial correlation. Notably, the analysis excludes variables such as mask use, testing intensity, or lockdown timing, which are endogenous to the pandemic's evolution. By relying exclusively on pre-pandemic structural characteristics, the study aims to identify deeper sources of national vulnerability and resilience.

To enhance interpretability, the authors report marginal effects that quantify the change in cases or deaths, expressed as a percentage of the sample average, associated with a one-standard-deviation increase in each explanatory variable. This framing facilitates a more intuitive assessment of the practical importance of different country-level determinants.

While Chang et al. [1] serve as the primary analytical framework in this section, we do not suggest that their study is exhaustive. Where appropriate, we complement

Fig. 3.1 (**a**) Number of COVID-19 confirmed cases reported to WHO (cumulative total). (**b**) Number of COVID-19 deaths reported to WHO (cumulative total). The number of confirmed COVID-19 cases and deaths across the globe reported to the World Health Organisation (WHO) as of 7 December 2025. *Panel* (**a**) illustrates the worldwide distribution of confirmed COVID-19 cases. Circle size reflects the cumulative number of confirmed cases in each country, with larger circles indicating higher case counts. The United States reports the highest number of confirmed cases, at approximately 103.4 million, followed by China with 99.4 million and India with 45.1 million. Globally, the total number of confirmed cases reaches approximately 779 million. *Panel* (**b**) depicts the global distribution of COVID-19 deaths, again using circle size to represent cumulative fatalities. The United States records the highest number of reported deaths at approximately 1.2 million, followed by Brazil with 704,000 deaths and India with 534,000 deaths. Total global COVID-19 deaths reported worldwide amount to approximately 7.1 million. (Both panels are reproduced from the World Health Organisation COVID-19 Dashboard https://data.who.int/dashboards/covid19)

their findings with evidence from other comparative studies to highlight areas of consensus, divergence, and extension. After presenting the core results from this cross-country framework, the chapter broadens the discussion by surveying additional international evidence. This broader synthesis helps contextualise the findings and sets the stage for Sect. 3.2.6, where insights from the broader literature are distilled into practical policy implications to strengthen pandemic preparedness and resilience.

3.2 Structural Determinants of COVID-19 Morbidity and Mortality

Figures 3.2 and 3.3 jointly illustrate how a common set of structural country characteristics shaped both COVID-19 morbidity and mortality. Although the magnitude of effects differs between infections and deaths, a consistent pattern emerges. Countries that faced greater demographic pressure, higher social interaction, and weaker institutional capacity experienced worse outcomes across both dimensions. In contrast, those with stronger health systems, prior epidemic experience, and favourable environmental conditions were more resilient.

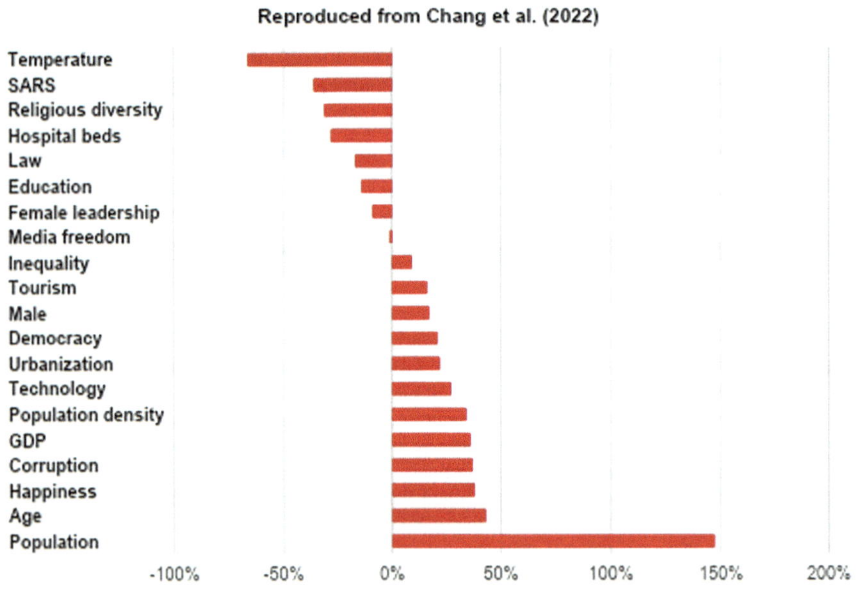

Fig. 3.2 Marginal effects of a one-standard-deviation change in determinants of confirmed cases effect (%). (Reproduced from Chang et al. [1])

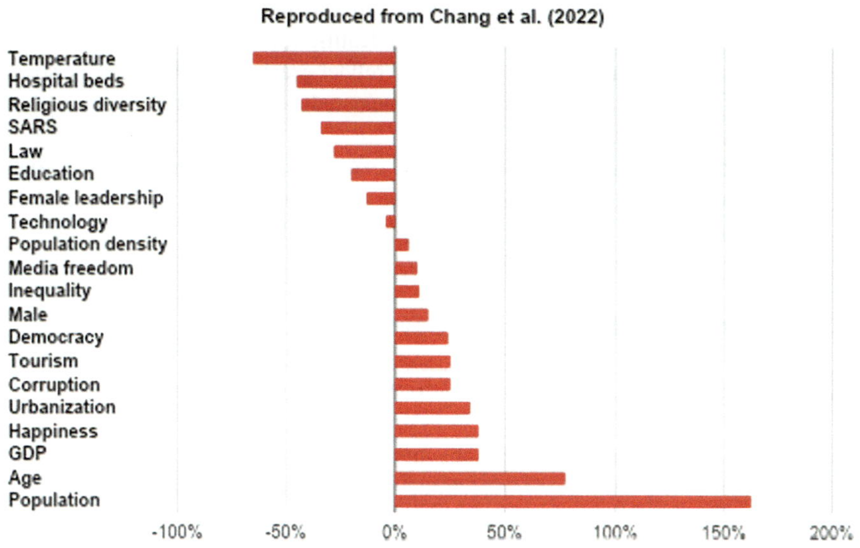

Fig. 3.3 Marginal effects of a one-standard-deviation change in determinants of COVID-19 deaths (%). (Reproduced from Chang et al. [1])

3.2.1 Demographic Factors

Demographic factors exert the strongest and most consistent influence across both confirmed cases and deaths.

- *Population size* dominates both figures, increasing confirmed cases by 147% and deaths by 162% for each one-standard-deviation increase. Larger populations posed inherent challenges for testing, contact tracing, and enforcement and also placed a heavier strain on healthcare systems as infections surged.
- *The population age* structure further amplified vulnerability. Median age raises infection rates by 43%. Still, it increases deaths by an even larger 77%, reflecting the disproportionate clinical severity of COVID-19 among older individuals and the concentration of risk within institutional care settings. The sharper mortality effect highlights how demographic ageing primarily operates through disease severity rather than exposure alone.

3.2.2 Socioeconomic Conditions and Social Behaviour

A second set of determinants includes socioeconomic conditions and social behaviour.

- *Higher national happiness, gross domestic product per capita, and urbanisation* are all linked to increases in both cases and deaths. These relationships may seem counterintuitive at first, but they probably reflect greater mobility, denser social networks, and increased international connectedness in more prosperous and socially active societies.
- The fact that wealth and life satisfaction exacerbate rather than mitigate pandemic outcomes underscores that economic development does not automatically translate into systemic resilience during global health shocks.

3.2.3 Institutional Quality and Governance

The institutional quality and governance further differentiate national outcomes.

- *Corruption* increases both infections and deaths, suggesting that weak institutions undermine policy implementation, coordination, and compliance.
- *Stronger legal systems* are associated with substantially lower mortality, even when infection levels remain elevated.

The above asymmetry indicates that governance quality may matter more for preventing fatal outcomes than for preventing transmission, particularly through effective enforcement of emergency measures and protection of healthcare delivery.

3.2.4 Environmental and Health System Factors

Environmental and health systems consistently mitigate both morbidity and mortality.

- *Temperature* emerges as the single most protective factor in both figures, reducing confirmed cases by 66% and deaths by 65%. This result aligns with evidence on viral stability, seasonality, and behavioural adaptation in warmer climates.
- *Healthcare capacity* also plays a critical role. Greater hospital bed availability reduces infections modestly but lowers deaths by 45%, highlighting that system readiness primarily saves lives once transmission occurs.
- *Prior experience* with severe acute respiratory syndrome (SARS) reduces both cases and deaths, demonstrating the enduring value of institutional memory, established protocols, and public familiarity with outbreak management.

3.2.5 Social Capital, Education, and Leadership Characteristics

Social capital, education, and leadership contribute meaningfully to resilience.

- *Education.* Higher levels of education reduce both infections and deaths by improving health literacy and adherence to guidance.

middle-income countries, while strategies aimed at achieving herd immunity raised both. Countries affected early in the pandemic experienced higher mortality, reflecting limited experience and constrained medical capacity. The authors argue that improving air quality and addressing chronic health risks are essential components of long-term pandemic preparedness.

Taken together, this broader literature complements the structural emphasis of Chang et al. [1] by showing that climate risk, inequality, governance, trust, and policy effectiveness jointly shape cross-national pandemic outcomes. Structural conditions determine baseline vulnerability, while institutions and policies influence how societies translate exposure into health consequences.

3.2.7 Policy Implications

The evidence summarised in this chapter suggests several important lessons for public policy:

1. *Invest in Prevention, Not Just Response*

Structural factors such as education, health capacity, and institutional trust had significant effects on pandemic outcomes. These cannot be built overnight and require consistent investment.

2. *Equity Is a Health Imperative*

Socioeconomic inequality, poor education, and weak governance amplified the risks posed by COVID-19. Addressing these issues is not just a moral obligation because it also improves societal resilience.

3. *Preserve Institutional Memory*

Countries with experience managing earlier outbreaks fared better. This underlines the importance of retaining expertise, maintaining response protocols, and conducting preparedness drills.

4. *Leadership and Representation Matter*

Countries led by women saw better outcomes, potentially reflecting leadership styles that emphasised transparency, empathy, and communication. This highlights the value of inclusive governance.

5. *Don't Assume Wealth Equals Safety*

High GDP per capita was not a safeguard. Policymakers in developed nations must remain vigilant and avoid complacency.

3.2.8 Summary/Conclusion

COVID-19 has served not only as a pandemic but also as a mirror, exposing both strengths and vulnerabilities within national systems. The findings from Chang et al. [1] make clear that many of the most critical determinants of pandemic success or failure were in place long before the virus appeared.

The wider cross-country evidence reviewed in this chapter reinforces this conclusion, showing that governance quality, public trust, inequality, environmental conditions, and the effectiveness of vaccination and non-pharmaceutical interventions played critical roles in shaping outcomes across countries. Together, these studies highlight that resilience depends not only on wealth but also on institutional capacity, social cohesion, and preparedness.

Structural preparedness, such as spanning healthcare, education, governance, and leadership, is not an optional extra. It is the core of a resilient society. To prepare for future pandemics, nations must move beyond reactive responses and invest in the systems that quietly but powerfully protect lives.

References

1. Chang D, Chang X, He Y, Tan KJK. The determinants of COVID-19 morbidity and mortality across countries. Sci Rep. 2022;12:5888; Springer Nature. https://doi.org/10.1038/s41598-022-09783-9.
2. Nojković A, Arsić M, Milošević E. Cross-country determinants of COVID-19 mortality and the manipulation of death data in autocratic regimes. Empirica. 2025;52(4):839–62. https://doi.org/10.1007/s10663-025-09660-4.
3. Sun MW, Troxell D, Tibshirani R. Public health factors help explain cross-country heterogeneity in excess death during the COVID-19 pandemic. Sci Rep. 2023;13:16196. https://doi.org/10.1038/s41598-023-43407-0.
4. Ozkan A, Ozkan G, Yalaman A, Yildiz Y. Climate risk, culture and the Covid-19 mortality: a cross-country analysis. World Dev. 2021;141:105412. https://doi.org/10.1016/j.worlddev.2021.105412.
5. Zhou C, Wheelock ÅM, Zhang C, Ma J, Li Z, Liang W, Gao J, Xu L. Country-specific determinants for COVID-19 case fatality rate and response strategies from a global perspective: an interpretable machine learning framework. Popul Health Metrics. 2024;22:10. https://doi.org/10.1186/s12963-024-00330-4.
6. Davies JB. Economic inequality and Covid-19 death rates in the first wave: a cross-country analysis. CESifo Working Paper No. 8957.
7. Farzanegan MR, Hofmann HP. A matter of trust? Political trust and the Covid-19 pandemic. CESifo Working Paper Series. No. 9121.
8. da Silva RE, Novaes MRCG, de Oliveira C, Guilhem DB. National governance and excess mortality due to COVID-19 in 213 countries: a retrospective analysis and perspectives on future pandemics. Glob Health. 2023;19:80. https://doi.org/10.1186/s12992-023-00982-1.
9. Agyapon-Ntra K, McSharry PE. A global analysis of the effectiveness of policy responses to COVID-19. Sci Rep. 2023;13:5629. https://doi.org/10.1038/s41598-023-31709-2.
10. Bretschger L, Grieg E, Welfens PJJ, Xiong T. COVID-19 infections and fatalities developments: empirical evidence for OECD countries and newly industrialised economies. IEEP. 2020;17(4):801–47. https://doi.org/10.1007/s10368-020-00487-x. Reviewed 4/1/2026.

Current Detection and Mitigation Windows Used for Detecting SARS-CoV-2 Infection

4

Ananda P. Dasanayake, Ranawaka A. P. M. Perera, and Lakhsman Samaranayake

4.1 Introduction

The initial clinical data from individuals with a confirmed diagnosis of SARS-CoV-2 (originally called 2019-nCoV) infection emerged in Wuhan, China, in December 2019, with most patients having direct exposure to a source at the Wuhan seafood market [1]. The RNA genome of the SARS-CoV-2 virus, which was later identified as the cause of the disease, is the largest known among RNA viruses [2], with a size ranging from 26 to 32 kb in length [3].

Since the Wuhan outbreak, the infection has developed into a global pandemic. As of September 2025, over 775 million people have been infected with either the original strain or a later variant; over 7 million have died from the infection; and more than 13.5 billion doses of COVID-19 vaccine have been administered worldwide [4]. However, global surveillance has decreased, leading to an underestimation of recent totals. The pandemic has severely affected the world socially, politically, and economically, with opportunists spreading discourse for political and financial gains, and conflicting private and public responsibilities splitting the global population into various camps, including those who refuse vaccination.

Dentistry was among the fields affected by the virus. During COVID-19, dental practices experienced significant drops in procedure volume, especially among patients covered by public insurance or living in underserved areas [5]. Except for scheduled orthodontic appointments or emergency care, all other practices were

A. P. Dasanayake (✉)
Department of Epidemiology, New York University College of Dentistry, New York, NY, USA

R. A. P. M. Perera
Department of Microbiology, University of Pennsylvania School of Medicine and Veterans Affairs, Philadelphia, PA, USA

L. Samaranayake
Faculty of Dentistry, University of Hong Kong, Hong Kong, China

S. R. Prabhu et al. (eds.), *COVID-19 in Dental Practice*,
https://doi.org/10.1007/978-3-032-26000-0_4

largely halted. Given this context, it is wise to critically review current preventive and mitigation strategies for this pandemic within dental settings. There are several unanswered questions, including the duration of viral shedding from the start to the end of both asymptomatic and symptomatic illness, the onset and decline of antibody responses, and the best methods, timing, and quarantine periods for virus detection based on current. Developing a general timeline that illustrates these windows is challenging because of differences in viral strains and variations among susceptible subgroups. Burn et al. have shown that, generally, aged males with comorbidities like diabetes tend to experience worse clinical outcomes from COVID-19 than other subgroups [6]. This chapter critically examines these various windows in relation to current mitigation practices. Conclusions should be coupled with the latest CDC and other guidelines [7].

4.2 Incubation Period

Since the start of the pandemic, several notable variants have emerged, including alpha, beta, delta, and omicron. The CDC is presently concentrating on omicron and its subvariants B.1.1.529, BA.1, BA.1.1, BA.2, BA.3, BA.4, BA.5, and variants such as JN.1, along with more recent lineages like XFG (78% of cases), NB.1.8.1 (14%), and LP.8.1 (3%).

In general, the symptomatic and transmissible phase of SARS-CoV-2 occurs around 3–7 days after initial viral entry for these variants and appears to be age-related, with shorter incubation times observed with recent variants, averaging 3–4 days for omicron lineages and 3–5 days for JN.1 descendants [8]. Disease symptoms appear as soon as 2 days after the initial exposure and most people show symptoms by day 12, and rarely after day 14. The very high infectivity during the incubation period of the omicron variant remains a formidable challenge for controlling the disease [9].

4.3 Clinical Phase

A person with COVID-19 is generally considered infectious starting 2 days before they develop symptoms or 2 days before the date of their positive test if they do not have symptoms [7]. The period between exposure and symptom onset ranges from about 5 days for early variants to 4 days for the Delta variant and approximately 3 days for the omicron variant. The first omicron variant emerged at the end of 2021 and was named B.1.1.529. This strain quickly overtook the alpha, beta, and delta variants. Following this initial variant, others such as BA.1, BA.2, BA.3, BA.4, and BA.5 appeared in subsequent waves. The mean incubation period of these omicron variants was estimated to be around 3.42 days (95% CI, 2.88–3.96 days) [10], with similar or slightly shorter periods (3–5 days) for 2024–2025 JN.1 lineage variants like XEC and KP 3.1.1, which are shorter than the incubation periods of alpha, beta, and delta variants. However, the incubation periods of the most recent JN.1 lineage variants, such as XEC and KP 3.1.1, have yet to be determined.

4.4 Antigen Detection Periods and Sensitivity

In general, COVID-19 diagnostic tests detect either viral antigens, which indicate a current infection, or host immune responses (i.e., specific antibodies). This could mean either an antibody response to the infection itself or due to vaccination (i.e., induction of natural or artificial immunity, respectively). Positive viral antigen tests show that the individual has the infection at the time of testing, such as Nucleic Acid Amplification Tests (NAAT) [7].

The antigen detection period for SARS-CoV-2 is now known to be approximately 3–10 days after initial exposure. The most sensitive tests to detect these antigens are Abbot/Healgen, R-biopharm, and Roche SD biosensor which are >95% sensitive but are considered inferior to PCR testing in low viral load scenarios [11]. The sensitivity and specificity of seven different commercial tests have shown that the sensitivity range of most tests overlapped with SARS-CoV-2 viral loads typically observed in the first week of symptoms, which marks the infectious period in most patients [11]. In addition, another study reported that tests from six manufacturers had an overall sensitivity of 75–100%, while four tests from other manufacturers had a sensitivity of 50–71.43%, with specificities consistently >99% [12].

4.5 Window of PCR Positivity and the Usefulness of PCR Testing

Polymerase chain reaction (PCR), which detects amplified viral genetic material, can test positive for 3–40 days after initial exposure. However, infectiousness diminishes substantially, to negligible levels, by around 8 days after symptom onset [13]. A pooled analysis of seven published studies evaluating RT-PCR performance in relation to time since symptom onset or SARS-CoV-2 exposure, (using upper respiratory tract samples (n = 1330), and employing a Bayesian hierarchical model to estimate the false-negative rate by day since exposure and symptom onset), found that Kucirka et al. examined false-negative RT-PCR results on different days. The chance of a false-negative result in an infected person drops from 100% (95% CI, 100–100%) on day 1–67% (CI, 27–94%) on day 4. On the day of symptom onset, the median false-negative rate was 38% (CI, 18–65%). This decreased to 20% (CI, 12–30%) by day 8 (3 days after symptom onset), then began to rise again, from 21% (CI, 13–31%) on day 9–66% (CI, 54–77%) by day 21 [14]. These patterns are consistent for the latest variants, although PCR positivity may diminish slightly (up to 30 days) due to faster viral clearance. Nevertheless, even if someone tests PCR-positive, they may not transmit the virus to close contacts. This is often overlooked when setting quarantine durations and making travel and work-related decisions. Additionally, unnecessarily prolonged quarantine periods may undermine their purpose and increase the risk of healthy individuals becoming infected within quarantine centres.

4.6 Cost of Unwanted and Ineffective Screening and Detection in Relation to Prevention

Most SARS-CoV-2 tests are worthless 10 days after symptom onset because transmission may be absent or minimal during that period in mild to moderate cases. The countries that impose a 21-day quarantine apparently ignore this scientific basis. Furthermore, there could be transmission within overcrowded quarantine facilities when people are kept simply because they are PCR-positive. For instance, in the face of declining omicron infections in New York, New York University College of Dentistry decided not to require testing or proof of vaccination for high-aerosol-generating procedures, effective Monday, February 7, 2022, aligning with the CDC's shift to symptom-based approaches rather than routine testing. The only circumstance in which patients will be required to show proof of a negative COVID-19 test within 72 h, regardless of vaccination status, will be for those undergoing sedation and/or general anaesthesia. As these rules may change, in the face of new omicron infections, clinicians must be cognizant of the most recent CDC quarantine and other COVID-related guidelines and updates and also of the natural history of the disease.

Despite the availability of rapid, sensitive tests for antigen and antibody detection, there appears to be a scarcity of reports summarising the window periods for viral detection at different disease stages described above. Fig. 4.1, prepared using the existing literature, indicates various endpoints related to SARS-CoV-2 from the date of initial exposure and is an attempt to construct these windows. The cascades

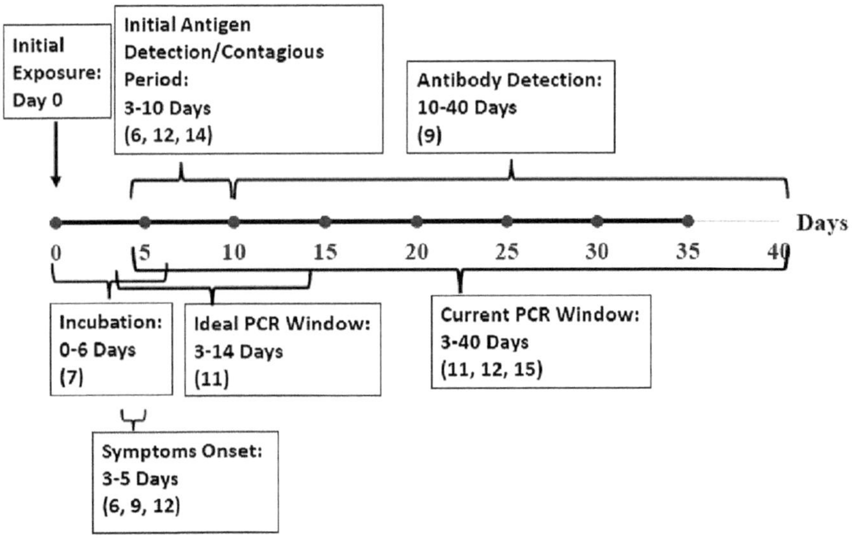

Fig. 4.1 Various diagnostic and clinical endpoint windows of the SARS-CoV-2 from the date of initial exposure

of clinical and humoral events that occur after the initial exposure may provide clinicians, public health practitioners, and policymakers with better guidelines for mitigating activities.

4.7 Clinical Stages of SARS-CoV-2 Infection

Dos Santos et al. describe three stages of the natural history of COVID-19 based on disease severity [15]. The first is related to the disease onset. It is generally characterised by the development of influenza-like symptoms such as fever, cough, runny nose, shortness of breath, fatigue, headache, loss of taste/smell, and/or diarrhoea. In the second phase, pneumonia-like symptoms are detected as lung opacities on chest radiography or as glass opacities on computed tomography. In stage 3, characterised by hyperinflammation and sepsis of the lungs, patients require management in intensive care units, and most of the affected eventually succumb to the disease [15]. However, window periods need to be constructed for each of these stages using data from large cohorts, accounting for variant-specific differences, e.g., faster progression of JN.1 lineages.

4.8 Window of Initial Antibody Response, Methods of Detection, and the Usefulness

Protective neutralising antibody response starts 10–14 days after the initial infection. A considerable antibody response can be detected within 9–10 days, with full seroconversion in 30–40 days, though antibody levels wane after 6–12 months post-infection or vaccination. Positive tests for antibodies indicate that the subject was infected with the virus in the past. Windows during which these antibody or serology tests are done may not overlap with the window during which the subject is infectious.

The gold standard for detecting these antibodies is the plaque neutralisation assay. Using this method, one can assess the duration of neutralising antibodies after infection. Usually, these antibody levels decrease after 6 months. Lau et al. tested 293 sera from an observational cohort of 195 confirmed SARS-CoV-2 cases, collected between 0 and 209 days after symptom onset [16]. Of the 115 sera collected ≥61 days after the onset of illness tested using plaque reduction neutralisation (PRNT) assays, 99.1% remained seropositive for both 90% (PRNT90) and 50% (PRNT50) neutralisation endpoints. They estimated that it takes at least 372, 416, and 133 days for PRNT50 titres to drop to the detection limit of 1:10 for severe, mild, and asymptomatic patients, respectively. In general, 6–12 months after the second dose seems to be the appropriate time to administer a booster to boost the antibody response and prevent reinfection, with adults >65 years receiving two doses for optimal protection.

4.9 Conclusion

In oral health care settings, including academic institutions and dental offices alike, current COVID-19 mitigation practices often rely on PCR negativity. A critical review of the natural history casts doubt on this approach, which may be questionable and misleading. A novel strategy, such as combining rapid antigen tests, symptom screening, and infection history, may be required to overcome this impasse, aligned with 2024–2025 CDC and ADA guidelines emphasising risk-based measures.

References

1. Huang C, Wang Y, Li X, et al. Clinical features of patients infected with 2019 novel coronavirus in Wuhan, China. Lancet. 2020;395(10223):497–506.
2. Brian DA, Baric RS. Coronavirus genome structure and replication. Curr Top Microbiol Immunol. 2005;287:1–30.
3. Lu R, Zhao X, Li J, et al. Genomic characterisation and epidemiology of 2019 novel coronavirus: implications for virus origins and receptor binding. Lancet. 2020;395(10224):565–74.
4. JHU Corona Virus Resource Center. 2022.. https://coronavirus.jhu.edu/map.html. Accessed 1 Feb 2022.
5. Choi SE, Simon L, Basu S, Barrow JR. Changes in dental care use patterns due to COVID-19 among insured patients in the United States. J Am Dent Assoc. 2021;152(12):1033–1043.e3.
6. Burn E, Tebe C, Fernandez-Bertolin S, et al. The natural history of symptomatic COVID-19 during the first wave in Catalonia. Nat Commun. 2021;12(1):777.
7. CDC COVID-19 Testing: What You Need to Know. Centers for Disease Control 2022.. https://www.cdc.gov/coronavirus/2019-ncov/symptoms-testing/testing.html. Accessed 1 Feb 2022.
8. Tan WYT, Wong LY, Leo YS, Toh M. Does incubation period of COVID-19 vary with age? A study of epidemiologically linked cases in Singapore. Epidemiol Infect. 2020;148:e197.
9. Yu P, Zhu J, Zhang Z, Han Y. A familial cluster of infection associated with the 2019 novel coronavirus indicating possible person-to-person transmission during the incubation period. J Infect Dis. 2020;221(11):1757–61.
10. Wu Y, Kang L, Guo Z, et al. Incubation period of COVID-19 caused by unique SARS-CoV-2 strains: a systematic review and meta-analysis. JAMA Netw Open. 2022;5(8):e2228008.
11. Corman VM, Haage VC, Bleicker T, et al. Comparison of seven commercial SARS-CoV-2 rapid point-of-care antigen tests: a single-centre Laboratory Evaluation Study. Lancet Microbe. 2021;2(7):e311–e19.
12. Abusrewil Z, Alhudiri IM, Kaal HH, et al. Time scale performance of rapid antigen testing for SARS-CoV-2: evaluation of 10 rapid antigen assays. J Med Virol. 2021;93(12):6512–8.
13. Perera R, Tso E, Tsang OTY, et al. SARS-CoV-2 Virus culture and subgenomic RNA for respiratory specimens from patients with mild coronavirus disease. Emerg Infect Dis. 2020;26(11):2701–4.
14. Kucirka LM, Lauer SA, Laeyendecker O, Boon D, Lessler J. Variation in false-negative rate of reverse transcriptase polymerase chain reaction-based SARS-CoV-2 tests by time since exposure. Ann Intern Med. 2020;173(4):262–7.
15. Dos Santos WG. Natural history of COVID-19 and current knowledge on treatment therapeutic options. Biomed Pharmacother. 2020;129:110493.
16. Lau EHY, Tsang OTY, Hui DSC, et al. Neutralizing antibody titres in SARS-CoV-2 infections. Nat Commun. 2021;12(1):63.

Impact of the COVID-19 Pandemic on Global Oral Health Services

5

Matt Hopcraft

5.1 Introduction

Oral health is crucial for maintaining overall health, and regular, timely access to dental care is essential for early detection, prevention, and treatment of oral diseases. When the pandemic began in early 2020, there was a perception that the dental profession faced increased risks of both virus transmission from patient to patient and from patients to dental staff, as most dental procedures generate aerosols [1]. It was widely believed that droplet and aerosol transmission of SARS-CoV-2 were the main concerns in the dental setting because it is difficult to avoid producing large amounts of aerosols and droplets mixed with the patient's saliva, as well as the patient's cough and breathing [2]. It was assumed that droplet particles and aerosols could remain airborne for an extended period before settling onto surfaces or entering the respiratory tract, making fomite transmission a potential risk. Another challenge was that the viral load was known to peak around the time of symptom onset, posing a risk of unknowingly coming into contact with an infectious asymptomatic patient [3].

As a result, routine dental care was suspended or restricted in many countries as governments, regulatory bodies and dental professional associations grappled with the emerging science regarding the risk of virus transmission via aerosols generated during dental procedures. These restrictions on the provision of dental services were deemed necessary to minimise the risk of COVID-19 transmission in the dental setting and were designed to protect both patients and staff. However, the chronic and progressive nature of dental disease means that limiting or deferring access to dental care is likely to contribute to poorer oral health and long-term problems for many people globally.

M. Hopcraft (✉)
Melbourne Dental School, University of Melbourne, Melbourne, VIC, Australia
e-mail: m.hopcraft@unimelb.edu.au

S. R. Prabhu et al. (eds.), *COVID-19 in Dental Practice*,
https://doi.org/10.1007/978-3-032-26000-0_5

5.2 Provision of Dental Services

Dentistry services are provided through both public and private clinics, depending on funding and the priorities of each country. Early in the pandemic, dental services were suspended, either due to government mandates or voluntary decisions by dental practices and patients. The decline in dental attendance was partly caused by patients' reluctance to visit the dentist for routine care and concerns among dental practitioners about the risk of COVID-19 transmission through aerosols.

A global study involving 36 countries evaluated the impact of the early stages of the pandemic from May to August 2020 on public and private dental services [4]. Although most dental practitioners reported offering some face-to-face care during this period, only emergency care was available in 13 countries across both public and private practices. Conversely, 14 countries continued to provide routine dental care. Several nations, including Egypt, Nigeria, Malaysia, Pakistan, and the United Kingdom, offered only urgent care in public dental clinics and hospitals, while routine care remained accessible in the private sector. This contrasts with other studies that found closures were more frequent in the private sector than in public clinics, resulting in a greater effect on the business and financial aspects of dentistry [5].

Where dental care was provided, it was often limited to urgent or emergency treatment. To facilitate this, telehealth and phone triage were used to prioritise access to care, although their use varied from less than 15% in countries including Albania, Romania, Russia, Nigeria (where the proportion continuing face-to-face treatment remained high), to more than 80% in Switzerland, the Netherlands, Germany, Belgium, Spain, and Pakistan [4].

The greatest impact on dental services occurred during the early months of the pandemic, with several studies reporting a decline in patient activity during this period. In the United States, it was reported that weekly visits to dental practices were 33% lower from March to August 2020, and in some states, the decrease was as high as 53% [6]. Although there was a notable rebound in patient appointments by June, they were still approximately 20% lower in August 2020 compared to the same period in the previous year. In Australia, there was a reduction of over 52% in the number of dental treatments provided to children between March and May 2020 compared with previous years [7]. A second wave of the pandemic in Victoria resulted in a 60% decrease in services across August and September 2020.

Data from the National Health Service in England showed a 98% decline in dental services utilised by children, adults, and older adults during the initial lockdown period [8]. As a result, there were reports of dental infections requiring emergency hospital treatment and instances of 'do it yourself' dentistry.

Access to dental care was often treated differently from medical care, and in the United States, dental utilisation decreased more rapidly during 'shelter-in-place' periods than for comparable medical services, rebounding more slowly after reopening [9]. Concerns about the impact of mitigation strategies in Germany led to a modelling study which showed a large reduction in the utilisation of all dental services, with the most severe impacts observed in prevention, with a reduction of 80% [10].

This reduced access to dental care negatively affected oral health outcomes for patients. A nationally representative survey revealed that nearly half of all adults in the United States delayed visiting the dentist or receiving dental treatment during the early months of the pandemic [6]. Deferred care increases the risk of dental diseases remaining undiagnosed and worsening over time, or planned treatments being compromised. Several studies document the impact of reduced dental care provision on oral health outcomes [10–12]. The decrease in access to dental services led to adverse effects on oral health. In Greece, children experienced an increase in dental caries prevalence, requiring more complex dental treatments after the lockdown ended [13]. The adult dental clinic at the University of Madrid reported that 59% of treatments were not carried out, mostly involving conservative or restorative dentistry and periodontal treatment, which raised the risk of tooth loss [14]. Delayed access to care meant patients underwent more invasive procedures and faced higher levels of stress-related dental conditions, such as bruxism and cracked teeth, along with increased demand for oral surgery services and a decline in preventive dental care [9]. There are also significant impacts on quality of life, with orthognathic patients who had their planned treatments temporarily cancelled reporting distress related to their appearance, self-confidence, and ability to eat and chew [15].

5.3 Increase in Inequalities

Poor oral health is closely associated with socioeconomic disadvantage, and many marginalised groups, including those who are homeless or unemployed, encounter barriers in accessing dental care. While it was well understood that overall health inequalities worsened during the pandemic, there was less research on how it impacted oral health.

Several studies highlighted how oral health inequalities widened during the pandemic. For example, patients in the least deprived areas of England accessed dental care at a rate 1.27 times higher than those in the most deprived areas immediately before the pandemic, but this increased to 1.83 times in the first half of 2020 [16]. This access gap did not return to pre-pandemic levels until the first half of 2022. Similarly, when non-urgent dental services resumed in October 2020, there was a higher uptake among children from the least deprived areas than from the most deprived [8]. In Scotland, relative inequalities in dental visits widened in early 2022, with a slow return to pre-pandemic levels afterwards [17].

The proportion of dentists treating patients with a disability, and the number of such patients seen weekly, decreased significantly worldwide, with reduced access to sedation and general anaesthesia services [18]. These studies highlight the unequal way in which the pandemic was experienced, not only across countries but also within different population groups within those countries. They also show that, although in many cases access to dental care was only restricted for a few months, the effects on disadvantaged populations lasted much longer.

5.4 Economic Impact

The suspension or restricted access to dental care caused a significant economic impact on dental practices during the pandemic. This was most acutely felt in private practices, with fewer patient visits, less treatment provided, and consequently, lower revenue. However, factors beyond the restrictions on dental practices contributed to further economic uncertainty and upheaval.

Once the significance of the pandemic became apparent, there was a global rush to acquire personal protective equipment (PPE). The worldwide supply chain was severely disrupted, restricting access to various protective supplies and equipment [19]. This led to a shortage that greatly increased the prices of these items. For example, the cost of face masks peaked at 11 times higher than pre-pandemic levels in March 2020, with the average price for N95 masks eight times higher and disposable gowns nearly 14 times higher in Chicago, USA [20]. In Brazil, it was reported that the expense of infection control measures was nearly 10 times greater during the pandemic [5]. Dental practitioners faced the dilemma of passing those costs onto patients or absorbing the expenses themselves. Factors that increased the cost of providing dental care led some patients to postpone treatment, creating additional financial difficulties for dental practices [5].

At the same time, dental practices were required to adopt new infection control protocols, including longer appointment times and the introduction of fallow periods between patients to ensure proper dispersion of aerosols and decrease transmission risk [21]. This led to fewer patients being treated each day, further impacting practice revenue. The decrease in daily patient numbers ranged from less than 20% in countries such as Pakistan, Albania, Macedonia, Lithuania, and Romania to over 60% in Egypt, El Salvador, Georgia, Tunisia, Venezuela, Argentina, Brazil, Colombia, Peru, Serbia, Chile, China, Malaysia, Saudi Arabia, Spain, Australia, Belgium, Germany, the Netherlands, Switzerland, and the United States [4]. Countries with higher gross national incomes generally experienced a greater reduction in the number of patient visits by dentists.

Dental practices also had to contend with the severe economic recession and widespread job losses affecting many parts of the world. Individuals and families faced uncertainty and financial hardship, forcing them to make difficult decisions about their disposable income and spending priorities [19]. While the dental profession argued that oral health care was essential, patients found it increasingly difficult to access and afford that care [22].

In some countries like Australia, significant safety net payments were provided to many employees to compensate for their inability to work, serving as a form of economic stimulus. Coupled with effective enforced savings during lockdown periods when travel was restricted, the dental profession experienced a robust recovery once restrictions were lifted.

5.5 Medication Prescribing

One consequence of suspending routine dental treatment was a greater dependence on pharmacological interventions to manage dental issues. This increases concerns about antimicrobial resistance, a significant global health problem that contributes to rising morbidity and mortality through resistant infections. It is estimated that antimicrobial resistance directly causes about 1.27 million deaths worldwide each year, with a further 4.95 million deaths indirectly linked. Dentistry is reported to account for roughly 10% of global antibiotic use in primary care settings [23].

Several studies reported changes in pharmaceutical prescribing patterns during the pandemic. In South Africa, there was an increase in antibiotic prescriptions by oral health practitioners despite fewer in-person consultations [24]. Antibiotics were most frequently prescribed for a painful tooth (58.7%), with amoxicillin and metronidazole being the antibiotics of choice, although in a significant proportion of cases, these were not actually indicated.

In contrast, Australia experienced a significant 18% decrease in dental prescriptions in April 2020 compared to April 2019, with a 16% drop for antibiotics and an 18% decrease for opioid analgesics [25]. When lockdowns ended, there was a rise in June 2020 in prescriptions of amoxicillin with clavulanic acid (20%), tramadol (46%), and oxycodone (73%), suggesting that the continued postponement of routine dental treatment contributed to a deterioration in oral health for many patients. Canada also observed a decrease in prescriptions for antibiotics and opioids between March and May 2020, although the average supply increased marginally [26]. This rise in medication supply per patient increased the risk of antimicrobial resistance and opioid dependence.

5.6 Mental Health and Well-Being of Practitioners

The suspension of dental services not only affected finances but also caused a hidden mental health toll on many dental practitioners. In the early stages of the pandemic, uncertainty surrounded the risk of transmission in dental settings, with media reports claiming that dentistry was among the highest risk professions. This heightened stress and anxiety, especially in the absence of clear evidence about the potential hazards for those infected.

In Norway, despite high vaccination coverage and a widespread sense of preparedness, many dental practitioners were concerned about infection—72.6% feared contracting it and 72.6% feared infecting others [27]. Female dentists expressed more concern about infection, while those with more extensive clinical experience were less worried about instability, leading to a notable psychological burden.

The evidence on the impact of the pandemic on stress and mental health issues among dental practitioners was mixed [28–31]. In Australia, by the end of 2021, self-reported psychological distress among dental practitioners was high, with 32% rated as experiencing moderate or severe psychological distress and 59.4% having a high likelihood of minor (or more severe) psychological distress [30]. One in four showed symptoms consistent with burnout, with one in ten reporting a current diagnosis of depression and one in eight having a current diagnosis of anxiety disorder. Alarmingly, 17.6% reported thoughts of suicide in the previous 12 months [32].

Dentists in the United Kingdom reported lower levels of psychological distress during a period of national lockdown compared with pre-pandemic measures, while dentists in Wales reported high levels of stress [28, 31].

Stress during the pandemic was associated with poor sleep quality, decreased physical activity, and increased maladaptive behaviours such as alcohol consumption, use of mood-enhancing medications, and nicotine use [30, 31]. In Australia, around one in six dental practitioners reported potentially hazardous or risky alcohol intake. Many dentists attended work despite not feeling mentally well enough, which raises concerns about their capacity to provide care [31].

5.7 Dental Education and Dental Students

The global closure of dental services greatly impacted the delivery of dental education and students. While dental schools managed to shift from face-to-face didactic teaching to online learning, dental education still depends heavily on preclinical simulation training and supervised direct dental treatments to allow students to demonstrate competence and ensure they can provide safe care.

Students in their final years of study felt the impact most, as reduced clinical experience raised concerns about their competence and confidence for new graduates [33]. Many worried they would not be able to graduate on time, increasing financial stress [34]. There was also fear of contracting COVID-19 while treating patients and potentially transmitting it to family and friends. Consequently, students experienced greater stress and mental health issues during the pandemic [34].

5.8 Conclusion

The COVID-19 pandemic significantly impacted dental services worldwide, as many procedures were suspended and concerns about potential risks affected both patients and dental practitioners. This led to fewer patients receiving care, resulting in a decline in oral health. Efforts to combat this may have heightened the risk of antimicrobial resistance. Dental practitioners and students experienced high levels of psychological and financial stress due to the uncertainty caused by the pandemic and the drop in patient numbers.

Oral health and dental care are regarded as separate and often private responsibilities, and decision-makers and health planners frequently do not include oral health care as an essential part of health services when devising pandemic scenarios. This is despite the significant burden of oral diseases worldwide and the impact of poor oral health on overall health, well-being, and the broader economy.

References

1. Coulthard P, Thomson P, Dave M, Coulthard FP, Seoudi N, Hill M. The COVID-19 pandemic and dentistry: the clinical, legal and economic consequences – part 2: consequences of withholding dental care. Br Dent J. 2020;229(12):801–5.
2. Peng X, Xu X, Li Y, Cheng L, Zhou X, Ren B. Transmission routes of 2019-nCoV and controls in dental practice. Int J Oral Sci. 2020;12(1):9.
3. Melo P, Barbosa JM, Jardim L, Carrilho E, Portugal J. COVID-19 management in clinical dental care. Part I: epidemiology, public health implications, and risk assessment. Int Dent J. 2021;71(3):251–62.
4. Campus G, Diaz Betancourt M, Cagetti MG, Giacaman RA, Manton DJ, Douglas GVA, et al. The COVID-19 pandemic and its global effects on dental practice. An International survey. J Dent. 2021;114:103749.
5. Farrokhi F, Farrokhi F, Mohebbi SZ, Khami MR. A scoping review of the impact of COVID-19 on dentistry: financial aspects. BMC Oral Health. 2024;24(1):945.
6. Kranz AM, Chen A, Gahlon G, Stein BD. 2020 trends in dental office visits during the COVID-19 pandemic. J Am Dent Assoc. 2021;152(7):535–41.e1.
7. Hopcraft M, Farmer G. Impact of COVID-19 on the provision of paediatric dental care: analysis of the Australian Child Dental Benefits Schedule. Commun Dent Oral Epidemiol. 2021;49(4):369–76.
8. Stennett M, Tsakos G. The impact of the COVID-19 pandemic on oral health inequalities and access to oral healthcare in England. Br Dent J. 2022;232(2):109–14.
9. Choi SE, Mo E, Sima C, Wu H, Thakkar-Samtani M, Tranby EP, et al. Impact of COVID-19 on dental care utilization and oral health conditions in the United States. JDR Clin Trans Res. 2024;9(3):256–64.
10. Schwendicke F, Krois J, Gomez J. Impact of SARS-CoV2 (Covid-19) on dental practices: economic analysis. J Dent. 2020;99:103387.
11. Scherrer C, Naavaal S, Lin M, Griffin SO. COVID-19 pandemic impact on US childhood caries and potential mitigation. J Dent Res. 2022;101(10):1147–54.
12. Danagoulian S, Wilk TA. Locking out prevention: dental care in the midst of a pandemic. Health Econ. 2022;31(9):1973–92.
13. Angelopoulou MV, Seremidi K, Papaioannou W, Gizani S. Impact of the COVID 19 lock down on the oral health status of paediatric dental patients in Greece. Int J Paed Dent. 2023;33(3):246–53.
14. Gómez-Costa D, Ramírez JM, García Guerrero I, Giovannini G, Rojo R, Gómez-de DR. A retrospective study on the effect of the COVID-19 pandemic on dental treatments in adults. BMC Oral Health. 2022;22(1):122.
15. Wemyss C, Benington P, Chung L, El-Angbawi A, Ayoub A. Impact of the COVID-19 pandemic on orthognathic patients: what have we learned? Br J Oral Maxillofac Surg. 2022;60(5):629–34.
16. O'Connor R, Landes D, Harris R. Trends and inequalities in realised access to NHS primary care dental services in England before, during and throughout recovery from the COVID-19 pandemic. Br Dent J. 2023;235(6):343.
17. Aminu AQ, McMahon AD, Clark C, Sherriff A, Buchanan C, Watling C, et al. Inequalities in access to NHS primary care dental services in Scotland during the COVID-19 pandemic. Br Dent J. 2023;24:1–6.
18. Mac Giolla Phadraig C, van Harten MT, Diniz-Freitas M, Limeres Posse J, Faulks D, Dougall A, et al. The impact of COVID-19 on access to dental care for people with disabilities: a global survey during the COVID-19 first wave lockdown. Med Oral Patol Oral Cir Bucal. 2021;26(6):e770–e7.
19. Akbari A, Khami MR, Beymouri A, Akbari S. Dental service utilization and the COVID-19 pandemic, a micro-data analysis. BMC Oral Health. 2024;24(1):16.

20. Patel R, Ali M, Bleasdale SC, Mena Lora AJ. Cost of personal protective equipment during the first wave of the coronavirus disease 2019 (COVID-19) pandemic. Infect Control Hosp Epidemiol. 2023;44(11):1897–9.
21. Mukonoweshuro R, Mulhearn K, Ablal M. Endodontics and COVID-19 – where are we now? BDJ Pract. 2022;35(2):12–3.
22. Benzian H, Beltrán-Aguilar E, Mathur MR, Niederman R. Pandemic considerations on essential oral health care. J Dent Res. 2021;100(3):221–5.
23. World Health Organisation. Antimicrobial resistance World Health Organisation. Geneva; 2023. Available from: https://www.who.int/news-room/fact-sheets/detail/antimicrobial-resistance. Accessed 22 Oct 2025.
24. Pillay L, Rikhotso RE. Antibiotic prescribing pattern of oral health practitioners before and during the COVID-19 pandemic at Wits Oral Health Centre. Br J Oral Maxillofac Surg. 2024;62(7):619–25.
25. Mian M, Teoh L, Hopcraft M. Trends in dental medication prescribing in Australia during the COVID-19 pandemic. JDR Clin Trans Res. 2021;6(2):145–52.
26. Immel R, Bohlouli B, Amin M. The impact of the COVID-19 pandemic on pattern of antibiotic and opioid prescriptions by dentists in Alberta, Canada. Clin Exp Dent Res. 2024;10(4):e913.
27. Shabestari M, Ansteinsson VE, Hovden EAS, Stangvaltaite-Mouhat L, Mdala I, Skudutyte-Rysstad R, et al. One year of COVID-19 in dental health services in Norway: psychological impact, risk perceptions and vaccination status. BMC Health Services Res. 2023;23(1):972.
28. Collin V, O'Selmo E, Whitehead P. Psychological distress and the perceived impact of the COVID-19 pandemic on UK dentists during a national lockdown. Br Dent J. 2021:1–8. https://doi.org/10.1038/s41415-020-2592-5.
29. Eldridge LA, Estrich CG, Gurenlian JR, Battrell A, Lynch A, Vujicic M, et al. United States dental health care workers' mental health during the COVID-19 pandemic. J Dent Hyg. 2022;96(4):9–11.
30. Hopcraft MS, McGrath R, Stormon N, Parker G. Mental health, psychological distress and burnout in Australian dental practitioners. Aust Dent J. 2023;68(3):160–70.
31. Owen C, Seddon C, Clarke K, Bysouth T, Johnson D. The impact of the COVID-19 pandemic on the mental health of dentists in Wales. Br Dent J. 2022;232(1):44–54.
32. Hopcraft MS, Stormon N, McGrath R, Parker G. Factors associated with suicidal ideation and suicide attempts by Australian dental practitioners. Community Dent Oral Epidemiol. 2023;51(6):1159–68.
33. Hill EB, Mastny-Jensen C, Loch C. Before and after: COVID-19 impacts on dental students' well-being, clinical competency and employment opportunities. Eur J Dent Educ. 2024;28(2):522–9.
34. Gunewardena NP, Hironaka ST, Khan HJ, Rassam TM, Kroon J. Impact of COVID-19 on depression, anxiety and stress of dental students: a systematic review. Eur J Dent Educ. 2025;29(1):29–35.

6 Effects of the COVID-19 Pandemic on Global Dental Education

Shilpi Ajwani and Vesna Miletic

6.1 Introduction

The COVID-19 pandemic had a significant impact on dental education worldwide, and the unprecedented challenges, along with its rapidly evolving nature, forced educational institutions to adapt and innovate. Globally, dental schools faced the closure of clinics and preclinical labs, the suspension of face-to-face teaching, and a shift to online modalities. These changes affected not only academic delivery but also student well-being, research, and institutional operations. The chapter discusses the global perspectives, challenges, adaptations, and preparedness for the future.

6.2 Disruption of Clinic-Based Training

The COVID-19 pandemic caused substantial disruption to dental education worldwide, particularly in teaching and clinical training [1]. As dentistry is a hands-on profession, the development of clinical skills through preclinical and clinical training is a cornerstone of dental education. A vast majority of dental procedures generate aerosols and involve close patient contact for extended periods. To minimise the risk of transmission, severe restrictions were placed on face-to-face patient contact and the undertaking of aerosol-generating procedures. As a result, most dental schools restricted clinical activities to emergency care only, and schools that had

S. Ajwani
Sydney Dental Hospital and Oral Health Services, Sydney Local Health District, NSW Health, Sydney, NSW, Australia

V. Miletic (✉)
Faculty of Medicine and Health, Sydney Dental School, The University of Sydney, Surry Hills, Sydney, NSW, Australia
e-mail: vesna.miletic@sydney.edu.au

S. R. Prabhu et al. (eds.), *COVID-19 in Dental Practice*,
https://doi.org/10.1007/978-3-032-26000-0_6

collaborations with public dental services suspended their clinical placements completely. This led to the immediate suspension of clinical teaching in dental schools worldwide [2].

In the UK, paediatric dentistry trainees experienced significant disruption, with outpatient clinics, inpatient assessments, and sedation- or general anaesthesia-based treatments all suspended. According to the American Dental Education Association (ADEA), dental school clinics experienced a 50% drop in patient visits between April and December 2020 compared to the same period in 2019. As a result, clinical training was halted, and students were sent home, with only faculty and residents providing emergency care. This severely limited students' opportunities for hands-on training [3].

The Dental Board of Australia, in collaboration with the Australian Dental Council (ADC-2020), acknowledged widespread disruption to clinical placements, exams, and training programmes. Many students were unable to complete essential clinical rotations [4].

Not only was clinical teaching affected, one of the earliest and most widespread impacts of the pandemic was the cessation of in-person instruction. Dental schools worldwide closed their doors to students and faculty, halting lectures, seminars, and preclinical/practical sessions [5]. In Europe, the Association of Dental Education in Europe (ADEE) reported that a vast majority of dental schools transitioned to online pedagogical tools, including live-streamed lectures, virtual meetings, and digital resources [6]. Similarly, in Pakistan, all educational and research activities were suspended, and even emergency care was limited to a few setups [7]. Students in China were instructed not to return to campuses, and all teaching was moved online [8]. Without a doubt, the impacts of COVID-19 on clinical-based training were quite severe. They raised serious concerns about the competency of graduating students, especially those in their final years who missed critical hands-on experiences [9].

6.3 Rapid Shift to Online Learning

The COVID-19 pandemic forced dental schools worldwide to transition rapidly to digital platforms. This shift was essential to maintain educational continuity but was implemented unevenly across regions due to differences in infrastructure, policy, and preparedness.

European dental schools, particularly the UK and Ireland, were relatively well-prepared for the transition. Many had already begun integrating blended learning and simulation technologies into their curricula before the pandemic. Blended learning combines synchronous and asynchronous online instruction with limited face-to-face sessions, allowing flexibility while maintaining educational standards [10]. UK dental schools were recognised for their digital innovation, having already invested in simulation-based education before the pandemic. They leveraged augmented reality (AR) and haptic simulators to replicate clinical scenarios. These tools enabled students to experience standardised cases and meet learning outcomes despite the suspension of in-person training. The Dental Schools Council and Association for Dental Education in Europe (ADEE) supported collaborative efforts to maintain quality and consistency in online education across member institutions [11].

In Latin America and Southern Europe, the shift to online learning was seen by faculty as an opportunity for growth, but students faced significant challenges. A scoping review of online active learning in dental education found that while problem-based learning, case-based learning, and flipped classrooms were widely adopted, students reported demotivation, cognitive overload, and difficulty engaging with clinical content. Students from lower socioeconomic backgrounds struggled with access to devices and stable internet, exacerbating educational inequalities. This was reported by students in other parts of the world, e.g., Egypt and India [12, 13]. Staff in Costa Rica and Italy expressed optimism about the long-term potential of digital education. Still, it acknowledged that online platforms could not fully replicate the tactile and interpersonal aspects of dental training [14].

Australian dental schools responded quickly to the crisis, implementing online tools and remote learning strategies [15]. However, the transition exposed disparities in digital access and readiness, particularly in rural and remote areas. The Australian Ministry of Health noted that while urban institutions adapted well, students in regional and remote communities faced challenges due to limited infrastructure and connectivity. Stakeholders emphasised the need for locally adaptable strategies, infrastructure investment, and flexible workforce models to ensure equitable access to dental education [16]. The pandemic prompted national discussions around integrating digital innovation into the next National Oral Health Plan, with a focus on sustainable and inclusive education models [17].

The rapid shift to online learning in dental education during the COVID-19 pandemic showcased both resilience and disparity. While some regions leveraged existing digital infrastructure to maintain continuity, others struggled with access, engagement, and pedagogical effectiveness. The experience has catalysed a global re-evaluation of dental education, emphasising the need for blended learning, simulation, and equitable digital access.

6.4 Adaptations

Most institutions turned to technological innovations and tele-dentistry to maintain educational continuity, ensure patient care, and support student learning. These tools not only helped bridge the gap during lockdowns but also laid the foundation for long-term transformation in dental education. A scientometric analysis of global tele-dentistry research during COVID-19 revealed widespread adoption in countries such as the United States, China, Italy, Japan, and the United Kingdom. Platforms like WeChat, WhatsApp, Attend Anywhere, and Mouthwatch TeleDent were used for communication, data storage, and remote consultation. Decision-making algorithms and AI-supported tools were also introduced to enhance diagnostic accuracy [18]. Students commonly used platforms like WhatsApp and Zoom to communicate with patients, discuss symptoms, and provide guidance. While the majority of patients reported effective communication and satisfaction with the process, students acknowledged the need for further training, especially in managing complex cases [19].

To compensate for the loss of hands-on training, many dental schools adopted simulation technologies, including virtual reality (VR) and haptic feedback systems. These tools allowed students to practice procedures in a controlled, virtual environment, receiving real-time feedback on technique and outcomes. VR simulators were equipped with tactile feedback mechanisms that mimicked the sensation of working on real teeth. This innovation helped students develop manual dexterity, hand-eye coordination, and reflective skills—critical components of clinical competence. In Germany, for instance, dental schools reorganised curricula to include up-to-date teaching methods and interdisciplinary simulation models, such as 3D-printed tooth replicas for endodontic training. The use of computer-generated simulations allowed students to repeatedly practice procedures without supervision, supporting skill acquisition during lockdowns [20].

Beyond tele-dentistry, dental education embraced a wide range of digital learning platforms and dental curricula that had long relied on face-to-face lectures and hands-on clinical training and was rapidly restructured to accommodate remote learning. Many institutions adopted hybrid models, combining online theoretical instruction with limited, socially distanced practical sessions. Tools like Moodle, Microsoft Teams, and Google Classroom were used to deliver lectures, host discussions, and manage assessments. Educators adopted flipped classrooms, problem-based learning, and interactive webinars to engage students remotely. In Egypt, for example, dental schools implemented a hybrid learning model that combined online theoretical instruction with limited in-person practical sessions. This approach minimised physical interaction while ensuring students acquired essential competencies. Video lectures, online exams, and virtual case presentations became standard components of the curriculum [21].

Traditional assessment methods, such as Objective Structured Clinical Examinations (OSCEs) and live-patient licensure exams, were disrupted. Dental schools responded by introducing online exams, virtual case discussions, and alternative competency assessments [22]. In India, faculty emphasised the need to reform the curriculum to include digital competencies and crisis preparedness. In Europe, some institutions extended training programmes to compensate for lost clinical time, while others adopted pass/fail grading systems to accommodate the limitations of online assessments.

Accrediting bodies, such as the Commission on Dental Accreditation (CODA) in the US and the Commission on Dental Accreditation of Canada (CDCA), maintained rigorous standards but allowed for temporary modifications to ensure students could progress and graduate. Australia's dental education sector underwent significant adjustments in both assessment and accreditation to ensure the continuity of training while maintaining public safety and professional standards. The Australian Dental Council (ADC), in collaboration with all dental practitioner program providers and endorsed by the Dental Board of Australia, has released a set of

COVID-19 accreditation principles to guide these changes. Education providers were encouraged to be flexible and use a variety of assessment methods, including simulation activities, remote assessments, and alternative clinical experiences, to determine whether students had achieved the required competencies [23]. While simulation was recognised as valuable, it was also acknowledged that it could not fully replace chair-side clinical experience.

The COVID-19 pandemic forced dental education to undergo rapid curriculum reform and faculty development. Through the adoption of hybrid models, the integration of technology, and investment in faculty upskilling, dental schools maintained educational continuity and prepared students for the evolving demands of the profession.

6.5 Regional Considerations

The literature offers complementary perspectives on the impact of COVID-19 on dental education, focusing on both local and global contexts [12, 13, 24–27]. These papers illustrate both the shared global challenges and the diverse adaptations in dental education during the pandemic.

Immediate challenges faced by U.S. dental schools included suspending clinical activities except for dental emergencies and focusing on preclinical training with social distancing, online learning, and OSCE-type examinations [24]. This article emphasised the importance of institutional agility, technological adaptation, and mental health support for students and faculty, as well as the role of national bodies in guiding policy and accreditation during the crisis.

A broader international lens compared the effects of the pandemic across countries, including the USA, Jordan, Brazil, France, Italy, China, Saudi Arabia, India, Pakistan, and Hong Kong [25]. This review underscored the universal disruption to the three learning domains, cognitive, psychomotor, and affective, and the varied responses based on local infrastructure and policy. For instance, while some countries invested in virtual reality and haptic technologies, others relied on simpler tools like manikins for home-based training. Given a similar approach to dental education worldwide, it is not surprising to see similar effects of the pandemic on dental education, from disrupted clinical and in-person teaching and assessments to the psychological toll on students [25].

Two cross-sectional studies, one from Egypt (337 dental students) and one from India (404 dental students), investigated dental students' perceptions of online education during the COVID-19 pandemic. Both cohorts recognised the flexibility and convenience of e-learning but reported significant challenges, including poor internet connectivity, reduced interaction, and insufficient clinical skill development. Consequently, students from both regions advocated for a blended or hybrid learning model that integrates online theoretical teaching with in-person clinical training to enhance educational effectiveness [12, 13].

Contrary to the above, a European study surveyed 879 dental students from 34 European countries did not report issues with internet connectivity related to online learning [26]. This study found that 50% reported spending less time on education during COVID-19, while 30% spent more time, with teaching methods ranging from online simulations to hybrid models. Satisfaction with education was mixed: 44% were satisfied or very satisfied, and 31% were unsatisfied. Communication from schools was a major source of dissatisfaction, while concerns centred on the loss of clinical experience and skills. Students generally supported some role for online teaching in the future, but emphasised the need for better organisation, more transparent communication, and strategies to compensate for reduced hands-on training [26].

6.6 Discipline-Related Impact

A few papers looked into discipline-related impacts COVID-19 pandemic had on teaching and learning. These approaches offered a chance to deep-dive into teaching discipline-specific modalities, providing more in-depth analyses than the broad overview offered in most of the literature. For example, anatomy teaching was hindered by the disruption of cadaveric dissection, a cornerstone of medical education, with merging methods (video-based learning, online resources, social media, 3D printing, augmented reality, and virtual reality) used instead [28]. While acknowledging the effectiveness of digital tools in enhancing engagement and understanding, it is emphasised that cadaveric dissection remains irreplaceable for its ethical, tactile, and spatial learning benefits. Prosection and plastination, based on demonstration of the authentic anatomic structures, rather than students performing dissections, could be in-person alternatives when social distancing and other preventive measures can be effectively implemented. The authors recommended a blended approach that integrates technology with traditional methods to ensure resilience and innovation in anatomy education [28]. Another example is the COVID-19 pandemic's impact on orthodontics and paediatric dentistry, showing that e-learning via platforms such as Moodle and WebCT, and virtual simulations, was generally well received and effective for these disciplines, particularly when used as a supplement to traditional teaching [29].

Irrespective of discipline-specific teaching aspects, blended learning and pedagogical flexibility in response to pandemic-induced disruptions improved students' learning experience. A broader shift in health education toward hybrid models that leverage digital innovation while preserving essential tactile and ethical dimensions of clinical training seems to be the best approach moving forward. There is, however, a need for ongoing research into the long-term impacts of these changes, particularly in assessing learning outcomes, student engagement, and professional preparedness across disciplines.

6.7 Equity and Access Challenges in Dental Education

Existing inequities in dental education worldwide were exposed and exacerbated during the COVID-19 pandemic. While the rapid shift to online learning was necessary to maintain educational continuity, it also highlighted disparities in access to technology, infrastructure, and support systems. These challenges were particularly pronounced in low- and middle-income countries, rural and remote areas, and among socioeconomically disadvantaged students. Equity in dental education, defined as fair access to learning opportunities and resources, was significantly compromised during the pandemic. Availability of stable internet connectivity and power outages severely hindered students' ability to participate in online classes and assessments [9, 12, 13] and significant variations were observed in the quality and availability of the networks, software, and hardware utilised by faculty and students [15]. Moreover, the cost of simulation technologies and digital platforms created barriers for many institutions. While some universities in North America and Europe could invest in advanced tools, others struggled to maintain basic educational services.

The pandemic disproportionately affected students from lower socioeconomic backgrounds. Many in developing countries lacked access to personal computers, quiet study spaces, and financial resources to purchase simulation tools or attend online tutorials. Even in developed countries, while many dental schools provided laptops and Wi-Fi hotspots to students in need, the demand often exceeded supply. Additionally, students who relied on campus facilities for internet access and study spaces were left without alternatives during lockdowns [5].

Equity challenges extended to clinical training, a core component of dental education. The suspension of in-person clinical rotations disproportionately affected students in their final years, who were preparing for licensure and practice. In Australia, educators expressed concern that students from disadvantaged backgrounds might not be able to afford additional training or simulation tools to compensate for lost clinical hours. In the UK, some dental schools extended training programmes to ensure students met competency requirements, but this was not feasible for all institutions. Students in less-resourced schools faced uncertainty about graduation timelines and career progression [30].

6.8 Mental Health and Well-Being

Mental health challenges faced by dental students during the COVID-19 pandemic were highlighted in several papers using different methodologies [31–33]. Together, they paint a comprehensive picture of the psychological toll of the pandemic on this population.

Gender (particularly being female), year of study, and living circumstances were identified as significant variables influencing depression, anxiety, and stress, with gender-associated social expectations of male self-reliance and resilience in the face of adversity being attributed to the finding of increased stress in females [31].

Final-year students and those with limited clinical exposure were particularly vulnerable, attributing increased levels of stress to increased clinical workloads and demands to meet clinical requirements [31].

A meta-analysis estimated a pooled depression prevalence of 37% among dental students during the pandemic, with higher rates observed in Asian countries; however, there was no significant variation in depression rates based on gender, age, or response rate [32]. Regional and educational system differences were identified as key contributors [32]. The educational differences were drawn from a study by Perry et al. (2017), who reported more prevalent use of haptic simulators and simulation clinics compared to European and American schools [34]. This does not, however, account for significantly affected clinical exposure and clinical teaching in the latter schools due to the pandemic.

The scoping review by Ramachandran et al. (2022) broadened the scope by identifying stressors and mental health issues from 55 studies involving over 31,000 participants [33]. It identifies three major categories of stressors: educational (e.g. transition to online learning and clinical skill deficits), infection-related (e.g. fear of contracting or transmitting COVID-19), and social isolation. The review also notes that female students were generally more affected, though some studies reported higher distress in males. Financial concerns, career and job outcomes, and personal and professional relationships were identified as additional, emerging stressors. [33]

There is a consensus that dental students are particularly vulnerable during the pandemic, mainly due to disruptions in clinical training and social isolation. The studies collectively underscore the urgent need for dental schools to implement comprehensive mental health strategies [31–33]. This includes not only immediate support during crises but also long-term structural changes in curriculum design, clinical training, supportive learning environments, and student well-being initiatives, including coping strategies and resilience-building programmes. The importance of targeted interventions and mental health support within dental institutions has been highlighted, warning that failure to address these issues could result in long-term consequences for the dental workforce [31]. The findings advocate for proactive, evidence-based approaches to foster resilience and ensure the sustainability of the dental profession.

6.9 Students' Self-Assessed Preparedness for Clinical Practice

Significant educational disruptions caused by the pandemic raised concerns about students' and recent graduates' clinical readiness and self-confidence. A nationwide cross-sectional survey in Malaysia used the Dental Undergraduates Preparedness Assessment Scale (DU-PAS) to assess perceived preparedness among final-year students and recent graduates [35]. Their findings revealed that while overall preparedness scores were satisfactory, final-year students scored significantly lower than recent graduates, which was attributed to new graduates being less affected by the pandemic and having prior work experience as dental assistants. Specialist clinical skills like endodontics on multirooted teeth, fixed prosthodontics, and orthodontics, as well as drug prescription, received the lowest preparedness scores. On the other side of the preparedness spectrum, students reported satisfactory skills in taking patients' history and obtaining consent, removing caries, placing direct aesthetic restorations, and performing non-surgical periodontal procedures. The study highlighted higher reported preparedness of students from public institutions and those who engaged in dental-related activities during the waiting period between graduation and mandatory government employment [35]. In contrast, another study focused on a single dental school in Serbia and compared the self-confidence levels of final-year students graduating during the pandemic (2020) with those from the pre-pandemic cohort (2019) [36]. Using a 40-item Likert-scale questionnaire, a statistically significant decline in self-confidence was reported across most clinical domains, especially in periodontology and endodontics. The study attributed this decline to the cessation of clinical training and the shift to online learning. Notably, students reported higher confidence in procedures they had completed before the lockdown, such as restorative dentistry and removable prosthodontics, suggesting that the timing of these procedures within the curriculum was critical [36].

6.10 Long-Term Implications

The disruption of teaching and training during the COVID-19 pandemic has prompted a re-evaluation of dental education models. Institutions are now providing hybrid curricula that combine online theoretical instruction along with in-person clinical training. The integration of VR, haptics, and tele-dentistry is expected to continue, though challenges in accessibility and scalability remain.

Educators are also advocating for curriculum amendments to include topics such as infectious disease control, crisis management, and digital literacy. The pandemic has underscored the need for resilience, adaptability, and innovation in dental education.

Possible measures to address reduced clinical readiness and confidence among dental students in a pandemic-interrupted learning environment could include extended clinical rotations and supplementary skills programmes to compensate for lost patient contact. Greater use of simulation-based learning through haptic devices and virtual reality can help build and maintain procedural competence. Mentorship and peer-assisted learning can provide both educational and emotional support. Competency-based assessments and reflective practice can help identify and address individual skill gaps.

The lessons from the pandemic must be preserved and serve as a foundation for any future curricular disruptions. This may be achieved through consultation between institutions and the sharing of information. Curriculum reforms should integrate digital literacy, tele-dentistry, and crisis preparedness, supported by faculty development in blended teaching and remote supervision, to ensure pandemic preparedness and sustained clinical competence in the post-pandemic era.

References

1. Farrokhi FMS, Farrokhi F, Khami MR. Impact of COVID-19 on dental education- a scoping review. BMC Med Educ. 2021;21(1):587.
2. Hattar S AA, Sawair FA, Alraheam IA, El-Ma'aita AW, Fouad K. Impact of COVID-19 pandemic on dental education: online experience and practice expectations among dental students at the University of Jordan. BMC Med Educ. 2021;21(1):151.
3. Escontrías OAIE, Flores S, Stewart DCL. Operational and financial impact of the COVID-19 pandemic on U.S. dental school clinics. J Dent Educ. 2021;85(12):1863–9.
4. Australian Government, Ahpra and National Boards, Forum HPAC. National principles for clinical education during the COVID-19 pandemic. 2020. https://www.ahpra.gov.au/Resources/COVID-19/National-principles-for-clinical-education-during-COVID-19.aspx?utm_source=chatgpt.com.
5. Alkadi L. Dental education in the COVID-19 era: challenges, solutions and opportunities. Open Dent J. 2021;15:17.
6. Quinn B FJ, Gorter R, Akota I, Manzanares MC, Paganelli C, et al. COVID-19: the immediate response of european academic dental institutions and future implications for dental education. Eur J Dent Educ. 2020;24(4):811–4.
7. Alzahrani SBAA, Aldossary MS. Impact of COVID-19 pandemic on dental education, research, and students. Int J Health Sci Res. 2020;10(6):207–12.
8. Meng LHF, Bian Z. Coronavirus disease 2019 (COVID-19): emerging and future challenges for dental and oral medicine. J Dent Res. 2020;99(5):481–7.
9. Li BCL, Wang H. Challenges and opportunities for dental education from COVID-19. Dent J (Basel). 2022;10(10):188.
10. Kavadella A. Are dental schools prepared for the "new normal"? Organisational and educational challenges in integrating e-learning into the curriculum. ADEE; 2020.
11. BDJ. Blended learning and simulation: the future of dental education in a post-COVID era. Br Dent J. 2022;233(6):490.
12. Hassan R, Khalifa AR, Elsewify T, Hassan MG. Perceptions of clinical dental students toward online education during the COVID-19 crisis: an Egyptian multicenter cross-sectional survey. Front Psychol. 2021;12:704179.
13. Karmakar S, Kar M, Francis DL, Reddy SSP, Modak B. From classroom to screen: dental students' perceptions of distance learning during COVID-19 pandemic in India. BMC Med Educ. 2025;25(1):1334.
14. Chavarría-Bolaños DG-FA, Dittel-Jiménez C, Montero-Aguilar M. E-learning in dental schools in the times of COVID-19: a review and analysis of an educational resource in times of the COVID-19 pandemic. Odovtos Int J Dent Sci. 2020;22(3):69–86.
15. Peres KG, Reher P, Castro RD, Vieira AR. COVID-19-related challenges in dental education: experiences from Brazil, the USA, and Australia. Pesqui Bras Odontopediatria Clín Integr. 2020;20:e0131.
16. Australia K. Increasing dental and oral health training in rural and remote Australia: feasibility study. 2022. https://www.health.gov.au/sites/default/files/2022-12/increasing-dental-and-oral-health-training-in-rural-and-remote-australia-feasibility-study-final-report.pdf.
17. Building the evidence base for the next National Oral Health Plan [press release]. 2024.
18. Mahdavi AAR, Naemi R. Teledentistry during COVID-19 pandemic: scientometric and content analysis approach. BMC Health Serv Res. 2022;22(1):1111.
19. Jin-Yu MLMC, Si Jin JL, Babar MG, Mahdi SS. Practical applications of teledentistry during the Covid-19 pandemic in ASEAN member states—a systematic review. BMC Oral Health. 2024;24(1):421.
20. Clemente MPMA, Pinto JC, Amarante JM, Mendes J. The challenge of dental education after COVID-19 pandemic – present and future innovation study design. Inquiry. 2021;58:469580211018293.

21. Hassan MGAH. Dental education in the time of COVID-19 pandemic: challenges and recommendations. Front Med (Lausanne). 2021;8:648899.
22. Salawu YK, Stewart D, Daud A. Structures, processes and outcomes of objective structured clinical examinations in dental education during the COVID-19 pandemic: a scoping review. Eur J Dent Educ. 2023;27(4):802–14.
23. Council AD. COVID-19 dental practitioner program accreditation principles. 2020.
24. Iyer P, Aziz K, Ojcius DM. Impact of COVID-19 on dental education in the United States. J Dent Educ. 2020;84(6):718–22.
25. Trivandrum Anandapadmanabhan L RP, Ramadoss R, Panneerselvam S, Sundar S. Effect of COVID-19 on dental education: a review. Cureus. 2022;14(4):e24455.
26. Coughlan J, Timus D, Crnic T, Srdoc D, Halton C, Dragan IF. Impact of COVID-19 on dental education in Europe: the students' perspective. Eur J Dent Educ. 2022;26(3):599–607.
27. Di Giacomo P, Di Paolo C. COVID-19 AND DENTAL DISTANCE-BASED EDUCATION: students' perceptions in an Italian University. BMC Med Educ. 2021;21(1):414.
28. Iwanaga J, Loukas M, Dumont AS, Tubbs RS. A review of anatomy education during and after the COVID-19 pandemic: revisiting traditional and modern methods to achieve future innovation. Clin Anat. 2021;34(1):108–14.
29. Patano ACN, Beretta M, Plantamura P, Inchingolo AD, Inchingolo AM, et al. Education technology in orthodontics and paediatric dentistry during the COVID-19 pandemic: a systematic review. Int J Environ Res Public Health. 2021;18(11):6056.
30. Deery C. The COVID-19 pandemic: implications for dental education. Evid Based Dent. 2020;21(2):46–7.
31. Gunewardena NP, Hironaka ST, Khan HJ, Rassam TM, Kroon J. Impact of COVID-19 on depression, anxiety and stress of dental students: a systematic review. Eur J Dent Educ. 2025;29(1):29–35.
32. Santabarbara JO-EN, Idoiaga N, Olaya B, Bueno-Novitol J. Meta-analysis of prevalence of depression in dental students during COVID-19 pandemic. Medicina (Kaunas). 2021;57(11):1278.
33. Ramachandran SSM, Brondani M. Stressors and mental health impacts of COVID-19 in dental students: a scoping review. J Dent Educ. 2023;87(3):326–42.
34. Perry SBM, Leung WK, Bridges SM. Simulation and curriculum design: a global survey in dental education. Aust Dent J. 2017;62(4):453–63.
35. Pandarathodiyil AKMS, Ghani WMN, Ramanathan A, Talib R, Zamzuri AT. Preparedness of recent dental graduates and final-year undergraduate dental students for practice amidst the COVID-19 pandemic. Eur J Dent Educ. 2023;27(1):78–86.
36. Ilic J RK, Savic-Stankovic T, Popovac A, Miletic V, Milic Lemic A. The effect of COVID-19 pandemic on final year dental students' self-confidence level in performing clinical procedures. PLoS One. 2021;16(10):e0257359.

The Impact of the COVID-19 Pandemic on the Global Economy

7

Ananda P. Dasanayake, Nuwan Indika, Neeky Yassari, Suresha Bandara, and Dennis Fernando

7.1 Introduction

The coronavirus disease 2019 (COVID-19) pandemic, first identified in late 2019, rapidly evolved into a global public health emergency with unprecedented social and economic consequences. As of 2025, more than 7 million deaths had been reported worldwide, with over 1.2 million deaths recorded in the United States alone [1]. While morbidity and mortality figures capture the immediate health burden, they represent only a fraction of the pandemic's true impact. Broader consequences include loss of productive years of life, rising healthcare expenditures, disruptions to education and labour markets, and long-lasting economic instability. We examined the multifaceted economic effects of the COVID-19 pandemic, focusing on global output, employment and income, trade and supply

A. P. Dasanayake (✉)
Department of Epidemiology, New York University College of Dentistry, New York, NY, USA
e-mail: ad75@nyu.edu

N. Indika
College of Business, Loyola University New Orleans, New Orleans, LA, USA
e-mail: nimillag@loyno.edu

N. Yassari
New York University College of Dentistry, New York, NY, USA
e-mail: ny685@nyu.edu

S. Bandara
Infectious Diseases Practitioner, Detroit, MI, USA

D. Fernando
Medmark, Chantilly, VA, USA
e-mail: DennisFernando@medmarc.com

S. R. Prabhu et al. (eds.), *COVID-19 in Dental Practice*,
https://doi.org/10.1007/978-3-032-26000-0_7

chains, fiscal and monetary responses, inflation and debt, sectoral shifts, inequality, mental health–related economic costs, impacts on the healthcare industry, and long-term structural legacies.

7.2 Methodological Approach

This chapter draws on global surveillance data, peer-reviewed literature, and policy analyses from international organisations, including the World Health Organization (WHO), World Bank, International Monetary Fund (IMF), International Labour Organization (ILO), Organisation for Economic Co-operation and Development (OECD), United Nations agencies, and The Lancet Global Burden of Disease (GBD) studies. Evidence published through December 2025 was prioritised to ensure relevance to both the acute and post-acute phases of the pandemic. Given the breadth and heterogeneity of available data, a narrative synthesis approach was adopted to integrate epidemiological, economic, and health-systems perspectives across countries and income settings.

To remain accessible for a global, primarily clinical readership, the chapter emphasises cross-country patterns and illustrative examples from large economies such as the United States, China, and India, rather than presenting detailed macroeconomic tables for any single country. This more balanced, summary-orientated approach is intended to convey the direction and scale of disruption relevant to health and dental professionals without overburdening the narrative with country-specific economic detail.

7.3 Global Morbidity, Mortality, and Economic Context

By December 2025, COVID-19 had caused more than 1.28 million deaths in the United States, with COVID-19 listed as the underlying cause in approximately 87% of cases [1]. Globally, reported cases exceeded 778 million, with more than 7.1 million deaths [2] (see Table 7.1).

These figures underestimate the total burden, as excess mortality analyses suggest substantial indirect mortality attributable to disrupted health services, delayed

Table 7.1 COVID-19 mortality summary (December 2025)

Year	COVID-19 deaths	All-cause deaths	% expected deaths	Pneumonia/Influenza/COVID deaths
2020	385,676	3,390,079	119%	565,242
2021	463,267	3,471,742	122%	616,484
2022	247,192	3,289,353	116%	411,918
2023	76,054	3,101,010	109%	244,307
2024	47,532	3,082,196	108%	221,988
2025	19,151	2,786,278	98%	189,888
Total	1,238,872	19,120,658	–	2,249,827

Deaths Involving COVID-19, Pneumonia, and Influenza United States (Data as of 12/11/2025)

diagnosis of chronic conditions, and reduced access to emergency care. Economic impacts must therefore be interpreted alongside health outcomes, incorporating healthcare spending, productivity losses, long-term disability, and post-COVID conditions that reduce labour-force participation.

7.4 Global Macroeconomic Impact

COVID-19 produced one of the most far-reaching economic shocks since the Second World War. Global GDP contracted by approximately 3.1% in 2020, representing the deepest peacetime recession in decades. More than 90% of countries experienced negative GDP growth, marking the most synchronised global downturn in over a century [3, 4]. Employment and income losses were unprecedented. The International Labour Organization estimated that the equivalent of 255 million full-time jobs was lost globally in 2020—four times the losses observed during the 2009 global financial crisis [3]. Global labour income declined by 8.3%, equivalent to US $3.7 trillion, with disproportionate impacts on informal workers and low-income households. Global trade volumes fell by approximately 8–9% in 2020 due to factory closures, transportation bottlenecks, and port congestion. Shipping delays and container shortages persisted into 2021–2022, significantly increasing logistics costs [5]. Governments deployed more than US $20 trillion in fiscal support globally, while central banks implemented near-zero interest rates and large-scale asset purchases [6]. As demand rebounded amid constrained supply, inflation surged to multi-decade highs during 2021–2022. Global public debt reached approximately 98% of GDP in 2020, with nearly 60% of low-income countries facing high debt distress by 2022 [6]. International tourism experienced an unprecedented collapse, with global arrivals declining by 74% in 2020 and export revenue losses estimated at US $1.3 trillion [7]. Conversely, digital commerce, telework, and digital payments expanded rapidly, accelerating long-term structural shifts in the global economy [8]. The pandemic exacerbated global inequality. The World Bank estimates that 70–150 million people were pushed into extreme poverty in 2020, reversing decades of progress [9]. Although global GDP surpassed pre-pandemic levels by 2022, recovery has remained uneven, particularly among low- and middle-income economies [6].

7.5 Employment, Income, and Labour Markets

Employment losses during the early phase of the pandemic were unprecedented. Low-wage workers, women, young adults, ethnic minorities, and informal-sector workers were disproportionately affected [3]. While fiscal transfers mitigated some household income shocks in high-income countries, coverage gaps persisted in many low- and middle-income economies. The pandemic accelerated structural labour-market changes, including remote and hybrid work, automation, digital platform employment, and shifting worker preferences toward flexibility and work–life balance. These changes continue to reshape labour supply, productivity, workforce participation, and geographic distribution of employment.

7.6 Trade and Supply Chains

The COVID-19 pandemic generated the most severe disruption to global trade and supply chains since the Second World War. Widespread factory shutdowns, transportation bottlenecks, port congestion, and labour shortages produced cascading effects across production networks and international markets [1, 2]. Global trade volumes declined by roughly 8–9% in 2020, with commercial services trade experiencing far sharper contractions than merchandise trade [3–5].

World trade contracted across all major regions, but the magnitude and composition of the shock varied by country and income level. In China, relatively rapid containment of early outbreaks, combined with strong external demand for medical supplies, electronics, and other manufactured goods, supported an earlier rebound in merchandise exports, even as contact-intensive services remained subdued. In India, stringent lockdowns and large informal-sector employment led to a sharper contraction in both goods and services trade, with particularly pronounced effects on small firms and lower-income workers. Many low- and middle-income economies also faced steep declines in tourism receipts and remittances, underscoring that the trade shock was global rather than concentrated in a single high-income country.

Commercial services exports were far more affected than goods, as border closures and mobility restrictions froze international travel, hospitality, and other face-to-face activities [5]. In value terms, global commercial services exports declined by approximately 21% in 2020, while the contraction in merchandise trade was notably smaller. Quarterly monitoring highlights this divergence: services trade fell by roughly 24% year-on-year in the third quarter of 2020 (following a 30% decline in the second quarter), even as goods trade began to stabilise and show early signs of rebound [5].

Maritime logistics constituted a central channel for the transmission of the trade shock. From late 2020 through 2021, freight rates for containerised and dry bulk shipping reached record highs, reflecting equipment shortages, port congestion, labour constraints, and imbalanced trade flows according to the United Nations Conference on Trade and Development (UNCTAD). These disruptions raised shipping costs, increased delivery times, and heightened the risk of price pass-through, particularly for small island developing states (SIDS) and least developed countries (LDCs) that rely heavily on maritime transport for essential imports and export earnings.

At the firm level, the pandemic prompted a reassessment of global value chain (GVC) design. Firms diversified suppliers, selectively re-shored or near-shored critical inputs, expanded inventory buffers, and invested in digital tools to improve supply-chain visibility [1, 6, 7]. Model-based evidence from multilateral institutions indicates that diversification across suppliers and regions generally provides greater resilience at lower economic cost than broad-based reshoring strategies, especially in complex, internationally fragmented production networks [8].

7.7 Fiscal and Monetary Responses

Governments and central banks worldwide implemented unprecedented fiscal and monetary interventions to mitigate the pandemic's economic fallout. The overall scale of fiscal support exceeded any previous peacetime response, with cumulative measures estimated at over US $20 trillion globally [4, 7]. These fiscal packages aimed to stabilise household incomes, preserve employment relationships, and prevent widespread business failures.

By 11 September 2020, discretionary fiscal measures worldwide totalled approximately US $11.7 trillion—equivalent to nearly 12% of global GDP—with roughly half in direct budgetary measures and foregone revenues and the remainder in liquidity support, guarantees, and quasi-fiscal interventions [8]. Central banks complemented fiscal interventions with extraordinary monetary accommodation, including near-zero interest rates, large-scale asset purchases, and extensive liquidity support measures to stabilise financial markets. In many African economies, central banks also cut policy rates and injected liquidity on an extraordinary scale, although the pace of easing slowed in the second half of 2020 [2]. While these measures prevented systemic collapse, subsequent assessments emphasised the difficulty of withdrawing extraordinary support in an environment of rising inflation and tightening global financial conditions. Table 7.2 provides an illustrative snapshot of the scale and composition of fiscal responses across selected regions, drawing on summaries from international financial institutions and regional reports.

Table 7.2 Regional fiscal responses to COVID-19

Region/ country	Total fiscal support (illustrative)	Types of measures	Target populations	Timeline	Outcomes reported (qualitative)
Global	Over US$20 trillion	Income support, wage subsidies, business grants/ loans, tax relief	Households and firms	2020–2021	Stabilised incomes and employment; contributed to higher public debt
Africa	Multiple regional and national packages	Budget support, health spending, liquidity, social protection	Health systems, vulnerable households	2020–2021	Larger deficits, higher debt; constrained fiscal space
England	Large, targeted measures	Job retention schemes, social transfers, temporary tax changes	Low-income households, workers, firms	2020–2021	Mitigated income loss but highlighted pre-existing inequalities

Table 7.3 Inflation and debt

Indicator	Value	Source
Global headline inflation (2022)	≈ 8.8%	IMF, *World Economic Outlook* (Oct 2022)
U.S. CPI inflation (May 2022, 12-month)	8.6%	BLS, CPI release
Total global debt (2020)	US$226 trillion (≈256% of world GDP)	IMF, global debt blog
Global public debt (2020)	≈ 99% of world GDP	IMF, global debt blog
EMDE government debt/ LIC distress (2020–2022)	EMDE debt around low-60s % of GDP; >½ of LICs in or at high risk of debt distress	World Bank, *Global Economic Prospects* (Jan 2022)

7.8 Inflation and Public Debt

The pandemic's economic disruptions generated severe inflationary pressures and unprecedented increases in public debt. As demand rebounded amid constrained supply, inflation surged to multi-decade highs during 2021–2022 [3, 7]. Supply constraints and energy price shocks were primary drivers of this inflation, compounded by rebounding demand as economies reopened [8].

Global headline inflation peaked at approximately 8.8% in 2022, driven by supply-chain disruptions, energy and food price shocks, and the interaction between strong post-pandemic demand and earlier accommodative macroeconomic policies. In the United States, consumer price inflation reached 8.6% year-on-year in May 2022, with energy and food prices making outsized contributions. In many emerging market and developing economies, including India and other large emerging market and developing economies (EMDEs), inflationary spikes were further amplified by currency depreciation and higher import costs for fuel and food (Table 7.3).

In parallel, public and private debt levels increased substantially. Total global debt rose to approximately US $226 trillion in 2020—about 256% of world GDP—while global public debt approached 99% of GDP. Among emerging market and developing economies (EMDEs), government debt ratios rose sharply, and more than half of low-income countries were assessed as being in debt distress or at high risk of it [9]. This build-up of debt was not confined to advanced economies; several large emerging markets, including China and India, also saw higher public-debt-to-GDP ratios, although with differing levels of market access and rollover risk.

7.9 Mental Health and Economic Costs

The COVID-19 pandemic caused significant mental health issues, leading to substantial and persistent economic impacts globally, both during the pandemic and in the post-pandemic recovery phase. Other concurrent factors, such as a surge in gun violence, increased war activities, and natural disasters, have also contributed to the rise in mental health crises during this period. However, the pandemic-related changes in social structure have posed unique challenges. The economic strain related to the COVID-19 pandemic resulted in both direct treatment costs and indirect costs related to decreased productivity and labour force changes.

The pandemic was associated, as expected, with a substantial increase in anxiety and depressive disorders worldwide, resulting in productivity losses, absenteeism, and reduced labour-force participation [11–14]. Health-worker burnout, early retirement, and post-COVID conditions further intensified economic strain. Mental health–related economic costs include direct treatment expenditures and indirect losses from reduced productivity, early retirement, and labour-market exit. Telehealth expansion and policy reforms partially mitigated care disruptions, particularly in underserved regions [11, 25].

Immediately, there was a surging demand for services. COVID-19 pandemic has shown a 27.6% increase in major depressive disorders and a 25.6% increase in anxiety disorders. It was estimated to have caused 137.1 additional disability adjusted life years per 100,000 population for major depressive disorders and 116.1 per 100,000 population for anxiety disorders [10]. COVID-19 is also associated with increased domestic violence contributed by stay-at-home orders, homeschooling, stress of child care, and male unemployment.

Then there was disrupted care. The increased demand coincided with severe disruptions to mental health services due to staff and infrastructure redeployment for COVID-19 relief, creating significant gaps in care. To counter the effect of disrupted care and the surging demand for services, several changes have been implemented in mental health services, including the utilisation of telehealth, the expansion of school-based mental health care, and the rollout of the 988 crisis line [10]. Expansion of telehealth due to health insurance policy reform, in response to COVID-19, has facilitated mental health outreach in remote areas, which previously tended to lack sufficient mental health care.

Mental health issues also directly impacted the workforce, contributing to substantial indirect costs: It led to reduced productivity and absenteeism. Mental health disorders significantly reduced worker productivity and increased sick leave, representing a substantial portion of the total expenditure related to mental health. The UK, for example, experienced a 30% increase in work absences due to mental health disorders [11].

The "Great Resignation" and burnout were other major factors**.** During the pandemic, the rate of job quitting in the United States has reached its highest in the twenty-first century, and this phenomenon is called "Great Resignation". This is likely due to pandemic-related factors, including increased stimulus payments, fear of infection, health concerns, childcare issues, and changing attitudes toward work. High levels of psychological distress, stress, and burnout, particularly among healthcare workers and those in direct customer-facing and heavily locked-down sectors, were likely to have also contributed to the "Great Resignation" [12].

Decreased Labour Force Participation (LFP) resulted in job loss and unemployment, which surged during the pandemic, and were strongly associated with a higher risk of depression and other mental health difficulties [13, 14]. LFP rates declined sharply and persistently, partially due to more people (especially women) leaving the workforce for caregiving responsibilities and an increase in early retirement due to health concerns, which are often exacerbated by mental distress [15]. Individuals with lower LFP during the pandemic faced a consistently increased short-term risk of depression [14]. The COVID-19 pandemic has resulted in increased demand and burden on healthcare workers, especially workers on the front line. Even after the acute risk of COVID-19 infection has subsided, the healthcare worker shortage has worsened. This continues to strain the healthcare system and continues to have a decline in recruitment [16]. Work absence due to COVID-19 has decreased compared to the initial pandemic stage, driven by changes in isolation recommendations, relaxation of workplace requirements, reduced testing, and declining prevalence. However, compared to the pre-pandemic stage, the work absence in the post-pandemic stage is comparable to that during flu season, which extended throughout the year [17].

Post-COVID-19 conditions are also known as long COVID. A significant minority (up to 25%) of people with persisting post-COVID symptoms, including mental health symptoms like anxiety, depression ("brain fog"), and PTSD, were reported as unable to work for some duration, adding a new layer of economic cost [18, 19]. PTSD occurs in patients who had a near-death experience and prolonged hospitalisation. Also, some people who have lost their loved ones have experienced Survivor's Guilt [19]. There was a disproportionate impact on vulnerable groups. The economic and mental health crises were interconnected, creating a vicious cycle, particularly for vulnerable populations. Economic uncertainty became a stressor. Increased economic uncertainty, job loss, and income insecurity were major stressors that led to mental health problems [10, 13]. Individuals who experienced household job loss were significantly more likely to report symptoms of anxiety and/or depression [8].

Young adults and lower-Income individuals: Young people and those in lower-income households reported the highest levels of anxiety and depression, with low-income households being far more likely to experience moderate-to-severe mental distress compared to high-income counterparts [20]. The pandemic altered the pay and the demographic of the workforce. The share of U.S. workers aged 16–24 shrank from 11.7% to 9.6% between May 2019 and May 2020 as young workers exited the workforce. Young workers returned to the workforce in 2023 as lockdowns eased and job opportunities increased [21]. There were exacerbated inequalities as well. Marginalised racial and ethnic groups, such as Latinx adults in the United States, were disproportionately affected by job loss and financial problems, which directly increased their risk for severe psychological distress [22].

7.10 Impact on the U.S. Health Insurance Industry

COVID-19 fundamentally altered the U.S. health insurance landscape. Reduced utilisation in 2020 led to unusually high insurer profits and significant medical loss ratio rebates, followed by cost surges as deferred care returned [23–25]. Medicaid enrolment increased to historic levels during pandemic-era continuous coverage

Table 7.4 Policy priorities and flagship guidance

Priority	Evidence-based takeaway	Source
Resilient GVCs	Diversification reduces exposure more efficiently than reshoring	IMF, *World Economic Outlook* (Apr 2022), Ch. 4
Support remote/ home work	Update labour standards, OSH, and portable benefits	ILO, *Working from Home: From invisibility to decent work*
Debt treatment	Use the G20 common framework and related DSSI architecture for tailored debt solutions	World Bank/IMF, Common Framework note
Post-COVID fiscal roadmap	Rebuild buffers; prioritise productivity-enhancing investment	IMF, *Fiscal Monitor* (Oct 2020)
EMDE outlook	Slower recoveries amidst debt and inflation pressures	World Bank, *Global Economic Prospects* (Jan 2022)

protections, followed by significant disenrollment during eligibility redeterminations, increasing market volatility [26, 27]. Telehealth utilisation increased more than 20-fold in 2020 and has since stabilised as a permanent component of care delivery [28]. Long COVID, behavioural health demand, provider wage inflation, and increased fraud risks have added complexity to actuarial modelling and regulatory oversight [23, 29, 30].

7.11 Long-Term Legacies and Policy Implications

The pandemic catalysed fundamental and potentially permanent changes across multiple dimensions of economic activity. Digital commerce, telework, and digital payments expanded rapidly, accelerating trends that might otherwise have taken years to unfold [3, 4]. Remote and hybrid work models became normalised, reshaping labour markets, urban form, and firm organisation [2]. Multilateral institutions highlight several priority domains for long-term policy reform (Table 7.4). By May 2020, Cambridge University estimated the cost to the global economy at $3.3 trillion to $82 trillion over 5 years, and in mid-2020, the UN estimated the cost to be $8.5 trillion over 2 years. Above, we discussed the economic implications within different sectors of the global economy. These lessons are valuable in preparing for future disasters of this nature which are likely to recur and may interact with other global risks such as climate change, geopolitical tensions, and future pandemics.

Acknowledgements The authors thank colleagues and reviewers who provided feedback on earlier drafts.

References

1. National Center for Health Statistics. Provisional COVID-19 death counts by week ending date and state. Atlanta: CDC; 2025.
2. Kaiser Family Foundation. Global COVID-19 tracker. San Francisco: KFF; 2025.

3. International Labor Organization. Uncertain and uneven recovery expected following unprecedented labor market crisis. Geneva: ILO; 2021.
4. Kose MA, Sugawara N. Understanding the depth of the 2020 global recession in five charts. World Bank Blogs; 2020.
5. Verschuur J, Koks EE, Hall JW. Implications of large-scale containment policies on global maritime trade. 2021. https://arxiv.org/abs/2010.15907.
6. International Monetary Fund. Fiscal monitor: strengthening the credibility of public finances. Washington, DC: IMF; 2021.
7. United Nations World Tourism Organization. Worst year in tourism history with one billion fewer international arrivals. UNWTO World Tourism Barometer. 2021;19(1).
8. Organization for Economic Co-operation and Development. E-commerce in the time of COVID-19. Paris: OECD Publishing; 2020.
9. World Bank. COVID-19 to add as many as 150 million extreme poor by 2021. Washington, DC: World Bank; 2020.
10. McKinsey Global Institute. Empty spaces and hybrid places. McKinsey & Company; 2020.
11. World Health Organization. Mental health and COVID-19: early evidence. WHO Scientific Brief; 2022.
12. Jiskrova GK. Impact of COVID-19 on the workforce. J Epidemiol Commun Health. 2022.
13. Melchior M, et al. Labor market participation and depression during COVID-19. Front Psychiatry; 2022.
14. Hellman SS, et al. Labor force participation and depression risk. Scand J Public Health. 2022.
15. Faria-e-Castro M. The COVID retirement boom. Federal Reserve Bank of St Louis; 2021.
16. Lee BEC, et al. Pandemic stress among healthcare workers. BMC Psychiatry. 2025.
17. Scully JM. Workforce absences post-pandemic. Yale School of Public Health; 2025.
18. Hou Y, et al. Global prevalence of long COVID. Open Forum Infect Dis. 2025.
19. Williamson L. Long COVID and mental health. American Heart Association News; 2023.
20. Lu X, Lin Z. COVID-19, mental health, and coping behaviors. Front Psychol. 2021.
21. Villafuerte V. COVID'S economic fallout and mental health risks. UCLA; 2022.
22. Panchal N, et al. Mental health and substance use implications of COVID-19. KFF; 2023.
23. Federal Reserve Bank of Chicago. Impact of COVID-19 on health insurers. Chicago Fed Lett; 2022.
24. Centers for Medicare & Medicaid Services (2023) Medical loss ratio requirements.. CMS.
25. American Academy of Actuaries. Telehealth and the ACA. AAA; 2022.
26. Musumeci M, et al. Medicaid enrollment and unwinding tracker. KFF; 2022.
27. Buettgens M, et al. Impact of COVID-19 PHE expiration. Urban Institute; 2022.
28. Mehrotra A, et al. Evolution of telehealth during COVID-19. RAND; 2021.
29. Reuters. Health insurer Centene reports surprise loss amid rising costs. 2025.
30. U.S. Department of Health and Human Services OIG. Telehealth program integrity risks. 2023.

Part II

Virology, Immunology and Diagnosis of COVID-19

8 Morphology and Pathogenesis of Severe Acute Respiratory Syndrome Coronavirus 2 (SARS-CoV-2)

Avinash Choudekar and Wajihul Hasan Khan

8.1 Introduction

Severe acute respiratory syndrome coronavirus 2 (SARS-CoV-2) is responsible for the most severe pandemic in history, profoundly impacting healthcare and related economic sectors [1, 2]. SARS-CoV-2 is the member of the genus *Betacoronavirus* and family *Coronaviridae*. It is linked to SARS-CoV and the Middle East respiratory syndrome coronavirus (MERS-CoV). SARS-CoV-2 has developed distinct genetic and structural modifications that facilitate its transmission and the infection of diverse tissues, despite its genome organization and replication mechanism being like other coronaviruses. SARS-CoV-2 is a single-stranded positive sense RNA virus with an envelope. Its genome is about 30 kb long. It can be either spherical or pleomorphic between diameter of 60 and 140 nm [3]. The RNA genome is surrounded by the nucleocapsid (N) protein inside the viral core. The viral envelope is made up of three primary structural proteins: the spike (S), the membrane (M), and the envelope (E). The envelope comes from the host cell membrane. The S glycoprotein is the most visible element of the surface. It is a trimeric class I fusion protein that makes the "corona" projections that may be viewed with an electron microscope [4]. The S protein is made up of two functional domains: S2 facilitates the fusion of viral and cellular membranes, and S1 has the receptor-binding domain (RBD) that interacts with the host angiotensin-converting enzyme 2 (ACE2) receptor [5]. The M protein is the fundamental structural portion of the virus. It shapes the viral envelope and controls how virions come together. Despite having a lower proportion, the E protein is essential for the virus to bud, release, and cause illness. The

A. Choudekar (✉) · W. H. Khan
Virology Laboratory, Department of Microbiology, All India Institute of Medical Sciences, New Delhi, Delhi, India

S. R. Prabhu et al. (eds.), *COVID-19 in Dental Practice*,
https://doi.org/10.1007/978-3-032-26000-0_8

N protein forms a ribonucleoprotein complex with genomic RNA to help the virus reproduce and package itself and present higher antigenicity to the host. Research employing cryo-electron microscopy and tomography has elucidated the three-dimensional structure of SARS-CoV-2, detailing the elements of the viral envelope's lipid bilayer and the adaptable arrangement of S trimers [3, 4, 6–8]. The S protein binds to the ACE2 receptor, which is found in significant proportion in the gastrointestinal tract, vascular endothelium, and respiratory epithelium [9, 10]. After binding to the receptor, host proteases such as furin, cathepsins, and transmembrane protease serine 2 (TMPRSS2) activate the S protein by cutting it at the S1/S2 and S2′ sites [11]. When the positive-sense RNA genome enters the host cell, it serves as a direct template for translation of viral proteins. The replication-transcription complex (RTC) is made up of two large polyproteins (pp1a and pp1ab) that are translated into non-structural proteins by viral proteases (Mpro and PLpro). This complex oversees making sub-genomic RNAs that code for structural and accessory proteins and copying the genome.

The virus replicates in the respiratory epithelium, where the infection begins, damaging the host cells, causing apoptosis, and rupturing the epithelial barrier. In severe cases, an uncontrolled inflammatory reaction known as a "cytokine storm" occurs, resulting in significant tissue damage.

In serious cases of COVID-19, the histological results show damage to the endothelium, thrombosis in the microvasculature, the formation of hyaline membranes, and major damage to the alveoli [12, 13]. Viral dissemination and systemic inflammation result in systemic manifestations, including myocarditis, acute renal injury, and neurological symptoms [12, 14]. SARS-CoV-2 may also alter innate immune signalling pathways, such as by inhibiting type I interferon responses [15], allowing the virus to persist in the body and exacerbate inflammation. Comprehension of the pathophysiology and structural biology of SARS-CoV-2 has been crucial for the advancement of diagnostic instruments, antiviral medications, and vaccines [16–22]. The structural characterization of the S protein facilitated the development of mRNA and vector-based vaccines aimed at targeting the prefusion conformation of the spike trimer [23]. Global efforts to monitor, prevent, and treat COVID-19 are being shaped by ongoing research on viral evolution, specifically spike protein changes in variations of concern. A comprehensive understanding of SARS-CoV-2 pathophysiology and structural characteristics enhances disease control and readiness in the preparation for emerging virus-based epidemics.

8.2 Genomic and Structural Features of SARS-CoV-2

SARS-CoV-2 has a genome of about 30 kb of positive-sense RNA that codes for 29 proteins. These include 4 structural proteins, S, E, M, and N, and 16 non-structural proteins (Nsps 1–16) that are necessary for the virus to replicate. The big open reading frame, ORF1ab (nucleotides 265–21,555), makes two polyproteins: pp1ab (which makes Nsps 1–16) and the shorter pp1a (which makes Nsps 1–11). This happens when a −1 ribosomal frameshift occurs. After then, either the papain-like protease (PLpro) or the major protease (Mpro) cuts these polyproteins into 16 mature non-structural proteins [24]. PLpro (Nsp3), 3C-like protease (Nsp5, Mpro), RNA-dependent RNA polymerase (Nsp12, RdRp), helicase (Nsp13), endoRNAse (Nsp15), and 2′-O-ribose-methyltransferase (Nsp16) are all Nsps that are like those found in other coronaviruses in terms of their sequences and functions. The last 3′ part of the genome codes for the structural proteins: S (a glycoprotein with a molecular weight of about 180 kDa), E (a protein with a molecular weight of 9–12 kDa), M (a protein with a molecular weight of 23–35 kDa), and N (a basic protein with a molecular weight of about 45.6 kDa that binds RNA). The 3′ end also has nine auxiliary proteins that help the virus replicate, assemble, and leave the cell. These proteins are ORF3a, ORF3b, ORF6, ORF7a, ORF7b, ORF8, ORF9b, ORF9c, and ORF10. They may also be used as antigenic targets.

The S protein produces trimers that give the virus its crown-like shape and is the viral antigen that is most exposed. This trimeric spike is the main protective antigen that causes substantial neutralizing antibody responses [25]. The spike glycoprotein has 1273 amino acids and is made up of two main parts: S1 (aa 14–685) and S2 (aa 686–1273). The S1 subunit has a signal peptide (SP) at the beginning (aa 1–3) and an N-terminal domain (NTD; aa 14–305) and an RBD; aa 319–541 at the end. The receptor-binding motif (RBM; aa 437–508) and the C-terminal domain (CTD) are in the middle. The RBD interacts only with the ACE2 receptor on host cells. The S2 subunit is responsible for membrane fusion and viral entry. It has functional parts such as the fusion peptide (FP; aa 788–806), heptad repeat 1 (HR1; aa 912–984), heptad repeat 2 (HR2; aa 1163–1213), transmembrane domain (TM; aa 1213–1237), and cytoplasmic tail (CT; aa 1237–1273). The spike protein is the main target of most SARS-CoV-2 vaccines, such as mRNA, DNA, and adenovirus vectored vaccines. In addition to the spike protein, other structural (N and M) and non-structural proteins, along with accessory proteins, may exhibit antigenic characteristics that render them viable vaccine candidates.

Immunoinformatic investigations have found multiple interesting B- and T-cell epitopes within SARS-CoV-2 proteins four in the M protein, eight in the N protein, and 13 in the S protein. Epitopes situated in M (aa 165–181 and 306–322), N (aa 314–330), and S (aa 817–833, 891–907, 897–913, and 1182–1209) are anticipated to be nonallergenic, nontoxic, and to possess a minimal likelihood of inducing autoimmune reactivity in roughly 87% of the global population [26]. These antigenic markers signify promising candidates for the formulation of next-generation SARS-CoV-2 vaccines. Figure. 8.1 and Table 8.1 shows the details about the structural and non structural proteins of the SARS-CoV-2.

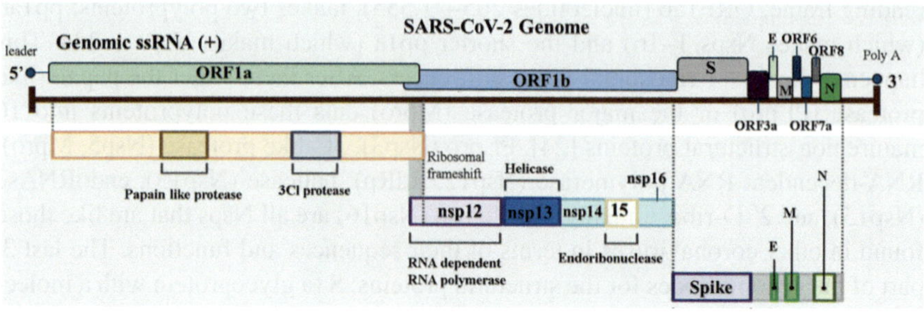

Fig. 8.1 SARS-CoV-2 genome structure and proteins: The genome of SARS-CoV-2 is around 30 kb long, with a 3′ poly(A) tail and a 5′ cap structure. SARS-CoV-2 genome encodes structural and non-structural proteins. The ORF1a and ORF1b are translated into the non-structural proteins (Nsps 1–16)

Table 8.1 Structural and non-structural proteins of SARS-CoV-2 and its important functions

Protein name	Size (kDa)	Amino acid length (aa)	Function
Structural proteins			
Spike (S) protein	~180–200	1273	Spike protein binds to ACE2 receptor for entry; target for neutralizing antibodies and vaccines development
Membrane (M) protein	~25–30	222	Most abundant protein, maintains viral shape and assists in assembly
Envelope (E) protein	~8–12	75	Smallest structural protein, acts as an ion channel and is involved in viral assembly & pathogenesis
Nucleocapsid (N) protein	~45–50	419	Binds viral RNA to form the ribonucleoprotein complex, assisting in replication & packaging
Non-structural proteins (Nsps)			
Nsp1	~17	180	Suppresses host mRNA translation, helps in evading to immune responses
Nsp2	~70	628	Modulates host cell processes and survival pathways
Nsp3 (PLpro)	~200	1922	Cleaves viral polyprotein; suppresses host immune responses (de-ubiquitination)
Nsp4	~50	500	Helps in double-membrane vesicle formation for viral replication
Nsp5 (3CLpro, Mpro)	~33	306	Main protease; cleaves polyprotein for replication
Nsp6	~36	390	Induces vesicle formation; limits autophagy to prevent virus degradation
Nsp7 & Nsp8	~9 & ~13	83 & 198	Forms complex with Nsp12 (RdRp) to enhance viral RNA replication
Nsp9	~13	113	Binds RNA to aid replication
Nsp10	~15	189	Activates Nsp14 (exonuclease) & Nsp16 (methyltransferase) for RNA proofreading

(continued)

Table 8.1 (continued)

Protein name	Size (kDa)	Amino acid length (aa)	Function
Nsp12 (RdRp)	~105	932	RNA-dependent RNA polymerase (RdRp); key enzyme for viral genome replication
Nsp13 (Helicase)	~67	601	Unwinds RNA during replication and transcription
Nsp14 (Exonuclease)	~60	527	Provides RNA proofreading to reduce mutations
Nsp15 (Endoribonuclease, NendoU)	~40	346	Cleaves viral RNA to evade immune detection
Nsp16 (Methyltransferase)	~35	298	Modifies viral RNA to mimic host mRNA and avoid immune detection
Accessory proteins			
ORF3a	~30	275	Ion channel; involved in inflammation and apoptosis
ORF6	~7	61	Suppresses host immune response
ORF7a	~11	121	Induces inflammation and immune evasion
ORF7b	~5	43	Possible role in virion assembly
ORF8	~14	121	Involved in immune evasion and virulence
ORF9b	~10	73	Disrupts host immune signalling
ORF10	~5	38	Possible role in host interaction, biological function uncertain

8.3 Morphological Study of SARS-CoV-2 Using Advanced Microscopic Technique

Transmission electron microscopy (TEM) and scanning electron microscopy (SEM) were the first tools used to see SARS-CoV-2 virions [4] (Fig. 8.2). The crown-like spike proteins on the surface of SARS-CoV-2 were found by TEM, which confirmed that the virus had a structure that is like other coronaviruses. SEM showed that the virus caused membranes to ruffle and vesicles to form on the surfaces of infected cells [27]. Cryo-EM showed the near-atomic structures of important viral proteins in their natural states, which changed the way scientists and researchers look at the structure of SARS-CoV-2. For example, high-resolution cryo-EM maps of the S glycoprotein have shown its prefusion and postfusion shapes. Cryo-EM has helped scientists figure out the structures of the viral RNA polymerase (nsp12-nsp7-nsp8), the nucleocapsid (N) protein, and the main protease (Mpro). Cryo-ET shows intact SARS-CoV-2 virions and infected cells in three dimensions at the nanoscale level [28]. Cryo-ET showed how spike proteins are spread out and ordered on virions, how the virus interacts with the ACE2 receptor, and how cells that are infected make double-membrane vesicles (DMVs). These results established a geographical and structural basis for the in situ examination of the viral life cycle. Super-resolution methods like stochastic optical reconstruction microscopy (STORM), photoactivated localization microscopy (PALM), and stimulated emission depletion (STED)

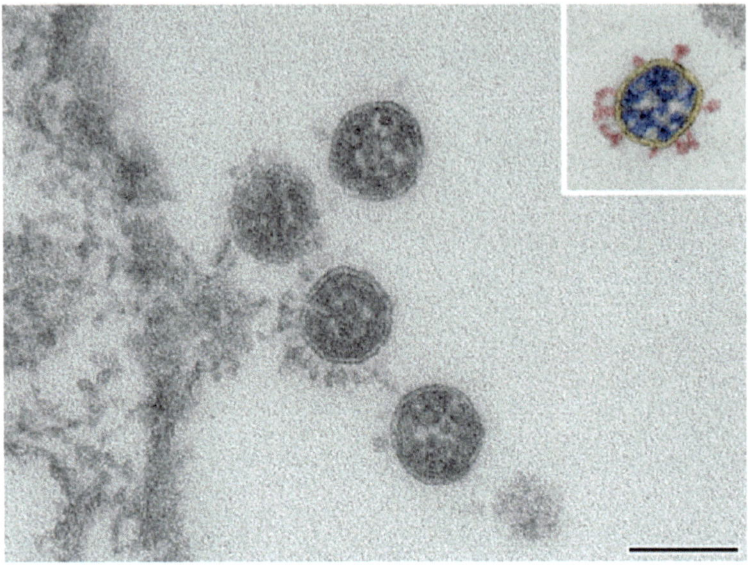

Fig. 8.2 An illustration of SARS-CoV-2 close to Vero cells using transmission electron microscopy at a 135,000X magnification. The spikes (red), the virus ribonucleoprotein (blue), and its enclosing membrane (yellow) are depicted in the inset as a coloured viral particle [4]

have made it possible to see parts of SARS-CoV-2 that are too small for light to see [29, 30]. These methods pinpointed viral proteins, RNA, and host cell receptors with nanoscale precision. STED microscopy has shown that ACE2 and TMPRSS2 cluster together on the membranes of host cells at the nanoscale. Correlative Light and Electron Microscopy (CLEM) combines the molecular sensitivity of fluorescence microscopy with the high resolution of electron microscopy to connect small structural features with dynamic events. Researchers studying SARS-CoV-2 have utilized CLEM to follow fluorescently tagged viral proteins during infection and EM to figure out where they fit into the ultrastructural images. This correlative method has revealed insights into the formation of viral replication compartments and the spatial relationships among host cell machinery. Atomic Force Microscopy (AFM) has allowed scientists to look at the mechanical properties and surface features of SARS-CoV-2. AFM has measured how stiff viral particles are, how strong the spike protein-ACE2 receptor bond is, and how stable spike protein mutations are [31]. Mechanical insights enhance structural and pharmacological data to elucidate viral infectivity and immune evasion.

8.4 Clinical Manifestation of SARS-Cov-2 Infection

The clinical presentation of SARS-CoV-2 infection continues to evolve, with new insights into its multisystem involvement, variant-specific features, and long-term sequelae. COVID-19 most frequently presents with fever, cough, fatigue, and dyspnea [32]. Other symptoms include myalgia, headache, sore throat, and gastrointestinal complaints such as nausea, vomiting, and diarrhoea. The disease spectrum ranges from asymptomatic to severe pneumonia and acute respiratory distress syndrome (ARDS), with a significant proportion of patients experiencing only mild or moderate symptoms [32, 33]. Imaging often reveals ground-glass opacities and bilateral lung involvement, even in some asymptomatic cases [34].

Acute and chronic neurological symptoms are increasingly recognized, including cognitive dysfunction, headache, autonomic dysfunction, chronic fatigue, anosmia, and ageusia. These symptoms can persist as part of post-acute sequelae (long COVID), with some evidence of structural changes in the brain. Neurological involvement is associated with poorer outcomes and may contribute to the risk of neurodegenerative diseases [35]. COVID-19 is also associated with a variety of cutaneous manifestations, including chilblain-like lesions and maculopapular, urticarial, vesicular, and livedoid rashes [36]. These can occur at any stage of illness and may be the presenting feature in some cases. Severe cases of cardiovascular, renal, and hepatic involvement, particularly in severe cases. Recent data indicate that while some symptoms (e.g., neurological) were more prevalent with earlier variants, they remain common with newer, less virulent strains [35, 37]. These diverse clinical manifestations highlight the importance of understanding the underlying pathogenesis of SARS-CoV-2, which involves viral entry and replication leading to direct cellular injury, endothelial dysfunction, and dysregulated immune responses across multiple organ systems. A deeper understanding of these mechanisms may help to elucidate the progression of disease severity, identify therapeutic targets, and improve strategies for prevention and management of both acute infection and its long-term complications.

8.5 Pathogenesis of SARS-CoV-2

The pathogenesis of SARS-CoV-2 represents a complex and dynamic interaction between the SARS-CoV-2 virus and host cellular and immune processes, resulting in a diverse spectrum of clinical manifestations that extend beyond the respiratory system. Infection begins when the virus enters human cells via its spike protein binding to ACE2 receptors, initially infecting nasal mucosa and lung epithelial cells [38]. This triggers an abnormal immune response characterized by a cytokine storm, with increased levels of inflammatory cytokines like IL-6, IL-10, and TNF-α, decreased lymphocyte counts, vascular injury and alveolar damage [1, 2]. As the disease progresses, the interplay between viral cytopathic effects and immune-mediated injury determines the extent of organ involvement, ranging from self-limited respiratory infection to severe multi-organ dysfunction [39, 40]. Gaining insights into this mechanism is crucial for developing targeted therapeutic strategies [41].

8.5.1 Human Host Cell Receptors

Various cellular receptors and coreceptors are implicated in viral entry, particularly for SARS-CoV-1 and SARS-CoV-2. ACE2 is the primary receptor for these coronaviruses on cells like epithelia, macrophages, platelets, and endothelial cells; it is also involved in regulating blood pressure via angiotensin II [42, 43]. Other molecules function as coreceptors or alternative entry points; for example, Neuropilin 1 (NRP1) acts as a coreceptor for SARS-CoV-2 following S-protein cleavage, while chondroitin sulfate contributes to the cell glycocalyx and acts as a coreceptor. It is concentrated in nerve cells of the brain and nasal cavity and in endothelial cells [43, 44]. The widely expressed CD147 (Basigin) is both a coreceptor and an activator of ACE2 [45]. GRP78 (BiP), a stress factor, also serves as a coreceptor on different cells [46]. Scavenger receptors show specific patterns: SR-B1 on proliferating cells, hepatocytes, macrophages, and adrenal cells; SR-H2 on macrophages and endothelial cells; CD209L (L-SIGN) on endothelial cells and alveolar epithelium; CD209 (DC-SIGN) on macrophages and dendritic cells; SR-E2 (Dectin-1) on myeloid cells like macrophages, monocytes, and neutrophils; and SR-E3 (mannose receptor 1) on macrophages, monocytes, and dendritic cells. DPP4 (CD26) is widespread, especially on the respiratory epithelium. ANPE is expressed on various epithelial cells and neutrophils, while ENPEP shares an expression pattern like ACE2 [47]. AXL is a putative alternative receptor highly expressed in the lungs [10]. Furthermore, DPP4 (CD26) is the main receptor for MERS-CoV and a possible SARS-CoV-2 alternative, and ANPE/ENPEP are also suggested as alternatives or coreceptors. ASGr1 is mainly found on hepatocytes, and KIM-1/TIM-1 is present on the epithelium of the lungs and kidneys [43, 48].

8.5.2 Human Host Cell Proteases

Human host cell proteases are critical for SARS-CoV-2 entry, facilitating the process through the cleavage and activation of the viral S protein [11]. The TMPRSS family, particularly TMPRSS2, expressed mainly in bronchial transient secretory cells, activates the S protein at the S2 site, enabling membrane fusion after binding to ACE2. TMPRSS4 expression in bronchial epithelial cells may be enhanced by smoking, increasing susceptibility [11, 48, 49]. Furthermore, the protease furin, a pro-protein convertase, cleaves the S protein at the unique S1/S2 site (PRRA) in SARS-CoV-2, which promotes viral entry, cell-to-cell fusion, and replication, with inhibitors being explored as treatment options [49, 50]. The ADAM family, notably ADAM-17, is involved in shedding the ACE2 ectodomain, a process potentially targeted pharmacologically [51]. Conversely, the endosomal protease Cathepsin L (CTSL), a lysosomal cysteine protease activated in low-pH environments, cleaves the S1 subunit, which is essential for late-pathway viral entry and fusion; CTSL inhibitors are effective, and drugs like fluoxetine and fluvoxamine might also limit infection by influencing intravesicular pH [52]. Host protein modifications, including ACE2 shedding, spike/ACE2 cleavage, and receptor polymorphisms, reflect the capacity of viruses to alter host protein function to its advantage [53].

8.5.3 Entry and Intracellular Replication of SARS-CoV-2 Virus

The S glycoprotein, particularly its RBD, binds to ACE2 with high affinity, enabling viral docking at the cell surface [40]. Following attachment, proteolytic activation of the spike protein by host enzymes is required to expose the fusion peptide and initiate membrane fusion or endocytosis [39, 41]. SARS-CoV-2 employs two main entry routes: direct fusion with the plasma membrane or clathrin-dependent or independent endocytosis [53, 54]. Both require proteolytic priming and depend on the

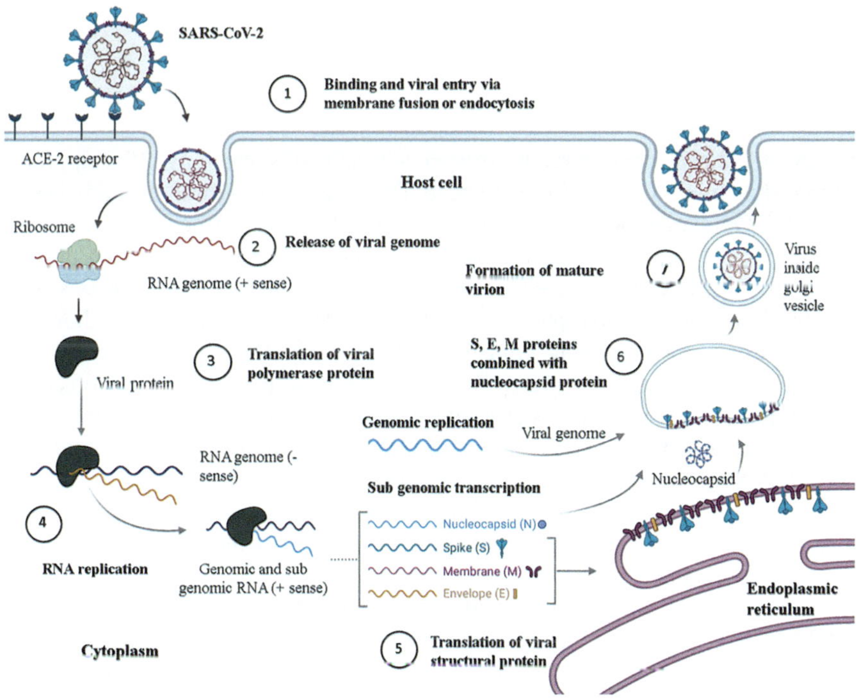

Fig. 8.3 SARS-CoV-2 infection and intracellular replication into host cell in the process of virions production

surrounding pH. Furin acts optimally at neutral pH, whereas cathepsin activity depends on endosomal acidification. This dual mechanism allows the virus to adapt to different cellular contexts and enhances its ability to infect diverse tissues [6, 9] (Fig. 8.3).

After entry, SARS-CoV-2 initiates replication within specialized membranous compartments that protect its RNA and facilitate efficient synthesis. Replication occurs predominantly in double-membrane vesicles (DMVs) derived from the endoplasmic reticulum (ER) [6, 9]. These structures shield viral RNA from cytosolic sensors such as RIG-I and MDA5, reducing interferon activation. The viral genome, a positive-sense RNA molecule, is directly translated to produce two polyproteins, pp1a and pp1ab, which are processed by the viral proteases PLpro (NSP3) and 3CLpro (NSP5) into a series of non-structural proteins (NSPs) [55]. The NSPs assemble to form the replication–transcription complex (RTC), responsible for both genome replication and transcription of sub-genomic RNAs. Core components include RNA-dependent RNA polymerase (NSP12), helicase (NSP13), and cofactors NSP7/8. The membrane-associated proteins NSP3, NSP4, and NSP6 anchor the complex to ER membranes. Subgenomic RNAs serve as templates for the synthesis of structural proteins: S, M, E, N and several accessory proteins that modulate host immune responses [15, 56].

8.5.4 Cell-to-Cell Spread and Membrane Fusion Processes

SARS-CoV-2 can spread directly between adjacent cells, enabling efficient propagation while minimizing exposure to neutralizing antibodies. Viral assembly begins in the ER-Golgi intermediate compartment (ERGIC), where structural proteins and genomic RNA combine to form complete virions. These are transported through vesicular pathways and released via exocytosis, lysosomal secretion, or, less commonly, plasma membrane rupture. Use of lysosomal trafficking pathways allows the virus to exit without causing immediate cell lysis, limiting immune recognition [57]. The S glycoprotein remains central to both viral egress and intercellular spread. Its fusogenic properties can induce syncytium formation, producing multinucleated cells formed by the fusion of infected cells with neighbouring uninfected cells [58]. Syncytia facilitate direct viral transfer, maintaining infection even in the presence of neutralizing antibodies. Host proteases such as furin and cathepsin L continue to cleave the spike protein during this process, demonstrating their ongoing role beyond initial entry [59].

Host cell lipid metabolism and endosomal transport also influence viral release. SARS-CoV-2 alters lipid biosynthesis to maintain membrane curvature and envelope integrity and modulates trafficking through the Golgi and endosomal systems to accelerate exocytosis [9, 54]. In secretory cell types, such as epithelial and endothelial cells, lysosome-mediated release complements classical exocytosis, providing an additional route for viral dissemination [43, 44]. Organ-specific patterns of spread reflect differences in cellular architecture and protease expression. Efficient cell-to-cell propagation has been demonstrated in respiratory, gastrointestinal, and neuronal tissues. In the respiratory tract, TMPRSS2 and furin facilitate fusion and syncytia formation [50]. In the nervous system, the virus can spread along the olfactory and possibly synaptic routes, supporting evidence for neuroinvasion [14].

8.5.5 Innate and Adaptive Immune Response and Hyperinflammation

The innate immune system acts as the first defence, activating neutrophils, macrophages, and endothelial cells that release pro-inflammatory cytokines like IL-6, IL-1β, and IFNs, NK cells, TNF, along with chemokines and other molecules, which intensify inflammation. The innate immune response to viral infection begins with the activation of resident macrophages, which detect pathogens through pattern recognition receptors (PRRs). These macrophages act as early antiviral defenders and release type I and type III interferons (IFNs) that signal nearby immune and epithelial cells. Plasmacytoid dendritic cells (pDCs) are subsequently recruited from adjacent lymphoid tissues to the infection site, where they also produce type I IFNs (IFN-α, IFN-β), amplifying antiviral signalling and activating both innate and adaptive immune pathways [15, 60, 61]. Natural killer (NK) cells are then drawn to the area under the influence of IFNs. They recognize and destroy infected host cells through necroptosis, helping to limit viral replication until cytotoxic $CD8^+$ T lymphocytes (CTLs) become active and provide a more specific antiviral response. However, during severe infections, interleukin-6 (IL-6) can suppress NK cell cytotoxicity, reducing their effectiveness. Interferons stimulate the transcription of hundreds of IFN-responsive genes, reinforcing the antiviral state and promoting a feedback loop that boosts immune activity (Fig. 8.4). These pathways also enhance macrophage secretion of pro-inflammatory cytokines (IL-1β, IL-6, IL-8, IL-12, and TNF) and anti-inflammatory cytokines (IL-10), recruiting more neutrophils and lymphocytes (Fig. 8.5a) [61]. On the other hand, the adaptive immune response involves T and B cells, but severe COVID-19 often features a reduction in T cells, particularly CD3+ T cells, and a high neutrophil-to-lymphocyte ratio, which is linked to worse outcomes. T cell responses to the virus are delayed by about 3 weeks, weakening early viral control and allowing excessive innate immune activation. Th17 cells, a type of CD4+ T cell that produces IL-17, play a significant role in worsening cytokine imbalances and inflammation by recruiting neutrophils and damaging tissue. The antibody response from B cells may also become overactive and contribute to inflammation, though this is less well understood [62].

The excessive activation of both immune responses leads to the hyperinflammation characteristic of severe COVID-19, which occurs due to an imbalance between innate immune overactivation and adaptive immune suppression [61] (Fig. 8.5b). A hyperinflammatory state is characterized by excessive cytokine and chemokine release, including IL-6, TNF-α, IL-1β, MCP-1, and IFN-γ, along with increased CCL2/MCP-1, CXCL10/IP-10, and CXCL8/IL-8, which promote leukocyte infiltration. An initially weak IFN-I response allows high viral replication and accumulation of viral RNA, triggering secondary activation of macrophages, monocytes,

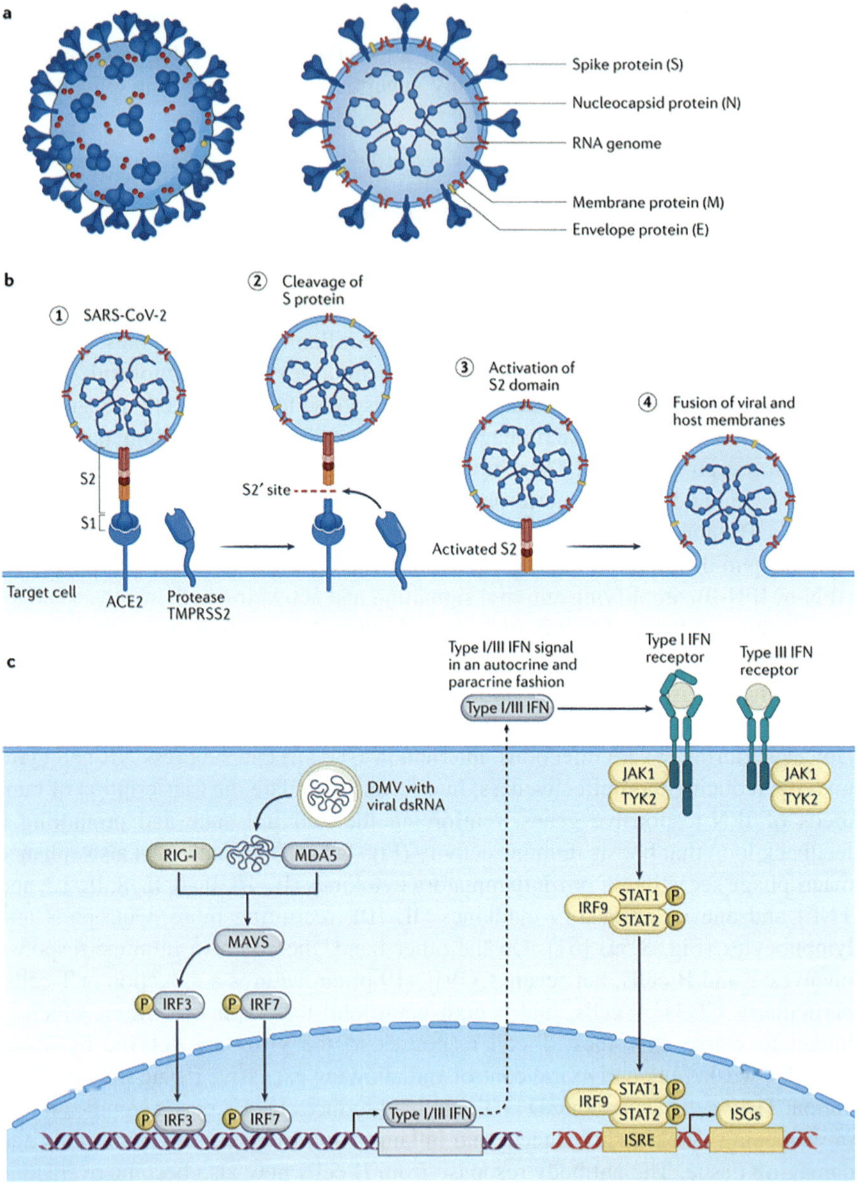

Fig. 8.4 SARS-CoV-2 virions contain structural proteins like spike, nucleocapsid, membrane, and envelope proteins (**a**). The S protein binds the host ACE2 receptor via its S1 domain, is cleaved by TMPRSS2, and activates S2 to fuse viral and host membranes, releasing the viral RNA genome (**b**). Viral replication produces dsRNA intermediates that trigger innate immune sensors (MDA5/RIG-I) and MAVS, inducing type I/III interferons. These IFNs activate the JAK–STAT pathway, leading to interferon-stimulated genes (ISGs) that exert antiviral effects (**c**). (Figure adapted from Lamers et al., "SARS-CoV-2 pathogenesis," Nature Reviews Microbiology, 2022, Springer Nature, with permission from the copyright holder [40])

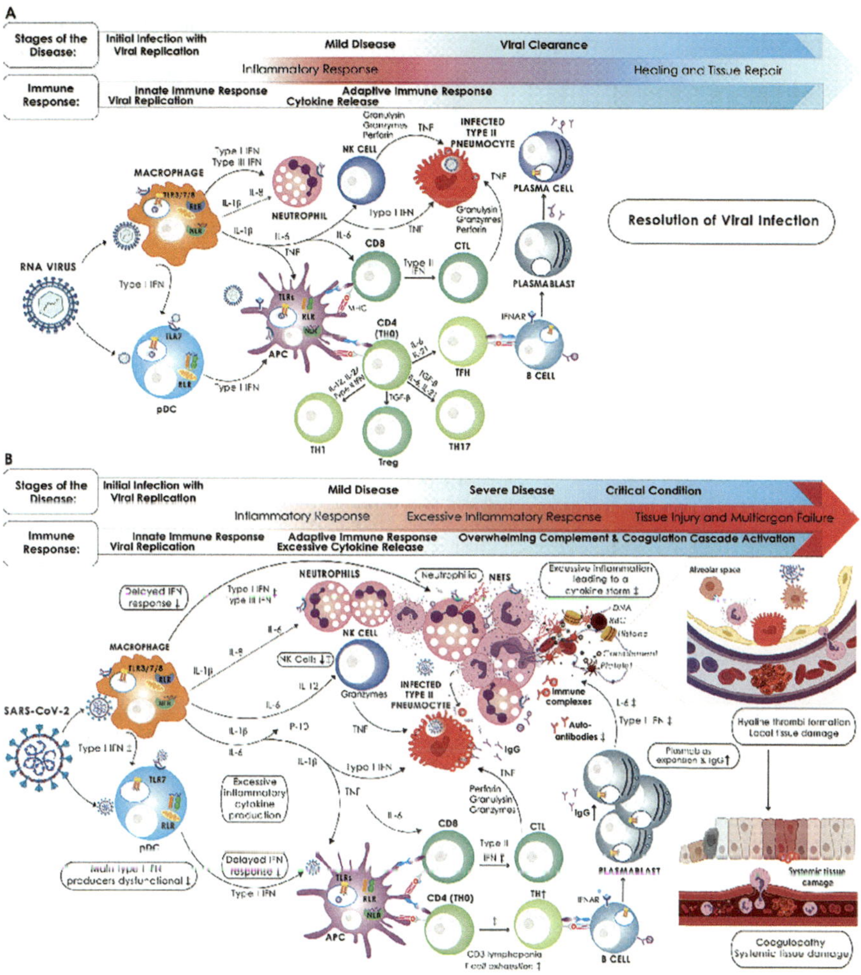

Fig. 8.5 (**a**) Innate and adaptive Immune response to SARS-COV-2. (**b**) Imbalance between the immune response, causing hyperinflammation and tissue damage [61]

and neutrophils [63, 64]. These myeloid cells secrete pro-inflammatory cytokines, driving systemic inflammation and endothelial activation. This cytokine storm is amplified by oxidative stress from reactive oxygen species (ROS), inflammasome activation (NLRP3), NETosis, complement system activation (C3/C5), and damage-associated molecular patterns like HMGB1. Concurrently, viral proteins and host factors such as CASP6, CASP8, and activin A further exacerbate immune and endothelial dysfunction, promoting a prothrombotic state marked by elevated D-dimer, CRP, ferritin, and other markers [65]. Endothelial dysfunction increases vascular permeability, favouring pulmonary oedema and multi-organ involvement. Anti-inflammatory cytokines, mainly IL-10, are also elevated but insufficient to counterbalance the pro-inflammatory state. IL-10 upregulation may additionally suppress

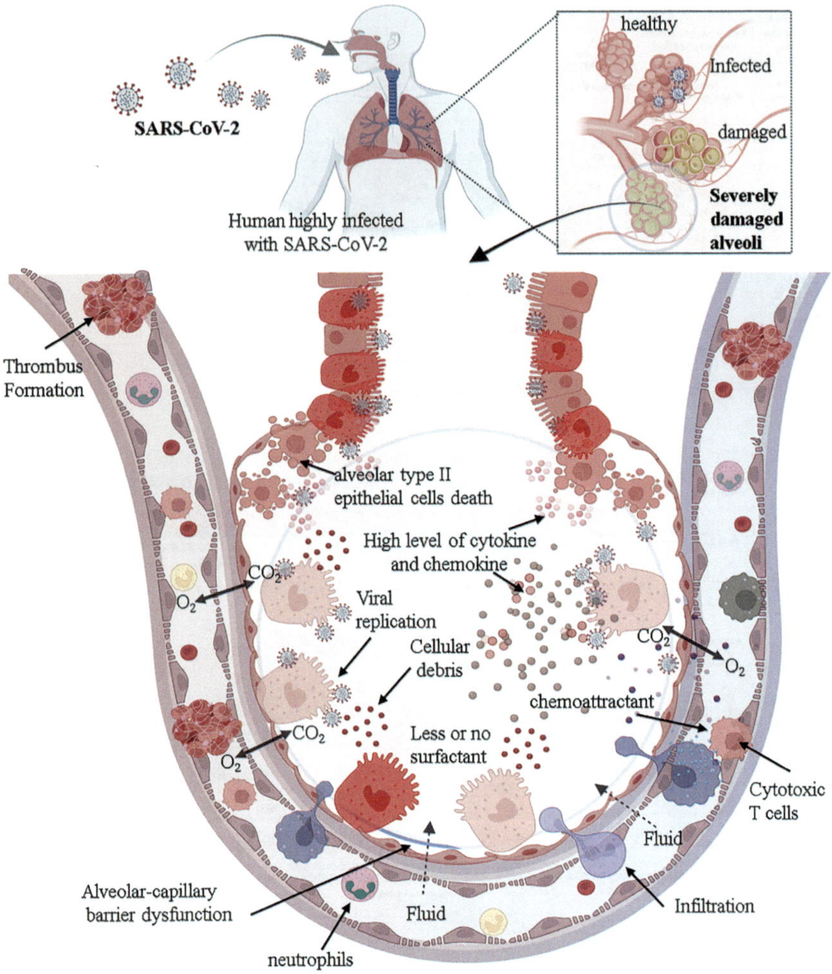

Fig. 8.6 SARS-CoV-2 infects airway epithelial cells and alveolar type 2 (AT2) cells, impairing interferon responses that promote viral spread, leading to alveolar flooding and microvascular thrombosis. Dysfunctional immune cells exacerbate inflammation, coagulation, and endothelial damage. The result is extensive damage to the alveoli, low oxygen levels, and acute respiratory distress syndrome (ARDS)

effective T-cell responses, further impairing viral clearance. Complement activation (C3a, C5a, C5b-9) and coagulation cascade engagement (tissue factor expression, platelet activation) occur in parallel, producing microthrombosis and immunothrombosis. These pathways contribute to acute lung injury and complications such as ARDS, acute renal failure, myocardial infarction, stroke, liver dysfunction, and multiorgan failure, which can be fatal [66].

8.5.6 Pathological Outcomes

SARS-CoV-2 primarily targets the lungs but can also affect multiple organ systems due to the widespread presence of ACE2 and TMPRSS2 receptors. This can lead to complications involving the lungs, kidneys, and liver. After severe COVID-19 infection, common lasting symptoms include fatigue, shortness of breath, cognitive problems, anxiety, depression, loss of smell, and loss of taste [14]. Milder cases often experience fatigue, muscle pain, headache, cough, and mucus production [67]. There is a greater risk of infection in both severe and mild cases (Fig. 8.6).

involving opportunistic pathogens and comorbidities [68–70]. Kidney damage may arise either directly from the virus or because of an overactive immune response, which causes infiltration of macrophages and complement proteins, resulting in tissue fibrosis. This damage impairs the kidney's ability to filter wastes and toxins, potentially causing kidney or liver failure [71]. Cardiovascular impacts include heart damage, myocardial injury, and heart rhythm disturbances that can develop into heart failure. These effects may result directly from viral infection or from an intensified immune reaction, leading to complications such as arrhythmias, deep vein thrombosis, pulmonary embolism, and decreased lung capacity. Individuals with existing heart conditions are prone to experience more severe symptoms [72].

Metabolic issues also occur, as the virus can cause insulin resistance, abnormal lipid levels, systemic inflammation, and hyperglycaemia through pancreas and liver dysfunction, which may contribute to new cases of diabetes [72]. Pulmonary complications are frequent and include fibrosis, respiratory failure, pulmonary embolisms, and bacterial pneumonia, caused either by viral damage or immune system reactions [73]. The gastrointestinal tract can be affected by damage to the gut lining, which triggers innate immune responses, impairing nutrient absorption and increasing intestinal permeability. Blood-related problems are common, such as low platelet counts, thrombosis, disseminated intravascular coagulation (DIC), and platelet dysfunction [74]. These may stem from antibody cross-reactivity or direct infection of platelet precursor cells in the bone marrow [75]. Neurologically, the virus may infect central nervous system cells, cross the blood-brain barrier, or damage nerves and sensory receptors, resulting in symptoms like cognitive impairment, encephalopathy, confusion, dizziness, and memory disturbances [76].

8.6 Conclusion

SARS-CoV-2 mainly affects the respiratory system via ACE2 receptors, causing inflammation, immunological dysregulation, and possible organ damage. Viral rep lication, immune evasion, and cytokine storms are the main factor which contributes to its pathogenic behaviour, and they can cause serious respiratory distress as well as systemic consequences. The long-term effects of COVID-19 must be monitored for any significant consequences in the future, and research must be made available to mitigate its impact on human health.

References

1. Kumar V, Doshi KU, Khan WH, Rathore AS. COVID-19 pandemic: mechanism, diagnosis, and treatment. J Chem Technol Biotechnol. 2021;96(2):299–308.
2. Naseer S, Khalid S, Parveen S, Abbass K, Song H, Achim MV. COVID-19 outbreak: impact on global economy. Front Public Health. 2022;10:1009393.
3. Laue M, Kauter A, Hoffmann T, Möller L, Michel J, Nitsche A. Morphometry of SARS-CoV and SARS-CoV-2 particles in ultrathin plastic sections of infected Vero cell cultures. Sci Rep. 2021;11(1):3515.
4. Hoffmann T, Michel J, Nitsche A, Mache C, Schulze J, Wolff T, et al. Electron microscopy images and morphometric data of SARS-CoV-2 variants in ultrathin plastic sections. Sci Data. 2024;11(1):1322.
5. Sun J, Liu M, Yang N. Insight into the origin of SARS-CoV-2 through structural analysis of receptor recognition: a molecular simulation study. RSC Adv. 2021;11(15):8718–29.
6. Li X, Yuan H, Li X, Wang H. Spike protein mediated membrane fusion during SARS-CoV-2 infection. J Med Virol. 2023;95(1):e28212.
7. Caldas LA, Carneiro FA, Higa LM, Monteiro FL, da Silva GP, da Costa LJ, et al. Ultrastructural analysis of SARS-CoV-2 interactions with the host cell via high resolution scanning electron microscopy. Sci Rep. 2020;10(1):16099.
8. Calder LJ, Calcraft T, Hussain S, Harvey R, Rosenthal PB. Electron cryotomography of SARS-CoV-2 virions reveals cylinder-shaped particles with a double layer RNP assembly. Commun Biol. 2022;5(1):1210.
9. Nejat R, Torshizi MF, Najafi DJ. S Protein, ACE2 and host cell proteases in SARS-CoV-2 cell entry and infectivity; is soluble ACE2 a two blade sword? A narrative review. Vaccines. 2023;11(2):204.
10. Peng R, Wu LA, Wang Q, Qi J, Gao GF. Cell entry by SARS-CoV-2. Trends Biochem Sci. 2021;46(10):848–60.
11. Zang R, Gomez Castro MF, McCune BT, Zeng Q, Rothlauf PW, Sonnek NM, et al. TMPRSS2 and TMPRSS4 promote SARS-CoV-2 infection of human small intestinal enterocytes. Sci Immunol. 2020;5(47):eabc3582.
12. Barth RF, Buja LM, Parwani AV. The spectrum of pathological findings in coronavirus disease (COVID-19) and the pathogenesis of SARS-CoV-2. Diagn Pathol. 2020;15(1):85.
13. Eckermann M, Frohn J, Reichardt M, Osterhoff M, Sprung M, Westermeier F, et al. 3D virtual pathohistology of lung tissue from Covid-19 patients based on phase contrast X-ray tomography. Elife. 2020;9:e60408.
14. Azhar A, Wali MA, Rashid Q, Khan WH, Al-Hosaini K, Owais M, et al. Crosstalk between SARS-CoV-2 infection and neurological disorders: a review. CNS Neurol Disord Drug Targets. 2023;22(5):643–58.
15. Nazir M, Mir IR, Lone SA, Muteeb G, Alam R, Fomda AB, et al. Innate immunity, therapeutic targets and monoclonal antibodies in SARS-CoV-2 infection. PeerJ. 2025;13:e19462.
16. Khan WH, Hashmi Z, Goel A, Ahmad R, Gupta K, Khan N, et al. COVID-19 pandemic and vaccines update on challenges and resolutions. Front Cell Infect Microbiol. 2021;11:690621.
17. Khan WH, Khan N, Mishra A, Gupta S, Bansode V, Mehta D, et al. Dimerization of SARS-CoV-2 nucleocapsid protein affects sensitivity of ELISA based diagnostics of COVID-19. Int J Biol Macromol. 2022;200:428–37.
18. Zeyaullah M, Khan N, Muzammil K, AlShahrani AM, Khan MS, Alam MS, et al. In-silico approaches for identification of compounds inhibiting SARS-CoV-2 3CL protease. PLoS One. 2023;18(4):e0284301.
19. Sharma S, Yakkala PA, Aboti J, Latief I, Ansari MA, Khan WH, et al. Design and synthesis of Michael acceptor-based peptidyl β-nitrostyrenes as 3CLpro inhibitors of SARS-CoV-2. ChemistrySelect. 2023;8(24):e202300912.

20. Chenna A, Khan WH, Dash R, Saraswat S, Chugh A, Rathore AS, et al. An efficient computational protocol for template-based design of peptides that inhibit interactions involving SARS-CoV-2 proteins. Proteins. 2023;91(9):1222–34.
21. Mishra A, Khan WH, Rathore AS. Synergistic effects of natural compounds toward inhibition of SARS-CoV-2 3CL protease. J Chem Inf Model. 2021;61(11):5708–18.
22. Zeyaullah M, AlShahrani AM, Muzammil K, Ahmad I, Alam S, Khan WH, et al. COVID-19 and SARS-CoV-2 variants: current challenges and health concern. Front Genet. 2021;12:693916.
23. Corbett KS, Edwards DK, Leist SR, Abiona OM, Boyoglu-Barnum S, Gillespie RA, et al. SARS-CoV-2 mRNA vaccine design enabled by prototype pathogen preparedness. Nature. 2020;586(7830):567–71.
24. Bhatt PR, Scaiola A, Loughran G, Leibundgut M, Kratzel A, Meurs R, et al. Structural basis of ribosomal frameshifting during translation of the SARS-CoV-2 RNA genome. Science (NY). 2021;372(6548):1306–13.
25. Grobben M, van der Straten K, Brouwer PJM, Brinkkemper M, Maisonnasse P, Dereuddre-Bosquet N, et al. Cross-reactive antibodies after SARS-CoV-2 infection and vaccination. Elife. 2021;10:e70330.
26. Mukherjee S, Tworowski D, Detroja R, Mukherjee SB, Frenkel-Morgenstern M. Immunoinformatics and structural analysis for identification of immunodominant epitopes in SARS-CoV-2 as potential vaccine targets. Vaccine. 2020;8(2):290.
27. Brahim Belhaouari D, Fontanini A, Baudoin JP, Haddad G, Le Bideau M, Bou Khalil JY, et al. The strengths of scanning electron microscopy in deciphering SARS-CoV-2 infectious cycle. Front Microbiol. 2020;11:2014.
28. Klein S, Cortese M, Winter SL, Wachsmuth-Melm M, Neufeldt CJ, Cerikan B, et al. SARS-CoV-2 structure and replication characterized by in situ cryo-electron tomography. Nat Commun. 2020;11(1):5885.
29. Raut P, Waters H, Zimmberberg J, Obeng B, Gosse J, Hess ST. Localization-based super-resolution microscopy reveals relationship between SARS-CoV2 spike and phosphatidylinositol (4,5)-bisphosphate. Proc SPIE Int Soc Opt Eng. 2022;11965:1196503.
30. Robb NC. Virus morphology: insights from super-resolution fluorescence microscopy. Biochim Biophys Acta Mol basis Dis. 2022;1868(4):166347.
31. Ray A, Simpson JD, Demir I, Gisbert VG, Gomes DB, Amadei F, et al. From viral assembly to host interaction: AFM's contributions to virology. J Virol. 2025;99(1):e0087324.
32. Parasher A. COVID-19: current understanding of its pathophysiology, clinical presentation and treatment. Postgrad Med J. 2021;97(1147):312–20.
33. Pizuorno A, Brim H, Ashktorab H. Gastrointestinal manifestations and SARS-CoV-2 infection. Curr Opin Pharmacol. 2021;61:114–9.
34. Xu X, Yu C, Qu J, Zhang L, Jiang S, Huang D, et al. Imaging and clinical features of patients with 2019 novel coronavirus SARS-CoV-2. Eur J Nucl Med Mol Imaging. 2020;47(5):1275–80.
35. Ocampo FF, Holroyd KB. Updates on the neurological manifestations of SARS-CoV-2 infection. Curr Opin Infect Dis. 2025;38(3):234–41.
36. Gisondi P, PIaserico S, Bordin C, Alaibac M, Girolomoni G, Naldi L. Cutaneous manifestations of SARS-CoV-2 infection: a clinical update. J Eur Acad Dermatol Venereol. 2020;34(11):2499–504.
37. Huynh T, Sanchez-Flores X, Yau J, Huang JT. Cutaneous manifestations of SARS-CoV-2 infection. Am J Clin Dermatol. 2022;23(3):277–86.
38. Afewerky HK. Pathology and pathogenicity of severe acute respiratory syndrome coronavirus 2 (SARS-CoV-2). Exp Biol Med (Maywood). 2020;245(15):1299–307.
39. Carvajal JJ, García-Castillo V, Cuellar SV, Campillay-Véliz CP, Salazar-Ardiles C, Avellaneda AM, et al. New insights into the pathogenesis of SARS-CoV-2 during and after the COVID-19 pandemic. Front Immunol. 2024;15:1363572.
40. Lamers MM, Haagmans BL. SARS-CoV-2 pathogenesis. Nat Rev Microbiol. 2022;20(5):270–84.

41. Sharma HN, Latimore COD, Matthews QL. Biology and pathogenesis of SARS-CoV-2: understandings for therapeutic developments against COVID-19. Pathogens. 2021;10(9):1218.
42. Pouremamali A, Babaei A, Malekshahi SS, Abbasi A, Rafiee N. Understanding the pivotal roles of ACE2 in SARS-CoV-2 infection: from structure/function to therapeutic implication. Egypt J Med Hum Genet. 2022;23(1):103.
43. Gusev E, Sarapultsev A, Solomatina L, Chereshnev V. SARS-CoV-2-specific immune response and the pathogenesis of COVID-19. Int J Mol Sci. 2022;23(3):1716.
44. Kyrou I, Randeva HS, Spandidos DA, Karteris E. Not only ACE2-the quest for additional host cell mediators of SARS-CoV-2 infection: Neuropilin-1 (NRP1) as a novel SARS-CoV-2 host cell entry mediator implicated in COVID-19. Signal Transduct Target Ther. 2021;6(1):21.
45. Wang K, Chen W, Zhang Z, Deng Y, Lian JQ, Du P, et al. CD147-spike protein is a novel route for SARS-CoV-2 infection to host cells. Signal Transduct Target Ther. 2020;5(1):283.
46. Carlos AJ, Ha DP, Yeh DW, Van Krieken R, Tseng CC, Zhang P, et al. The chaperone GRP78 is a host auxiliary factor for SARS-CoV-2 and GRP78 depleting antibody blocks viral entry and infection. J Biol Chem. 2021;296:100759.
47. Gadanec LK, McSweeney KR, Qaradakhi T, Ali B, Zulli A, Apostolopoulos V. Can SARS-CoV-2 virus use multiple receptors to enter host cells? Int J Mol Sci. 2021;22(3):992.
48. Behboudi E, Nooreddin Faraji S, Daryabor G, Mohammad Ali Hashemi S, Asadi M, Edalat F, et al. SARS-CoV-2 mechanisms of cell tropism in various organs considering host factors. Heliyon. 2024;10(4):e26577.
49. Bestle D, Heindl MR, Limburg H, Van Lam van T, Pilgram O, Moulton H, et al. TMPRSS2 and furin are both essential for proteolytic activation of SARS-CoV-2 in human airway cells. Life Sci Alliance. 2020;3(9):e202000786.
50. Cheng YW, Chao TL, Li CL, Chiu MF, Kao HC, Wang SH, et al. Furin inhibitors block SARS-CoV-2 spike protein cleavage to suppress virus production and cytopathic effects. Cell Rep. 2020;33(2):108254.
51. Morici N, Bottiroli M, Fumagalli R, Marini C, Cattaneo M. Role of von Willebrand factor and ADAMTS-13 in the pathogenesis of thrombi in SARS-CoV-2 infection: time to rethink. Thromb Haemost. 2020;120(9):1339–42.
52. Zhao MM, Yang WL, Yang FY, Zhang L, Huang WJ, Hou W, et al. Cathepsin L plays a key role in SARS-CoV-2 infection in humans and humanized mice and is a promising target for new drug development. Signal Transduct Target Ther. 2021;6(1):134.
53. Knyazev E, Nersisyan S, Tonevitsky A. Endocytosis and transcytosis of SARS-CoV-2 across the intestinal epithelium and other tissue barriers. Front Immunol. 2021;12:636966.
54. Seyedpour S, Khodaei B, Loghman AH, Seyedpour N, Kisomi MF, Balibegloo M, et al. Targeted therapy strategies against SARS-CoV-2 cell entry mechanisms: a systematic review of in vitro and in vivo studies. J Cell Physiol. 2021;236(4):2364–92.
55. Wu HY, Brian DA. Subgenomic messenger RNA amplification in coronaviruses. Proc Natl Acad Sci USA. 2010;107(27):12257–62.
56. Siu YL, Teoh KT, Lo J, Chan CM, Kien F, Escriou N, et al. The M, E, and N structural proteins of the severe acute respiratory syndrome coronavirus are required for efficient assembly, trafficking, and release of virus-like particles. J Virol. 2008;82(22):11318–30.
57. Harrison AG, Lin T, Wang P. Mechanisms of SARS-CoV-2 transmission and pathogenesis. Trends Immunol. 2020;41(12):1100–15.
58. Boson B, Legros V, Zhou B, Siret E, Mathieu C, Cosset FL, et al. The SARS-CoV-2 envelope and membrane proteins modulate maturation and retention of the spike protein, allowing assembly of virus-like particles. J Biol Chem. 2021;296:100111.
59. Gramberg T, Hofmann H, Möller P, Lalor PF, Marzi A, Geier M, et al. LSECtin interacts with filovirus glycoproteins and the spike protein of SARS coronavirus. Virology. 2005;340(2):224–36.
60. Boechat JL, Chora I, Morais A, Delgado L. The immune response to SARS-CoV-2 and COVID-19 immunopathology – current perspectives. Pulmonology. 2021;27(5):423–37.

61. Chau AS, Weber AG, Maria NI, Narain S, Liu A, Hajizadeh N, et al. The longitudinal immune response to coronavirus disease 2019: chasing the cytokine storm. Arthritis Rheumatol. 2021;73(1):23–35.
62. Primorac D, Vrdoljak K, Brlek P, Pavelić E, Molnar V, Matišić V, et al. Adaptive immune responses and immunity to SARS-CoV-2. Front Immunol. 2022;13:848582.
63. Blanco-Melo D, Nilsson-Payant BE, Liu WC, Uhl S, Hoagland D, Møller R, et al. Imbalanced host response to SARS-CoV-2 drives development of COVID-19. Cell. 2020;181(5):1036–45.e9.
64. Shah VK, Firmal P, Alam A, Ganguly D, Chattopadhyay S. Overview of immune response during SARS-CoV-2 infection: lessons from the past. Front Immunol. 2020;11:1949.
65. Silva MJA, Ribeiro LR, Gouveia MIM, Marcelino BDR, Santos CSD, Lima KVB, et al. Hyperinflammatory response in COVID-19: a systematic review. Viruses. 2023;15(2):553.
66. Wong CK, Lam CW, Wu AK, Ip WK, Lee NL, Chan IH, et al. Plasma inflammatory cytokines and chemokines in severe acute respiratory syndrome. Clin Exp Immunol. 2004;136(1):95–103.
67. Xu Z, Shi L, Wang Y, Zhang J, Huang L, Zhang C, et al. Pathological findings of COVID-19 associated with acute respiratory distress syndrome. Lancet Respir Med. 2020;8(4):420–2.
68. Azhar A, Khan WH, Khan PA, Alhosaini K, Owais M, Ahmad A. Mucormycosis and COVID-19 pandemic: clinical and diagnostic approach. J Infect Public Health. 2022;15(4):466–79.
69. Azhar A, Khan WH, Al-Hosaini K, Zia Q, Kamal MA. Crosstalk between SARS-CoV-2 infection and type II diabetes. Comb Chem High Throughput Screen. 2022;25(14):2429–42.
70. Khan WH, Ahmad R, Alam R, Khan N, Rather IA, Wani MY, et al. Role of ribosomal pathways and comorbidity in COVID-19: insight from SARS-CoV-2 proteins and host proteins interaction network analysis. Heliyon. 2024;10(9):e29967.
71. Kunutsor SK, Laukkanen JA. Renal complications in COVID-19: a systematic review and meta-analysis. Ann Med. 2020;52(7):345–53.
72. Ashraf O, Young M, Malik KJ, Cheema T. Systemic complications of COVID-19. Crit Care Nurs Q. 2020;43(4):390–9.
73. Lechowicz K, Drożdżal S, Machaj F, Rosik J, Szostak B, Zegan-Barańska M, et al. COVID-19: the potential treatment of pulmonary fibrosis associated with SARS-CoV-2 infection. J Clin Med. 2020;9(6):1917.
74. Carvalho A, Alqusairi R, Adams A, Paul M, Kothari N, Peters S, et al. SARS-CoV-2 gastrointestinal infection causing hemorrhagic colitis: implications for detection and transmission of COVID-19 disease. Am J Gastroenterol. 2020;115(6):942–6.
75. Rocke J, Hopkins C, Philpott C, Kumar N. Is loss of sense of smell a diagnostic marker in COVID-19: a systematic review and meta-analysis. Clin Otolaryngol. 2020;45(6):914–22.
76. Toscano G, Palmerini F, Ravaglia S, Ruiz L, Invernizzi P, Cuzzoni MG, et al. Guillain-Barré syndrome associated with SARS CoV 2. N Engl J Med. 2020;382(26):2574–6.

Immune Responses to Severe Acute Respiratory Syndrome Coronavirus-2

9

Himanshu Kaushal and Priyasi Mittal

Abbreviations

ACE2	Angiotensin-Converting Enzyme 2
ARDS	Acute Respiratory Distress Syndrome
COVID-19	Coronavirus Disease 2019
CTL	Cytotoxic T Lymphocyte
GM-CSF	Granulocyte–Macrophage Colony-Stimulating Factor
IFN	Interferon
ISG	Interferon-Stimulated Gene
mAb	Monoclonal Antibody
NET	Neutrophil Extracellular Trap
NK cell	Natural Killer Cell
PRR	Pattern Recognition Receptor
RBD	Receptor Binding Domain
SARS-CoV-2	Severe Acute Respiratory Syndrome Coronavirus-2
Tfh	T Follicular Helper Cell
TLR	Toll-Like Receptor

H. Kaushal (✉)
ICMR-National Institute of Virology, Pune, Maharashtra, India

Academy of Scientific and Innovative Research (AcSIR), Ghaziabad, India

P. Mittal
ICMR-National Institute of Virology, Pune, India

S. R. Prabhu et al. (eds.), *COVID-19 in Dental Practice*,
https://doi.org/10.1007/978-3-032-26000-0_9

9.1 Introduction

The emergence of Severe Acute Respiratory Syndrome Coronavirus 2 (SARS-CoV-2) in late 2019 led to the global COVID-19 pandemic, resulting in unprecedented levels of morbidity, mortality, and socioeconomic disruption. Within months, the virus had spread worldwide, prompting rapid scientific and public health responses. SARS-CoV-2 is an enveloped, positive-sense RNA virus belonging to the β-coronavirus genus. It primarily infects respiratory epithelial cells by binding to the angiotensin-converting enzyme 2 (ACE2) receptor via its spike (S) protein, a process facilitated by TMPRSS2-mediated priming [1, 2].

The host immune response is central to shaping the clinical spectrum of COVID-19, which varies from asymptomatic infection to severe respiratory failure and multi-organ dysfunction. A well-coordinated innate and adaptive immune response is vital for early viral control and recovery, while dysregulated or excessive immune activation can lead to severe disease features such as the cytokine storm and immunothrombosis [3, 4]. Understanding the dual nature of immunity—both protective and pathogenic—is key to decoding COVID-19 pathogenesis. Interferon-mediated antiviral responses and neutralising antibodies assist in clearing the virus. Conversely, hyper-inflammatory cascades and immune exhaustion may worsen tissue damage [5, 6]. This chapter offers an overview of the immune responses in SARS-CoV-2 infection, covering the body's innate and adaptive defences, harmful immune reactions, immune memory, host factors, and the ways the virus evades detection.

9.2 Innate Immune Responses to SARS-CoV-2

The innate immune system serves as the body's first defence against SARS-CoV-2 infection and significantly influences subsequent adaptive immune responses. Recognition of the virus by the host immune system begins when pathogen-associated molecular patterns (PAMPs) within the viral genome are identified by pattern recognition receptors (PRRs). Toll-like receptors (TLR3 and TLR7), NOD-like receptors (NLRs), and RIG-I-like receptors (RIG-I and MDA5) act as sensors for virus detection [7–9]. When stimulated, these receptors trigger intracellular signalling pathways that activate transcription factors such as IRF3, IRF7, and NF-κb. These regulators promote the production of type I and type III interferons (IFNs) along with pro-inflammatory cytokines, including IL-6, IL-1β, and TNF-α [10, 11].

The IFNs stimulate interferon-stimulated genes (ISGs) that limit viral replication and enhance antigen presentation, forming a vital part of the host's antiviral defence. However, SARS-CoV-2 has developed multiple strategies to evade these protective mechanisms. Viral non-structural proteins such as NSP1 and NSP13 inhibit interferon activation through different methods—NSP1 blocks host mRNA translation, while NSP13 interferes with TBK1 and IRF3 activation, thereby decreasing interferon signalling [12]. Additionally, ORF6 prevents the nuclear import of immune transcription factors, further reducing antiviral responses [13]. Importantly, nearly half of the 30 proteins of SARS-CoV-2 have been reported to target components of the interferon system, demonstrating the virus's extensive immune evasion strategies [14]. As a result, a delayed or weakened interferon response—often seen in severe COVID-19—leads to unchecked viral replication and heightened inflammatory reactions [7, 15].

Alongside interferon responses, various innate immune cells, including macrophages, monocytes, dendritic cells, neutrophils, and NK cells, support early antiviral defence. In mild COVID-19 infections, coordinated activation of these cells facilitates viral clearance and primes adaptive immunity. Conversely, prolonged activation of macrophages and neutrophils can lead to excessive cytokine release—commonly called the cytokine storm—marked by elevated levels of IL-6, IL-1β, TNF-α, IL-8, and IL-10 [11, 16, 17]. This hyperinflammatory state contributes to acute respiratory distress syndrome (ARDS), vascular injury, and multi-organ dysfunction [18]. Therefore, the innate immune response to SARS-CoV-2 is a double-edged sword—crucial for initial pathogen control but potentially harmful when dysregulated. Understanding these mechanisms offers key insights for developing targeted immunomodulatory therapies to restore immune balance and prevent severe COVID-19 outcomes.

9.3 Adaptive Immune Responses to SARS-CoV-2

The adaptive immune system offers pathogen-specific and long-lasting protection against SARS-CoV-2 through a carefully coordinated interaction of T- and B-cell responses. After viral infection, antigen-presenting cells such as dendritic cells process and display viral peptides via MHC molecules, activating both $CD4^+$ helper and $CD8^+$ T lymphocytes that help clear the virus and create immunological memory [19].

$CD4^+$ T cells differentiate into functional subsets—Th1, Th2, Th17, and T follicular helper (Tfh) cells—each contributing differently to the host response. Among these, Th1 and Tfh subsets are the most prominent in effective SARS-CoV-2 immunity, producing IFN-γ and IL-21 to enhance macrophage activation and drive B-cell antibody production [7, 19]. In contrast, dysregulated Th17 responses and excessive cytokine production can amplify inflammation, contributing to immunopathology in severe disease [16, 20, 21].

$CD8^+$ cytotoxic T lymphocytes (CTLs) play a crucial antiviral role by recognizing and eliminating infected cells through perforin- and granzyme-mediated cytotoxicity. SARS-CoV-2-specific $CD8^+$ T cells arise early in infection and are associated with milder disease and faster recovery [19]. However, chronic antigen exposure during severe infection may induce T-cell exhaustion, characterized by upregulation of inhibitory receptors such as PD-1 and TIM-3, resulting in diminished effector function [22]. Single-cell transcriptomic analyses further reveal dynamic remodelling of T-cell repertoires and peripheral lymphocyte populations in COVID-19, reflecting both protective and maladaptive immune reprogramming [23].

B cells form the humoral component of adaptive immunity, producing antibodies that target viral antigens—mainly the S and nucleocapsid (N) proteins. When activated, naïve B cells differentiate into plasma cells that produce virus-specific antibodies. Neutralising antibodies that target the receptor-binding domain (RBD) of the S protein prevent viral entry by blocking ACE2 binding, thus stopping infection [24, 25]. The antibody response follows a typical pattern, with an initial IgM response shifting to high-affinity IgG and secretory IgA, which are essential for mucosal protection at respiratory surfaces [26].

Studies show that nearly all individuals recovering from SARS-CoV-2 infection develop virus-specific antibodies, while about 90% generate measurable $CD8^+$ T-cell responses [27]. The spike protein acts as the primary immunogen for both neutralising antibodies and cytotoxic T-cell responses, forming the basis for current vaccine design [27, 28]. Notably, disease severity relates more to the quality rather than the magnitude of adaptive responses—mild cases display coordinated T- and B-cell immunity, whereas severe cases show dysregulated or exhausted lymphocyte responses [6, 29]. Although neutralising antibody titres naturally decline within months of infection, memory B cells and long-lived T cells remain and can quickly reactivate upon re-exposure, providing lasting protection against reinfection [28, 30]. Overall, an effective adaptive immune response—characterised by balanced and sustained T- and B-cell activity—is essential for viral clearance, recovery, and long-term immunity, while its dysregulation contributes to severe disease and poor outcomes.

9.4 Immunopathology of Severe COVID-19

Severe cases of COVID-19 are characterised not only by uncontrolled viral replication but, more critically, by an exaggerated and dysregulated host immune response that causes widespread inflammation, vascular injury, and multi-organ failure [16, 31]. This immunopathology results from an imbalance between antiviral defence and hyperinflammatory signalling, involving cytokine storms, lymphocyte exhaustion, and immune–coagulative interactions that lead to ARDS and systemic organ failure [32, 33].

A hallmark of severe COVID-19 is the cytokine storm, characterised by the uncontrolled release of pro-inflammatory cytokines such as IL-6, TNF-α, IL-1β, and IL-8. These mediators—mainly produced by activated macrophages, monocytes, and T cells—amplify systemic inflammation, endothelial permeability, and pulmonary oedema, leading to diffuse alveolar damage and hypoxaemia [7, 34]. Elevated serum IL-6 levels strongly correlate with disease severity and an unfavourable prognosis, offering a rationale for therapeutic targeting of IL-6 signalling [11].

Severe disease is also marked by innate immune dysregulation, including delayed interferon responses, lymphopenia, and neutrophilia [32, 35]. SARS-CoV-2 infection of pneumocytes and endothelial cells causes cell death through pyroptosis and apoptosis, releasing damage-associated molecular patterns (DAMPs) that further enhance inflammation [34]. Persistent antigenic stimulation results in T-cell exhaustion, with decreased cytotoxic function and impaired viral clearance, while prolonged activation of myeloid cells drives cytokine overproduction [36].

Additionally, the formation of neutrophil extracellular traps (NETs), which are DNA-protein web-like structures produced by activated neutrophils, contributes to pathogen capture and local immune defence. However, excessive NET formation promotes endothelial injury, platelet aggregation, and microvascular thrombosis [37]. These processes link innate immune activation to coagulation abnormalities. This interaction between inflammation and coagulation leads to immunothrombosis, a hallmark of severe and fatal COVID-19 [38]. The complement system, activated platelets, and tissue factor expression initiate fibrin deposition and microthrombi formation in pulmonary capillaries, causing vascular occlusion and impaired gas exchange [37]. Overall, these events—cytokine storm, NET-mediated vascular injury, and immunothrombosis—indicate a shift from a protective immune response to a harmful, self-perpetuating inflammatory state. This maladaptive immunity causes more tissue damage than the viral cytopathic effect itself [32].

9.5 Immune Memory and Long-Term Immunity

Following acute SARS-CoV-2 infection, the development of long-lasting immune memory is vital for ongoing protection and reduced disease severity upon re-infection. Long-term immunity results from the coordinated persistence of memory B cells, long-lived plasma cells, and memory T cells, which together enable rapid and strong recall responses during reinfection [28]. Memory B cells help sustain humoral immunity even as circulating antibody levels gradually decrease. These cells continue to undergo affinity maturation within germinal centres, producing antibodies with improved neutralisation against variants [30, 39]. Serum antibody levels generally decline 6–12 months after SARS-CoV-2 infection; however, memory B cells can rapidly expand upon re-exposure, producing high-affinity antibodies that bolster protection against the virus [28]. Notably, studies show that SARS-CoV-2–specific antibody responses decline over time, with long-lived plasma cells responsible for an extended antibody half-life exceeding 200 days [40, 41].

Memory T cells, including both $CD4^+$ helper and $CD8^+$ cytotoxic subsets, are equally vital for long-term immunity. These cells persist for months or even years after infection and show cross-reactivity with epitopes from other seasonal coronaviruses, indicating a role in broad antiviral defence [42, 43]. $CD4^+$ T helper cells provide crucial support to B cells for secondary antibody responses, while $CD8^+$ T cells directly recognise and eliminate infected cells via conserved epitopes that are less susceptible to mutational escape [19]. The maintenance of these polyfunctional memory T cells ensures a sustained ability for rapid antiviral responses even when antibody levels decline.

Recovered individuals consistently exhibit a coordinated memory response involving both humoral and cellular components—a hallmark of lasting immunity.

Moreover, hybrid immunity, which results from natural infection followed by vaccination, produces the most potent and broadest immune protection, enhancing antibody diversity and T cell cross-reactivity against multiple SARS-CoV-2 variants [39, 44]. SARS-CoV-2 immunity maintains detectable immune memory for at least 8 months after infection [40, 41]. These findings collectively confirm that SARS-CoV-2 infection creates a strong and enduring immune memory involving various cellular compartments. This long-term immunity—especially when boosted by vaccination—provides hope for sustained protection against reinfection and cross-protection against ongoing viral evolution.

9.6 Immune Evasion Strategies of SARS-CoV-2

SARS-CoV-2 has developed a range of sophisticated mechanisms to evade host immune surveillance, ensuring efficient replication, prolonged persistence, and increased transmissibility. These immune evasion strategies target both innate and adaptive immune pathways, resulting in delayed viral clearance and, in some cases, excessive immune activation and pathology [11, 45].

One of the main immune evasion strategies of SARS-CoV-2 involves the suppression of the IFN response, which is vital for early antiviral defence. The virus encodes several non-structural and accessory proteins—such as NSP1, NSP6, NSP8, NSP12–15, ORF3a, ORF6, ORF9b, and ORF10—that interfere with different stages of type I and type III IFN signalling [15, 45–48]. NSP1 inhibits host mRNA translation by binding to the 40S ribosomal subunit, thus globally reducing protein synthesis, including that of ISGs [45]. Likewise, ORF6 prevents nuclear translocation of STAT1 and STAT2, effectively blocking IFN-mediated transcriptional activation [15, 49]. Other viral proteins, including NSP13 and NSP14, impair RNA sensing by disrupting the RIG-I and MDA5 pathways, thereby reducing antiviral responses [47]. Overall, this complex suppression of interferon signalling allows SARS-CoV-2 to replicate efficiently before adaptive immunity is triggered.

SARS-CoV-2 also uses direct mechanisms to impair antigen presentation and recognition by CTLS. The N and ORF8 proteins have been shown to downregulate MHC-I expression on infected cells, hindering their detection and destruction by $CD8^+$ T cells [11, 50]. ORF8 facilitates this process by binding to MHC-I molecules and directing them for lysosomal degradation, effectively lowering cell-surface antigen display [51]. This immune evasion strategy enables the virus to persist within host tissues, especially in individuals with weakened immune systems.

Beyond IFN antagonism and antigen presentation blockade, SARS-CoV-2 alters multiple cellular processes to escape immune surveillance. The virus disrupts mitochondrial function via ORF9b and ORF10, which localise to mitochondria and suppress MAVS (mitochondrial antiviral signalling) activity, thereby reducing IFN induction and promoting ROS generation [51]. Furthermore, the virus has been reported to spread through tunnelling nanotubes between cells, enabling direct cell-to-cell transmission while avoiding exposure to neutralising antibodies [49]. In parallel, SARS-CoV-2 modulates innate immune sensors such as NLRs. Overactivation of NLRP3 inflammasome leads to excessive IL-1β and IL-18 production, fuelling cytokine storm development and tissue inflammation [52]. Thus, the virus not only suppresses antiviral signalling but also induces inflammatory dysregulation, contributing to immunopathology.

SARS-CoV-2 evolves under immune pressure within populations. Mutations in the spike glycoprotein—especially in the RBD and N-terminal domain—enable the virus to evade neutralising antibodies from infection or vaccination [39, 44]. Variants like Delta and Omicron possess substitutions (e.g., E484K, N501Y) that decrease antibody-binding affinity and undermine neutralisation. These antigenic changes highlight the virus's capacity to adapt to immune responses and continue to challenge vaccine and therapy development.

9.7 Impact of Host Factors on Immune Responses

Host-related factors, such as age, comorbidities, host genetics, and nutritional status, influence the magnitude, quality, and durability of immune responses to SARS-CoV-2 infection. These variables affect disease severity, susceptibility to infection, and recovery [7, 53]. Understanding them is crucial for predicting clinical outcomes across populations.

Age plays a significant role in COVID-19 severity. Older adults experience immunosenescence, a state of immune ageing characterised by a decline in naïve T-cell populations, impaired antigen presentation, reduced interferon production, and a chronic pro-inflammatory condition often called "inflammaging" [19]. These age-related changes result in delayed viral clearance and also heighten the risk of severe disease and death. Conversely, children and younger adults tend to mount stronger innate immune responses. They exhibit rapid interferon signalling and effectively recognise viruses. They also have lower levels of inflammatory cytokines. These factors may explain why they typically experience milder illness [7]. Besides age-related factors, chronic conditions such as obesity, diabetes, cardiovascular disease, and hypertension make COVID-19 more severe. These conditions promote low-grade inflammation and disrupt cytokine balance. They are characterised by metabolic disturbances and diminished immune cell signalling. Consequently, infections can provoke more intense inflammatory responses [7]. For example, obesity affects macrophage function and diminishes the interferon response, increasing the risk of cytokine storms and respiratory failure.

Furthermore, host genetic variation influences individual immune competence through intricate genetic and epigenetic mechanisms. Zhang et al. (2020) revealed that rare genetic defects in type I interferon pathways account for at least 3.5% of life-threatening COVID-19 cases, involving variants in eight key genes [53]. Made et al. (2022) further confirmed that monogenic risk factors affecting interferon-I signalling have an expected prevalence of 1–5% in young, previously healthy individuals with severe COVID-19 [54]. Srivastava et al. (2022) highlight that HLA gene variations significantly affect susceptibility to infectious diseases by modulating antigen presentation [55]. Additionally, Licciardi et al. (2012) emphasise that epigenetic modifications, such as histone deacetylase activity, can influence immune gene expression, adding another layer of immune system variability. These findings underscore the complex genetic architecture underlying individual immune responses [56].

Gut microbiota and nutritional status are crucial in determining how the immune system responds during COVID-19 infection. Diet and micronutrients are especially important for supporting immune defences against viruses. For example, dietary modifications and micronutrient levels influence immune system performance [57]. Vitamins D and A are essential components of the immune system, and deficiencies in these vitamins diminish antiviral defences [58]. Studies show that diet, gut microbiota, and immune function are intricately linked. Changes in nutrition affect the composition and function of gut microbiota, thereby impacting host immunity. Increasing evidence supports the idea that malnutrition is a significant risk factor for susceptibility to COVID-19 [59].

9.8 Immune Responses in Special Populations

Immune responses to SARS-CoV-2 can vary significantly in children, individuals with weakened immune systems, and those suffering from long COVID [60]. Understanding these differences is crucial for developing more effective prevention and treatment strategies. Children typically experience milder COVID-19 symptoms than adults, likely due to several factors. For instance, they have lower ACE2 levels in their airways, which may hinder the virus's ability to enter and replicate [61]. Their innate immune system is also more active, allowing rapid type I interferon responses that help control the virus early [62]. Additionally, children are more frequently exposed to seasonal coronaviruses, which might offer some cross-protection against SARS-CoV-2 [62]. Research indicates that children under five have fewer myeloid cells [63], and generally, children possess more regulatory T and B cells than adults [64]. These immune characteristics may help reduce the risk of severe inflammation during infection.

Individuals with weakened immune systems—including those undergoing chemotherapy, organ transplantation, or receiving immunosuppressive therapies—demonstrate reduced immune responses to SARS-CoV-2 infection. Such individuals experience longer viral shedding and delayed viral clearance due to impaired interferon signalling, decreased B-cell function, and suboptimal T-cell responses [28].

Long COVID is characterised by prolonged or relapsing symptoms such as fatigue, dyspnoea, cognitive dysfunction, and autonomic disturbances lasting weeks to months after acute COVID-19 infection. Immunologically, this condition is associated with sustained immune activation, inflammatory signalling, and autoreactive antibodies [65]. Impaired IFN responses and persistent viral antigens may perpetuate a chronic inflammatory environment, even in the absence of active viral replication [66]. Recent studies indicate that both adults and children with long COVID display immune exhaustion, altered T-cell phenotypes, and elevated pro-inflammatory cytokines [67]. These findings suggest a persistent immune imbalance that contributes to multi-organ symptoms and delayed recovery.

9.9 Conclusion

The global experience with COVID-19 highlights the vital importance of understanding host immune responses to SARS-CoV-2. Protective immunity depends on a carefully balanced interaction between the innate and adaptive systems; prompt interferon signalling, effective T- and B-cell activation, and immune memory enable viral clearance and long-term protection. Conversely, dysregulated responses—characterised by cytokine storms, immune exhaustion, and immunothrombosis—lead to severe disease and death.

Ongoing research into immune correlates of protection, how viruses evade immunity, and host factors will be crucial for improving vaccines, guiding treatments, and preparing for future coronavirus outbreaks. Specifically, future work should aim to identify specific immunological markers of long-term protection, understand how viruses adapt, and assess host genetic factors that affect disease outcomes. In the end, using these insights will help us better protect global health against current and emerging threats.

References

1. Hoffmann M, Kleine-Weber H, Schroeder S, Krüger N, Herrler T, Erichsen S, et al. SARS-CoV 2 cell entry depends on ACE2 and TMPRSS2 and is blocked by a clinically proven protease inhibitor. Cell. 2020;181(2):271–280.e8.
2. Senapati S, Banerjee P, Bhagavatula S, Kushwaha PP, Kumar S. Contributions of human ACE2 and TMPRSS2 in determining host–pathogen interaction of COVID-19. J Genet. 2021;100:21. Springer.
3. Bonaventura A, Vecchió A, Dagna L, Martinod K, Dixon DL, Van Tassell BW, et al. Endothelial dysfunction and immunothrombosis as key pathogenic mechanisms in COVID-19. Nat Rev Immunol. 2021;21(5):319–29.
4. Hiti L, Markovič T, Lainscak M, Farkaš Lainščak J, Pal E, Mlinarič-Raščan I. The immunopathogenesis of a cytokine storm: the key mechanisms underlying severe COVID-19. Cytokine Growth Factor Rev. 2025;82:1–17.
5. Tan LY, Komarasamy TV, RMT Balasubramaniam V. Hyperinflammatory Immune Response and COVID-19: a double edged sword. Front Immunol. 2021;12:742941. Frontiers Media S.A.
6. Mazzoni A, Salvati L, Maggi L, Annunziato F, Cosmi L. Hallmarks of immune response in COVID-19: exploring dysregulation and exhaustion. Semin Immunol. 2021;55:101508. Academic.
7. Schultze JL, Aschenbrenner AC. COVID-19 and the human innate immune system. Cell. 2021;184:1671–92. Elsevier B.V.
8. Schiuma G, Beltrami S, Bortolotti D, Rizzo S, Rizzo R. Innate immune response in SARS-CoV-2 infection. Microorganisms. 2022;10(3):501.
9. Sievers BL, Cheng MTK, Csiba K, Meng B, Gupta RK. SARS-CoV-2 and innate immunity: the good, the bad, and the "goldilocks". Cell Mol Immunol. 2024;21(2):171–83.

10. Newton AH, Cardani A, Braciale TJ. The host immune response in respiratory virus infection: balancing virus clearance and immunopathology. Semin Immunopathol. 2016;38(4):471–82.
11. Lowery SA, Sariol A, Perlman S. Innate immune and inflammatory responses to SARS-CoV-2: implications for COVID-19. Cell Host Microbe. 2021;29(7):1052–62.
12. Vazquez C, Swanson SE, Negatu SG, Dittmar M, Miller J, Ramage HR, et al. SARS-CoV-2 viral proteins NSP1 and NSP13 inhibit interferon activation through distinct mechanisms. PLoS One. 2021;16:e0253089.
13. Xia H, Cao Z, Xie X, Zhang X, Chen JYC, Wang H, et al. Evasion of type I interferon by SARS-CoV-2. Cell Rep. 2020;33(1):108234.
14. Lee JH, Koepke L, Kirchhoff F, Sparrer KMJ. Interferon antagonists encoded by SARS-CoV-2 at a glance. Med Microbiol Immunol. 2023;212:125–31.
15. Blanco-Melo D, Nilsson-Payant BE, Liu WC, Uhl S, Hoagland D, Møller R, et al. Imbalanced host response to SARS-CoV-2 drives development of COVID-19. Cell. 2020;181(5):1036–1045.e9.
16. Vabret N, Britton GJ, Gruber C, Hegde S, Kim J, Kuksin M, et al. Immunology of COVID-19: current state of the science. Immunity. 2020;52(6):910–41.
17. Han H, Ma Q, Li C, Liu R, Zhao L, Wang W, et al. Profiling serum cytokines in COVID-19 patients reveals IL-6 and IL-10 are disease severity predictors. Emerg Microbes Infect. 2020;9(1):1123–30.
18. Diamond MS, Kanneganti TD. Innate immunity: the first line of defense against SARS-CoV-2. Nat Immunol. 2022;23(2):165–76.
19. Sette A, Crotty S. Adaptive immunity to SARS-CoV-2 and COVID-19. Cell. 2021;184(4):861–80.
20. Pardiño-Vega MA, Herrera-González NE. Loss of regulation of T helper 17 cells: a definitive factor for critical cases of coronavirus disease 2019. Explor Immunol. 2023;3(5):490–9.
21. Kang YW, Lee SC, Jeon SM, Jo EK. Roles of interleukin-17 and th17 responses in covid-19. J Bacteriol Virol. 2021;51(3):89–102.
22. Minervina AA, Pogorelyy MV, Kirk AM, Crawford JC, Allen EK, Chou CH, et al. SARS-CoV-2 antigen exposure history shapes phenotypes and specificity of memory CD8+ T cells. Nat Immunol. 2022;23(5):781–90.
23. Zhang JY, Wang XM, Xing X, Xu Z, Zhang C, Song JW, et al. Single-cell landscape of immunological responses in patients with COVID-19. Nat Immunol. 2020;21(9):1107–18.
24. Yuan M, Liu H, Wu NC, Wilson IA. Recognition of the SARS-CoV-2 receptor binding domain by neutralizing antibodies. Biochem Biophys Res Commun. 2021;538:192–203.
25. Tai W, He L, Zhang X, Pu J, Voronin D, Jiang S, et al. Characterization of the receptor-binding domain (RBD) of 2019 novel coronavirus: implication for development of RBD protein as a viral attachment inhibitor and vaccine. Cell Mol Immunol. 2020;17(6):613–20.
26. Liu X, Wang J, Xu X, Liao G, Chen Y, Hu CH. Patterns of IgG and IgM antibody response in COVID-19 patients. Emerg Microbes Infect. 2020;9:1269–74.
27. Nielsen SCA, Yang F, Jackson KJL, Hoh RA, Röltgen K, Jean GH, et al. Human B cell clonal expansion and convergent antibody responses to SARS-CoV-2. Cell Host Microbe. 2020;28(4):516–525.e5.
28. Sette A, Crotty S. Immunological memory to SARS-CoV-2 infection and COVID-19 vaccines. Immunol Rev. 2022;310:27–46.
29. Qin C, Zhou L, Hu Z, Zhang S, Yang S, Tao Y, et al. Dysregulation of immune response in patients with coronavirus 2019 (COVID-19) in Wuhan, China. Clin Infect Dis. 2020;71(15):762–8.
30. Turner JS, O'Halloran JA, Kalaidina E, Kim W, Schmitz AJ, Zhou JQ, et al. SARS-CoV-2 mRNA vaccines induce persistent human germinal centre responses. Nature. 2021;596(7870):109–13.
31. Lucas C, Wong P, Klein J, Castro TBR, Silva J, Sundaram M, et al. Longitudinal analyses reveal immunological misfiring in severe COVID-19. Nature. 2020;584(7821):463–9.
32. Bordallo B, Bellas M, Cortez AF, Vieira M, Pinheiro M. Severe COVID-19: What have we learned with the immunopathogenesis? Adv Rheumatol. 2020;60(1):50.
33. Cao X. COVID-19: immunopathology and its implications for therapy. Nat Rev Immunol. 2020;20(5):269–70.

34. Li G, Fan Y, Lai Y, Han T, Li Z, Zhou P, et al. Coronavirus infections and immune responses. J Med Virol. 2020;92(4):424–32.
35. Gustine JN, Jones D. Immunopathology of Hyperinflammation in COVID-19. Am J Pathol. 2021;191(1):4–17.
36. Mazzoni A, Salvati L, Maggi L, Capone M, Vanni A, Spinicci M, et al. Impaired immune cell cytotoxicity in severe COVID-19 is IL-6 dependent. J Clin Invest. 2020;130(9):4694–703.
37. O'Donnell JS, Peyvandi F, Martin-Loeches I. Pulmonary immuno-thrombosis in COVID-19 ARDS pathogenesis. Intensive Care Med. 2021;47(8):899–902.
38. Laing AG, Lorenc A, Del Molino Del Barrio I, Das A, Fish M, Monin L, et al. A dynamic COVID-19 immune signature includes associations with poor prognosis. Nat Med. 2020;26(10):1623–35.
39. Wang Z, Muecksch F, Schaefer-Babajew D, Finkin S, Viant C, Gaebler C, et al. Naturally enhanced neutralizing breadth against SARS-CoV-2 one year after infection. Nature. 2021;595(7867):426–31.
40. Cohen KW, Linderman SL, Moodie Z, Czartoski J, Lai L, Mantus G, et al. Longitudinal analysis shows durable and broad immune memory after SARS-CoV-2 infection with persisting antibody responses and memory B and T cells. Cell Reports Med. 2021;2(7):100354.
41. Dan JM, Mateus J, Kato Y, Hastie KM, Yu ED, Faliti CE, et al. Immunological memory to SARS-CoV-2 assessed for up to 8 months after infection. Science. 2021;371(6529):eabf4063.
42. Loyal L, Braun J, Henze L, Kruse B, Dingeldey M, Reimer U, et al. Cross-reactive CD4+ T cells enhance SARS-CoV-2 immune responses upon infection and vaccination. Science. 2021;374(6564):eabh1823.
43. Mateus J, Grifoni A, Tarke A, Sidney J, Ramirez SI, Dan JM, et al. Selective and cross-reactive SARS-CoV-2 T cell epitopes in unexposed humans. Science. 2020;370(6512):89–94.
44. Barouch DH. Covid-19 vaccines—immunity, variants, boosters. N Engl J Med. 2022;387(11):1011–20.
45. Thorne LG, Bouhaddou M, Reuschl AK, Zuliani-Alvarez L, Polacco B, Pelin A, et al. Evolution of enhanced innate immune evasion by SARS-CoV-2. Nature. 2022;602(7897):487–95.
46. Lundrigan E, Toudic C, Pennock E, Pezacki JP. SARS-CoV-2 protein Nsp9 is involved in viral evasion through interactions with innate immune pathways. ACS Omega. 2024;9(24):26428–38.
47. Rashid F, Xie Z, Suleman M, Shah A, Khan S, Luo S. Roles and functions of SARS-CoV-2 proteins in host immune evasion. Front Immunol. 2022;13:1–12.
48. Lu Y, Michel HA, Wang PH, Smith GL. Manipulation of innate immune signaling pathways by SARS-CoV-2 non-structural proteins. Front Microbiol. 2022;13:1027015.
49. Bouayad A. Innate immune evasion by SARS-CoV-2: comparison with SARS-CoV. Rev Med Virol. 2020;30:1–9.
50. Vinjamuri S, Li L, Bouvier M. SARS-CoV-2 ORF8: one protein, seemingly one structure, and many functions. Front Immunol. 2022;13:1–8.
51. Rubio-Casillas A, Redwan EM, Uversky VN. SARS-CoV-2: a master of immune evasion. Biomedicines. 2022;10:1339. MDPI.
52. Tay MZ, Poh CM, Rénia L, MacAry PA, Ng LFP. The trinity of COVID-19: immunity, inflammation and intervention. Nat Rev Immunol. 2020;20(6):363–74.
53. Zhang Q, Liu Z, Moncada-Velez M, Chen J, Ogishi M, Bigio B, et al. Inborn errors of type I IFN immunity in patients with life-threatening COVID-19. Science. 2020;370(6515):eabd4570.
54. van der Made CI, Netea MG, van der Veerdonk FL, Hoischen A. Clinical implications of host genetic variation and susceptibility to severe or critical COVID-19. Genome Med. 2022;14(1):1–22.
55. Srivastava A, Hollenbach JA. The immunogenetics of COVID-19. Immunogenetics. 2023;75:309–20.
56. Licciardi PV, Karagiannis TC. Regulation of immune responses by histone deacetylase inhibitors. ISRN Hematol. 2012;2012:1–10.
57. Calder PC, Carr AC, Gombart AF, Eggersdorfer M. Optimal nutritional status for a well-functioning immune system is an important factor to protect against viral infections. Nutrients. 2020;12:1181. Multidisciplinary Digital Publishing Institute.

58. Renata RBN, Arely GRA, Gabriela LMA, Esther MLM. Immunomodulatory role of microelements in COVID-19 outcome: a relationship with nutritional status. Biol Trace Elem Res. 2023;201:1596–614. Springer.
59. de Hernández-Flores T J, Pedraza-Brindis EJ, Cárdenas-Bedoya J, Ruíz-Carrillo JD, Méndez-Clemente AS, Martínez-Guzmán MA, et al. Role of micronutrients and gut microbiota-derived metabolites in COVID-19 recovery. Int J Mol Sci. 2022;23:12324. MDPI.
60. Costagliola G, Spada E, Consolini R. Age-related differences in the immune response could contribute to determine the spectrum of severity of COVID-19. Immunity, Inflamm Dis. 2021;9(2):331–9.
61. Rotulo GA, Palma P. Understanding COVID-19 in children: immune determinants and post-infection conditions. Pediatr Res. 2023;94(2):434–42.
62. Dioguardi M, Cazzolla AP, Arena C, Sovereto D, Caloro GA, Dioguardi A, et al. Innate immunity in children and the role of ACE2 expression in SARS-CoV-2 infection. Pediatr Rep. 2021;13(3):363–82.
63. Neeland MR, Bannister S, Clifford V, Dohle K, Mulholland K, Sutton P, et al. Innate cell profiles during the acute and convalescent phase of SARS-CoV-2 infection in children. Nat Commun. 2021;12(1):1084.
64. Petrara MR, Bonfante F, Costenaro P, Cantarutti A, Carmona F, Ruffoni E, et al. Asymptomatic and mild SARS-CoV-2 infections elicit lower immune activation and higher specific neutralizing antibodies in children than in adults. Front Immunol. 2021;12:741796.
65. Adhikari A, Maddumage J, Eriksson EM, Annesley SJ, Lawson VA, Bryant VL, et al. Beyond acute infection: mechanisms underlying post-acute sequelae of COVID-19 (PASC). Med J Aust. 2024;221:S40–8.
66. Mohan A, Iyer VA, Kumar D, Batra L, Dahiya P. Navigating the post-COVID-19 immunological era: understanding long COVID-19 and immune response. Life. 2023;13(11):1–27.
67. Filippatos F, Tatsi EB, Michos A. Immune response to SARS-CoV-2 in children: a review of the current knowledge. Pediatr Investig. 2021;5:217–28.

COVID-19 Diagnostic Tests

10

Manohar Lal Choudhary

10.1 Introduction

Severe acute respiratory syndrome coronavirus 2 (SARS-CoV-2) is a respiratory pathogen that emerged in December 2019 and led to a global pandemic by March 2020, with over seven million deaths caused by Coronavirus Disease 2019 (COVID-19) worldwide as of September 2025.

Severe Acute Respiratory Syndrome Coronavirus 2 (SARS-CoV-2) is a respiratory pathogen that causes Coronavirus Disease 2019 (COVID-19). It emerged in December 2019 and led to a pandemic by March 2020. On 9 January 2020, the identification of this causative agent was publicly announced. The first genome sequence of the novel coronavirus was published on the Virological website on 10 January, and additional complete genome sequences uploaded by various research groups were released via the GISAID database on 12 January 2020 [1–3] (commonly referred to as the Wuhan-1 virus). This swift response enabled the rapid development of diagnostic tests, vaccines, and therapeutics. Initially unidentified, the virus manifested with pneumonia-like symptoms in patients and rapidly spread through the population [1]. By January 2020, the virus had been successfully isolated and identified as Severe Acute Respiratory Syndrome Coronavirus 2 (SARS-CoV-2) [4]. As of October 2025, more than 778 million infections and over seven million deaths due to COVID-19 have been documented globally on the WHO (World Health Organization) COVID-19 dashboard.

Diagnosis forms the basis for case identification, isolation, contact tracing, and quarantine strategies, all of which are vital for reducing the virus's transmission. Accurate diagnosis of SARS CoV-2 infection is essential for patient treatment, lowering transmission rates, and infection control measures in hospitals, as well as for public health initiatives. Symptomatic patients are the primary source of

M. L. Choudhary (✉)
ICMR-National Institute of Virology, Pune, Maharashtra, India

S. R. Prabhu et al. (eds.), *COVID-19 in Dental Practice*,
https://doi.org/10.1007/978-3-032-26000-0_10

transmission; undiagnosed asymptomatic cases heighten the risk of spread. Detecting SARS CoV-2 through laboratory or point-of-care tests is crucial because symptoms alone cannot reliably distinguish COVID-19 from other respiratory infections. Molecular and rapid antigen tests (RAT; also known as lateral flow assays) are the main diagnostic tools [5, 6].

The crucial challenges of the pandemic are that several individuals with SARS-Cov-2 infections are mildly symptomatic or asymptomatic and remain capable of transmitting the virus [7]. Therefore, diagnostic assays must be sensitive enough to detect these hidden infections early to prevent further transmission. Diagnostics provide critical data to understand disease prevalence, transmission dynamics, and the effectiveness of control measures, in addition to individual patient care. SARS-Cov-2 diagnostic methods are widely classified based on the targets detected, either viral genetic material or host immune response, into molecular and serological assays, respectively. Molecular diagnostic methods focus on detecting viral nucleic acids, generally through amplification-based techniques. Serological methods, on the other hand, detect antibodies produced by the immune system in response to infection. Each category of diagnostic method offers unique advantages and presents specific challenges regarding sensitivity, specificity, turnaround time, and applicability in various settings [8].

The clinical resemblance makes symptom-based diagnosis unreliable and emphasises the importance of laboratory confirmatory testing for accurate diagnosis [9]. Laboratory-based diagnostics play an important role in patient management and public health decision-making. This provides conclusive evidence of infection, differentiates COVID-19 from other diseases with similar clinical features, and supports surveillance systems. The usefulness of laboratory detection of viral aetiology depends not only on their accuracy but also on the speed of result delivery and the resources needed for their deployment [10].

Clinically, COVID-19 presents with signs and symptoms such as fever, cough, dyspnoea, and pneumonia. However, these symptoms often significantly overlap with other respiratory illnesses caused by various viral and bacterial agents. This clinical similarity makes symptom-based diagnosis unreliable and emphasises the importance of confirmatory laboratory testing for an accurate diagnosis [9]. Laboratory diagnostics are crucial in clinical management and public health decision-making. The usefulness of laboratory diagnostics depends not only on their accuracy but also on the speed at which results are delivered and the resources needed for their implementation [10].

10.2 Sample Types for Diagnosis

SARS-CoV-2 transmits via respiratory aerosols or fomites. Nasal or oropharyngeal samples, collected alone or in combination, are used for confirmation of viral infection. SARS-CoV-2 migrates from the upper to the lower respiratory tract, where it replicates. Bronchoalveolar lavage, tracheal aspirates, and stool samples contain the virus [11]. Viral load varies by sample type, with respiratory, serum, and stool samples showing broad variation in virus quantity. The spread of the virus from the respiratory tract to other organs and tissues is associated with the cell-specific expression of angiotensin-converting enzyme-2 (ACE2) receptors [12].

Three types of diagnostic assays are crucial for patient management and pandemic control: molecular or nucleic acid amplification tests (e.g., RT-PCR tests) that detect viral RNA; antigen tests that identify viral proteins (e.g., nucleocapsid or spike proteins); and serology assays that identify host antibodies in response to infection, vaccination, or both. The first two types of tests help diagnose acute infection, while serology tests offer only indirect evidence of infection 1–2 weeks after symptoms appear and are useful for surveillance.

10.2.1 Molecular Approaches for Detection of SARS-CoV-2 Infection

Molecular methods include the following: (1) nucleic acid amplification techniques (NAATs) are the main tests used in both research and clinical settings. These include real-time reverse transcriptase polymerase chain reaction (RT-qRT-PCR), sequencing, and digital PCR (dPCR). (2) Isothermal amplification methods include loop-mediated isothermal amplification (LAMP), recombinase polymerase amplification (RPA), and clustered regularly interspaced short palindromic repeats (CRISPR)-related amplification.

Nucleic acid amplification test (NAAT), usually carried out by reverse transcription polymerase chain reaction (RT-PCR), is the preferred laboratory diagnostic test for hospitalised patients because it is highly sensitive and specific, with a quick turnaround time. RT-PCR detects viral RNA in respiratory specimens such as oropharyngeal/nasopharyngeal swabs, sputum, tracheal aspirates, and bronchoalveolar lavage fluid, providing direct evidence of active infection. The gold standard for confirming SARS-CoV-2 infection has been molecular testing based on nucleic acid amplification. RT-PCR remains the most widely used method because of its high sensitivity and specificity. Specimens are subjected to RT-PCR testing targeting specific regions of the viral genome, including the envelope (E), spike (S), nucleoprotein (N), and ORF 1a/b genes, selected for their strong genetic conservation across virus strains. Before performing RT-PCR, viral RNA must be extracted from the specimen. Both manual extraction protocols, such as TRIzol reagent, and commercially available viral nucleic acid extraction kits can be used to isolate RNA effectively. The reverse transcriptase first converts viral RNA into DNA using specific primers, producing complementary DNA (cDNA). A fluorescently labelled, sequence-specific DNA probe monitors the amplification of DNA in real time.

To speed up screenings, pooling can provide surveillance for infected individuals [13]. If a pool is negative, all the individual samples are considered negative from that test. If a pool is positive, individual samples must be tested to identify the positive source. When choosing a cost-effective pooling strategy, we must consider disease prevalence in the population along with specificity, sensitivity, and test probability [14].

Real-time RT-PCR results using primers targeting different viral genome segments can be affected by sequence variation in viral RNA. Even a single mutation in a primer-probe sequence can compromise the sensitivity of RT-qPCR assays, leading to false-negative detection. Furthermore, false-negative results may occur due to viral evolution [15]. Despite these limitations, the RT-PCR test remains the gold standard for SARS-CoV-2 diagnosis. SARS-CoV-2 RT-PCR has been incorporated into most commercially available multiplex PCR respiratory panels. However, there are several caveats associated with NAAT. First, prolonged shedding of SARS-CoV-2 RNA can occur, and sporadic shedding can be detected even among immunocompetent patients for a few weeks after symptom onset [16]. Second, NAAT can only be performed in clinical laboratories equipped for molecular diagnostic testing. However, fully automated NAAT assays are now available, enabling NAAT at the point of care. Third, mutations at the target sites of the RT-PCR primers or probes can lead to false-negative results. For example, the Alpha variant contained a deletion at the spike protein amino acid residues 69 and 70, leading to the failure of some RT-PCR assays [17].

10.3 Test Sensitivity and Specificity

The analytical specificity of a molecular test is its ability to identify only the analyte it aims to detect in the presence of non-target templates or interfering substances under controlled laboratory conditions. The analytical sensitivity of an assay often refers to the lowest amount of analyte that can be precisely measured by the assay. Both adequate analytical sensitivity and specificity ultimately lead to optimal clinical performance. For molecular SARS-Cov-2 tests, the quality and abundance of RNA in collected samples—heavily dependent on the collection method and site—are crucial for the sensitivity of the assays [18].

10.3.1 Isothermal Amplification Approaches

An isothermal amplification test functions at a constant temperature throughout the reaction, as these assays amplify a target sequence at a single temperature. No thermocycler is needed to maintain the required temperature changes during the RT-PCR process. Although the sensitivity of isothermal amplification assays like RT-LAMP and RT-RPA is slightly lower than RT-PCR in samples with low viral load, they offer potential for low-cost point-of-care testing in resource-limited settings.

10.3.2 Reverse Transcription Loop-Mediated Isothermal Amplification (RT-LAMP)

RT-LAMP is a rapid, cost-effective, and highly sensitive method that complements traditional molecular diagnostics. Its suitability for portable formats and minimal equipment needs makes it especially valuable in low-resource environments and for field-level SARS CoV-2 surveillance. The principle of RT-LAMP relies on a specially designed set of multiple primers that recognise six to eight distinct regions within a target gene [10].

Despite these advantages, one of the main limitations of RT-LAMP is its dependence on multiple primers, which raises the chances of non-specific binding and mis-amplification. To reduce the risk of false-positive results, assays are generally designed with shorter run times, usually around 30 min, ensuring dependable performance while limiting non-specific amplification [19].

10.3.3 Recombinase Polymerase Amplification (RPA)

In the RPA diagnosis test, the recombinase enzyme interacts with primers to form a recombinase–primer complex. The primer checks its complementary sequence and binds to the target site, while the recombinase enzyme cuts the target strand. A single-stranded DNA binding protein stabilises the other strand, whereas DNA polymerase extends the cut strand. Further rounds of extension can still utilise the recombinase. In the RPA assay, results are obtained in 10–15 min, amplifying DNA sequences at 37–42 °c. RT-RPA is a more advanced version of the RPA assay for virus detection, which includes a reverse transcription step [20].

10.3.4 CRISPR-Based Detection Technique

The clustered regularly interspaced short palindromic repeats (CRISPR) method can identify RNA and DNA present in a sample. It has many advantages compared to conventional diagnostic assays. This method offers a rapid turnaround time, excellent specificity and sensitivity, and is cost-effective. Additionally, it does not require a thermocycler, making CRISPR suitable for POC testing [21]. The CRISPR technique relies on identifying the viral genome, which reduces the likelihood of false-negative results and enables early detection of infection. Broughton et al. [22] developed the SARS-Cov-2 DNA endonuclease-targeted CRISPR trans-reporter (DETECTR), a CRISPR-based detection method.

10.3.5 Sequencing for Diagnostic Purposes

The advantage of sequence-based identification is the capacity to monitor viral mutations in new strains. This method aids in the detection and classification of emerging new coronavirus variants [23]. Notable novel mutant variants include alpha (B.1.1.7), beta (B.1.351), gamma (P.1), and delta (B.1.617.2), which may heighten disease severity and speed up virus transmission [24–26]. High-throughput and portable rapid sequencing technologies have been developed for SARS CoV-2 diagnosis [27]. However, viral genome sequencing is not practical for quick detection in large populations due to its high costs.

10.4 Serological Methods

10.4.1 SARS CoV-2 Antigens Detection

Rapid diagnostic tests (RDTs) based on lateral flow technology are more affordable and used for point-of-care testing, although they are less sensitive than RT-qpcr. Rapid antigen test (RAT) is a suitable alternative when molecular testing is unavailable. RAT is highly specific, technically simple, and inexpensive, with results usually available within 15–20 min. Overall, RAT exhibits lower sensitivity than NAAT (60–70% versus 80–90%) [28, 29]. The WHO recommends antigen RDTs that meet the requirements of ≥80% sensitivity and ≥97% specificity compared to RT-qPCR assay, which could be used to diagnose SARS CoV-2 infection within the first 5–7 days after symptom onset. RAT sensitivity can exceed 80% within the first 5 days of illness for symptomatic individuals when viral load is at its peak [30, 31]. In this assay, antigen present in the clinical sample binds to antibodies affixed on a paper strip enclosed in a plastic casing. This reaction produces a visually detectable signal within 30 min. The detected antigens are only present if the virus is actively replicating, so the tests can only identify acute or early infections [32].

The working principle of LFA depends on capillary action, which moves a liquid sample across a nitrocellulose membrane strip that has been pre-treated with specific capture or detection antibodies. When a biological sample, such as a nasal or throat swab extract, is applied to the sample well, it migrates through the strip and encounters reagents stored in different zones [33]. Typically, coloured nanoparticles (often gold nanoparticles) are conjugated to antibodies and act as visible indicators. When they bind to the target antigen, a coloured band appears on the corresponding test line of the membrane, allowing detection even without complex equipment [34].

Serological assays identify antibodies produced by the immune system in response to SARS-CoV-2 infection. These tests are important for evaluating past exposure, immune status, and for population-level surveillance. Common serological techniques include enzyme-linked immunosorbent assays (ELISA), chemiluminescent immunoassays (CLIA), and lateral flow devices (LFDs). Each technique differs in sensitivity, throughput, and the need for laboratory infrastructure [35, 36].

Serological assays for SARS-CoV-2 typically detect antibodies against the N or spike protein. However, they should not be used to diagnose an acute infection because antibodies are generally not detectable within 8–10 days of symptom onset [37], and many people have now been infected and/or vaccinated. Therefore, serological tests might show high positivity rates in a population, which does not necessarily indicate current infection. In the early stages of the COVID-19 pandemic, serological tests were valuable for retrospective diagnosis, especially for contact tracing and identifying patients with immune-mediated complications of COVID-19, such as multisystem inflammatory syndrome in children, where the initial infection had gone undiagnosed. Serological assays were also used to measure seroprevalence and assess humoral immunity in populations. However, these assays should be used with caution; for instance, some individuals who previously contracted

SARS-CoV-2 may no longer have detectable antibody levels due to waning over time or may not produce antibodies at all, particularly in immunocompromised patients. When the specimen migrates across the strip, antibody-antigen interactions are visualised as coloured lines.

10.4.2 Enzyme Immunoassay (EIA) or Enzyme-Linked Immunosorbent Assay (ELISA)

Enzyme immunoassay (EIA), commonly known as enzyme-linked immunosorbent assay (ELISA), is one of the most widely used serological tools for detecting antibodies produced after viral infections [38, 39]. In relation to SARS-CoV-2, ELISA provides a relatively rapid, safe, and effective method of identifying the host immune response, mainly by detecting immunoglobulin classes such as IgA, IgM, and IgG in patient serum or plasma samples [39]. ELISA platforms target multiple SARS-Cov-2 antigens, including the nucleocapsid (N) protein, the spike (S) protein, its S1 subunit, and the receptor binding domain (RBD) [40].

10.4.3 Chemiluminescent Immunoassays (CLIA)

Chemiluminescent immunoassays (CLIA) represent an advanced generation of immunodiagnostic techniques that share the same basic principle as enzyme-linked immunosorbent assay (ELISA), in which antigen–antibody interactions are detected using an enzyme-labelled system [41, 42]. However, CLIA offers several operational advantages over traditional ELISA. Unlike ELISA, CLIA does not require a separate stop reagent to terminate the enzymatic reaction, thereby simplifying workflow and eliminating an extra processing step. Additionally, incubation times are significantly shorter, allowing for higher throughput testing and rapid turnaround, making CLIA more suitable for large-scale diagnostic applications [43]. In terms of analytical performance, CLIA is characterised by a wider dynamic range and higher sensitivity compared to conventional colourimetric ELISA assays. Overall, CLIA-based platforms such as Roche Elecsys® and Abbott Architect® have become essential tools for large-scale serosurveillance, vaccine evaluation, and monitoring immunity against SARS-CoV-2, providing rapid, sensitive, and scalable alternatives to conventional ELISA assays. A summary of all the methodologies, their principles, required samples, costs, and advantages is given in Table 10.1.

In summary, the COVID-19 pandemic has underscored the essential role of diagnostic testing in controlling infectious diseases. Molecular and serological assays, along with innovative biosensor technologies, offer a range of tools for detecting SARS-CoV-2 infection in various clinical and community settings. Ongoing innovations and improvements in test sensitivity, speed, accessibility, and affordability are vital to accurately identify both symptomatic and asymptomatic cases, reduce transmission, and ultimately manage and lessen the impact of COVID-19 worldwide.

Table 10.1 A summary of all the methodologies, their principles, samples needed, costs, and advantages

Methodologies	Test	Principle	Sample	Advantage	Cost
Molecular methods	Real time RT-PCR	Conversion of SARS CoV-2 RNA to cDNA via transcriptase enzyme, followed by real-time PCR for amplification of cDNA	Nasopharyngeal/ oropharyngeal swab	Gold standard test Sensitive	Expensive
	RT-LAMP	Conversion of SARS CoV-2 RNA to cDNA via transcriptase enzyme and is performed at a temperature between 60 and 65 °C	Nasopharyngeal/ oropharyngeal swab	Do not require thermal cycle Time efficient Does not need access to high-tech laboratory	Very cost-effective
	Nucleic acid hybridization using microarray	Conversion of SARS CoV-2 RNA to cDNA via transcriptase enzyme, followed by adding it in wells containing fixed SARS CoV-2 specific oligonucleotides followed washing the hybridized virus cDNA for remains and emitting signal for positive samples	Nasopharyngeal/ oropharyngeal swab	Sensitive	Expensive
	Amplicon-based metagenomic sequencing	Hypervariable regions of conserved genes or intergenic regions are amplified by PCR, evaluated by the next-generation sequencing (NGS), and the resulting sequences are compared against databases	Nasopharyngeal/ oropharyngeal swab	Diagnoses of the different coronavirus strains	Expensive
Serological methods	Enzyme linked immunosorbent assay (ELISA)	Binding antibody against SARS CoV-2 with coated antigen in ELISA plates to form complex and detect with labelled secondary antibody which produced colour or fluorescence	Blood serum or plasma	Rapid	Not very expensive
	Chemiluminescence immunoassay (CLIA)	Using chemical probes which could produce light emission through chemical reaction to label the antibody against SARS CoV-2	Blood serum or plasma	Sensitive Rapid	Expensive
	SARS CoV-2 antigen assay	Detection of SARS CoV-2 antigen with its specific antibody based on ELISA or CLIA	Blood serum or plasma	Rapid	Variable costs

Point-of-care detection of SARS CoV-2	Lateral flow assays	The antigens bind to the gold nanoparticle–antibody conjugates. The control and test lines appear	Nasopharyngeal/ oropharyngeal swab	High specificity Rapid Simple and easy to use No need for a laboratory	Cheap
	Biosensors	Based on the type of sensor, its principle varies	Upper respiratory Specimens or blood or urine	Sensitive Rapid Easy to use	Expensive
Nanotechnology-based approaches	The applications of nanoparticles in several methods, which are mentioned above	Based on the type of method, its principle varies	Upper respiratory	Sensitive	Expensive

References

1. Zhou P, Yang XL, Wang XG, Hu B, Zhang L, Zhang W, Si HR, Zhu Y, Li B, Huang CL, Chen HD, Chen J, Luo Y, Guo H, Jiang RD, Liu MQ, Chen Y, Shen XR, Wang X, Zheng XS, Zhao K, Chen QJ, Deng F, Liu LL, Yan B, Zhan FX, Wang YY, Xiao GF, Shi ZL. A pneumonia outbreak associated with a new coronavirus of probable bat origin. Nature. 2020;579(7798):270–3.
2. Wu F, Zhao S, Yu B, Chen YM, Wang W, Song ZG, Hu Y, Tao ZW, Tian JH, Pei YY, Yuan ML, Zhang YL, Dai FH, Liu Y, Wang QM, Zheng JJ, Xu L, Holmes EC, Zhang YZ. A new coronavirus associated with human respiratory disease in China. Nature. 2020;579(7798):265–9.
3. Gralinski LE, Menachery VD. Return of the coronavirus: 2019-nCoV. Viruses. 2020;12(2):135.
4. D'amico F, Baumgart DC, Danese S, Peyrin-Biroulet L. Diarrhea during COVID-19 infection: pathogenesis, epidemiology, prevention, and management. Clin Gastroenterol Hepatol. 2020;18(8):1663–72.
5. Fragkou PC, De Angelis G, Menchinelli G, Can F, Garcia F, Morfin-Sherpa F, Dimopoulou D, Mack E, de Salazar A, Grossi A, Lytras T, Skevaki C. ESCMID COVID-19 guidelines: diagnostic testing for SARS-CoV-2. Clin Microbiol Infect. 2022;28(6):812–22.
6. Fragkou PC, Moschopoulos CD, Dimopoulou D, Ong DSY, Dimopoulou K, Nelson PP, Schweitzer VA, Janocha H, Karofylakis E, Papathanasiou KA, Tsiordras S, De Angelis G, Thölken C, Sanguinetti M, Chung HR, Skevaki C. European Society of Clinical Microbiology and Infection Study Group for Respiratory Viruses. Performance of point-of care molecular and antigen-based tests for SARS-CoV-2: a living systematic review and meta-analysis. Clin Microbiol Infect. 2023;29(3):291–301.
7. Singh A, Shaikh A, Singh R, Singh AK. COVID-19: from bench to bed side. Diabetes Metab Syndr Clin Res Rev. 2020;14(4):277–81.
8. Eftekhari A, Alipour M, Chodari L, Maleki Dizaj S, Ardalan M, Samiei M, Sharifi S, Zununi Vahed S, Huseynova I, Khalilov R, Ahmadian E, Cucchiarini M. A comprehensive review of detection methods for SARS-CoV-2. Microorganisms. 2021;9(2):232.
9. Ishiguro T, Kobayashi Y, Uozumi R, Takata N, Takaku Y, Kagiyama N, et al. Viral pneumonia requiring differentiation from acute and progressive diffuse interstitial lung diseases. Intern Med. 2019;58(24):3509–19.
10. Kevadiya BD, Machhi J, Herskovitz J, Oleynikov MD, Blomberg WR, Bajwa N, et al. Diagnostics for SARS-CoV-2 infections. Nat Mater. 2021;20(5):593–605.
11. Zhang W, Du RH, Li B, Zheng XS, Yang XL, Hu B, Wang YY, Xiao GF, Yan B, Shi ZL, Zhou P. Molecular and serological investigation of 2019-nCoV infected patients: implication of multiple shedding routes. Emerg Microbes Infect. 2020;9(1):386–9.
12. Tsang NNY, So HC, Ng KY, Cowling BJ, Leung GM, Ip DKM. Diagnostic performance of different sampling approaches for SARS-CoV-2 RT-PCR testing: a systematic review and meta-analysis. Lancet Infect Dis. 2021;21(9):1233–45.
13. Cesselli D, Bulfoni M, Marzinotto S, Marcon B, Cmet S, Cussigh AR, Migotti A, Martinella R, Pipan C, Beltrami AP, Curcio F. Implementation and validation of a pooling strategy for a sustainable screening campaign for the presence of SARS-CoV-2. Preprint at medRxiv. 2020; https://doi.org/10.1101/2020.08.28.20174946.
14. Watkins AE, Fenichel EP, Weinberger DM, Vogels CBF, Brackney DE, Casanovas-Massana A, Campbell M, Fournier J, Bermejo S, Datta R, Dela Cruz CS, Farhadian SF, Iwasaki A, Ko AI, Grubaugh ND, Wyllie AL, Yale IMPACT Research Team2. Increased SARS-CoV-2 testing capacity with pooled saliva samples. Emerg Infect Dis. 2021;27(4):1184–7.
15. Shen Z, Xiao Y, Kang L, Ma W, Shi L, Zhang L, Zhou Z, Yang J, Zhong J, Yang D, Guo L, Zhang G, Li H, Xu Y, Chen M, Gao Z, Wang J, Ren L, Li M. Genomic diversity of severe acute respiratory syndrome-coronavirus 2 in patients with coronavirus disease 2019. Clin Infect Dis. 2020;71(15):713–20.
16. Barak N, Ben-Ami R, Sido T, Perri A, Shtoyer A, Rivkin M, Licht T, Peretz A, Magenheim J, Fogel I, Livneh A, Daitch Y, Oiknine-Djian E, Benedek G, Dor Y, Wolf DG, Yassour M,

Hebrew University-Hadassah COVID-19 Diagnosis Team. Lessons from applied large-scale pooling of 133,816 SARS-CoV-2 RT-PCR tests. Sci Transl Med. 2021;13(589):eabf2823.
17. Kidd M, Richter A, Best A, Cumley N, Mirza J, Percival B, Mayhew M, Megram O, Ashford F, White T, Moles-Garcia E, Crawford L, Bosworth A, Atabani SF, Plant T, McNally A. S-variant SARS-CoV-2 lineage B1.1.7 is associated with significantly higher viral load in samples tested by TaqPath polymerase chain reaction. J Infect Dis. 2021;223(10):1666–70.
18. Lieberman JA, Pepper G, Naccache SN, Huang ML, Jerome KR, Greninger AL. Comparison of commercially available and laboratory-developed assays for in vitro detection of SARS-CoV-2 in clinical laboratories. J Clin Microbiol. 2020;58(8):e00821–0.
19. Feng W, Newbigging AM, Le C, Pang B, Peng H, Cao Y, et al. Molecular diagnosis of COVID-19: challenges and research needs. Anal Chem. 2020;92(15):10196–209.
20. Wang G, Yang X, Dong H, Tu Z, Zhou Y, Rong Z, Wang S. Recombinase polymerase amplification combined with fluorescence immunochromatography assay for on-site and ultrasensitive detection of SARS-CoV-2. Pathogens. 2022;11(11):1252.
21. Javalkote VS, Kancharla N, Bhadra B, Shukla M, Soni B, Sapre A, et al. CRISPR-based assays for rapid detection of SARS-CoV-2. Methods. 2022;203:594–603.
22. Broughton JP, Deng X, Yu G, Fasching CL, Servellita V, Singh J, Miao X, Streithorst JA, Granados A, Sotomayor-Gonzalez A, Zorn K, Gopez A, Hsu E, Gu W, Miller S, Pan CY, Guevara H, Wadford DA, Chen JS, Chiu CY. CRISPR-Cas12-based detection of SARS-CoV-2. Nat Biotechnol. 2020;38(7):870–4.
23. Lu R, Zhao X, Li J, Niu P, Yang B, Wu H, Wang W, Song H, Huang B, Zhu N, et al. Genomic characterisation and epidemiology of 2019 novel coronavirus: implications for virus origins and receptor binding. Lancet. 2020;395:565–74.
24. Tang JW, Tambyah PA, Hui DS. Emergence of a new SARS-CoV-2 variant in the UK. J Infect. 2021;82:e27–8.
25. Makoni M. South Africa responds to new SARS-CoV-2 variant. Lancet. 2021;397:267.
26. Uraki R, Korber B, Diamond MS, Kawaoka Y. SARS-CoV-2 variants: biology, pathogenicity, immunity and control. Nat Rev Microbiol. 2026;24(1):8–28.
27. Lam C, Gray K, Gall M, Sadsad R, Arnott A, Johnson-Mackinnon J, Fong W, Basile K, Kok J, Dwyer DE, Sintchenko V, Rockett RJ. SARS-CoV 2 genome sequencing methods differ in their abilities to detect variants from low-viral-load samples. J Clin Microbiol. 2021;59(11):e0104621.
28. Serrano MM, Rodríguez DN, Palop NT, Arenas RO, Córdoba MM, Mochón MDO, Cardona CG. Comparison of commercial lateral flow immunoassays and ELISA for SARS-CoV-2 antibody detection. J Clin Virol. 2020;129:104529.
29. Hirabayashi E, Mercado G, Hull B, Soin S, Koshy-Chenthittayil S, Raman S, Huang T, Keerthisinghe C, Feliciano S, Dongo A, Kal J, Azizan A, Duus K, Else T, DeArmond M, Stone AEL. Comparison of diagnostic accuracy of rapid antigen tests for COVID-19 compared to the viral genetic test in adults: a systematic review and meta-analysis. JBI Evid Synth. 2024;22:1939–2002.
30. Drain PK. Rapid diagnostic testing for SARS-CoV-2. N Engl J Med. 2022;386(3):264–72.
31. Hayden MK, Hanson KE, Englund JA, Lee F, Lee MJ, Loeb M, Morgan DJ, Patel R, El Alayli A, El Mikati IK, Sultan S, Falck-Ytter Y, Mansour R, Amarin JZ, Morgan RL, Murad MH, Patel P, Bhimraj A, Mustafa RA. The Infectious Diseases Society of America guidelines on the diagnosis of COVID-19: antigen testing (January 2023). Clin Infect Dis. 2024;78:e350–84.
32. Frew E, Roberts D, Barry S, Holden M, Restell Mand A, Mitsock E, Tan E, Yu W, Skog J. A SARS-CoV-2 antigen rapid diagnostic test for resource limited settings. Sci Rep. 2021;11(1):23009.
33. Li Z, Yi Y, Luo X, Xiong N, Liu Y, Li S, et al. Development and clinical application of a rapid IgM-IgG combined antibody test for SARS-CoV-2 infection diagnosis. J Med Virol. 2020;92(9):1518–24.
34. Xiang J, Yan M, Li H, Liu T, Lin C, Huang S, et al. Evaluation of enzyme-linked immunoassay and colloidal gold-immunochromatographic assay kit for detection of novel coronavirus

(SARS-Cov-2) causing an outbreak of pneumonia (COVID-19). MedRxiv. 2020; https://doi.org/10.1101/2020.02.27.20028787.
35. Michel M, Bouam A, Edouard S, Fenollar F, Di Pinto F, Mège J-L, et al. Evaluating ELISA, immunofluorescence, and lateral flow assay for SARS-CoV-2 serologic assays. Front Microbiol. 2020;11:597529.
36. Sherman AC, Gray GE, Cao B, To KKW, Rouphael N, Henao-Restrepo AM, Gordon AC, Baden LR. Acute SARS-CoV-2 infection. Nat Rev Dis Primers. 2025;11(1):75.
37. To KK, Tsang OT, Leung WS, Tam AR, Wu TC, Lung DC, Yip CC, Cai JP, Chan JM, Chik TS, Lau DP, Choi CY, Chen LL, Chan WM, Chan KH, Ip JD, Ng AC, Poon RW, Luo CT, Cheng VC, Chan JF, Hung IF, Chen Z, Chen H, Yuen KY. Temporal profiles of viral load in posterior oropharyngeal saliva samples and serum antibody responses during infection by SARS-CoV-2: an observational cohort study. Lancet Infect Dis. 2020;20:565–74.
38. Meng Z, Guo S, Zhou Y, Li M, Wang M, Ying B. Applications of laboratory findings in the prevention, diagnosis, treatment, and monitoring of COVID-19. Signal Transduct Target Ther. 2021;6(1):316.
39. Hou H, Wang T, Zhang B, Luo Y, Mao L, Wang F, Wu S, Sun Z. Detection of IgM and IgG antibodies in patients with coronavirus disease 2019. Clin Transl Immunol. 2020;9(5):e01136.
40. Pisanic N, Randad PR, Kruczynski K, Manabe YC, Thomas DL, Pekosz A, et al. COVID-19 serology at population scale: SARS-CoV-2-specific antibody responses in saliva. J Clin Microbiol. 2020;59(1). https://doi.org/10.1128/jcm.02204-02220.
41. Infantino M, Grossi V, Lari B, Bambi R, Perri A, Manneschi M, Terenzi G, Liotti I, Ciotta G, Taddei C, Benucci M, Casprini P, Veneziani F, Fabbri S, Pompetti A, Manfredi M. Diagnostic accuracy of an automated chemiluminescent immunoassay for anti-SARS-CoV-2 IgM and IgG antibodies: an Italian experience. J Med Virol. 2020;92(9):1671–5.
42. Kholmanskikh O, Wang Y-M, Hersey S, Wadhwa M, Block K, Bandukwala A, et al. 2023 White paper on recent issues in bioanalysis: EU IVDR 2017/746 implementation/impact, IVD/CDx/CLIA approved assays, high dimensional cytometry, multiplexing technologies, LBA tissue analysis, vaccine study endpoints, cell-based assays for biomarkers, cell therapy and vaccines (PART 2–recommendations on development & validation of biomarkers, IVD, CDx, cell-based, flow cytometry, ligand-binding and enzyme assays; advanced critical reagents strategies). Bioanalysis. 2024;16(8):179–220.
43. Böger B, Fachi MM, Vilhena RO, Cobre AF, Tonin FS, Pontarolo R. Systematic review with meta-analysis of the accuracy of diagnostic tests for COVID-19. Am J Infect Control. 2021;49(1):21–9.

11 The Use of Telehealth During the Coronavirus (COVID-19) Pandemic

Matt Hopcraft

11.1 Introduction

The COVID-19 pandemic compelled the dental profession to reevaluate what constitutes urgent and essential dental care and how to deliver it safely to patients [1]. Dentistry was regarded as high risk due to the potential for spreading the COVID-19 virus through aerosols produced during dental procedures. The World Health Organisation advised that routine non-urgent oral health care, which typically includes oral health check-ups, dental cleanings, and preventive care, should be postponed until there has been a significant reduction in COVID-19 transmission rates from community spread to cluster cases or according to official guidelines at national, sub-national, or local levels [2].

In this context, urgent oral health care can be considered as interventions for oral diseases and conditions that are severe in terms of bleeding, infection, swelling, or pain, or that otherwise have significant consequences if left untreated, thereby necessitating treatment or referral without delay [1].

In many parts of the world, routine and non-urgent dental care was suspended to reduce transmission risk, and this was further worsened by genuine hesitancy from patients to visit the dentist. With the ability to provide care greatly reduced, both dental practitioners and patients had to rethink their approach to oral health care.

As the rest of the world moved to the virtual realm—with schools offering online learning and offices switching to virtual meetings—dentistry turned to telehealth as a way of staying connected with and providing essential healthcare to patients.

Although teledentistry technology existed before the pandemic, there was no well-established use-case, and adoption worldwide was inconsistent. Historically, this was partly due to technological and cost challenges, but also because of the perception that dental care could only be provided face-to-face. A review published

M. Hopcraft (✉)
Melbourne Dental School, University of Melbourne, Melbourne, VIC, Australia
e-mail: m.hopcraft@unimelb.edu.au

S. R. Prabhu et al. (eds.), *COVID-19 in Dental Practice*,
https://doi.org/10.1007/978-3-032-26000-0_11

before the pandemic noted that as information and communication technologies have continued to develop and become more affordable, clinicians are increasingly finding it both cheaper and easier to implement teledentistry [3].

11.2 What Is Teledentistry?

Teledentistry is defined as the remote delivery of dental care, advice, or treatment using information technology rather than through direct patient contact [4]. It can involve diagnosis, providing advice, or prescribing pharmaceutical treatments for a patient. It can also be utilised to obtain a second opinion from another clinician.

Broadly, there are two main teledentistry systems or methodologies: synchronous (live) and asynchronous (store and forward). A synchronous mode involves using video (or audio) for communication and consultation between relevant parties—usually a dental practitioner and patient. An asynchronous mode involves sharing written, photographic, radiological, or other patient data as a means of communication and consultation.

Increasingly, teledentistry is utilising smartphone-based applications and intraoral photography to improve the transfer of information from patient to clinician, or from clinician to clinician. Remote patient monitoring and mobile health are modalities that record data collected by patients, clinicians, or smart devices and allow clinicians to assess, monitor, and care for patients remotely by tracking their health status.

Teledentistry is primarily used for triage purposes, helping to identify whether treatment is needed and, if so, its priority or urgency. This is especially beneficial for patients in rural or isolated areas who are far from a dental practitioner. It also proved important during the pandemic when dental practitioners in many parts of the world were restricted from seeing routine patients.

11.3 Effectiveness

One of the major concerns with teledentistry is whether it is an appropriate mechanism to provide oral health care. Dental practitioners have a strong reliance on and bias to visual-tactile examination and the adjunctive use of radiographs in order to accurately diagnose dental conditions. They have previously expressed reluctance to use teledentistry due to concerns about inaccurate diagnosis and the medico-legal ramifications that might eventuate [5].

Effectiveness can be viewed as increasing access to services, improving clinical accuracy, reducing costs, saving time for patients and/or clinicians, and ensuring acceptability among end users. Before the pandemic, access barriers were mainly seen as geographic, such as patients from rural areas, or physical, like patients who were homebound or residing in residential aged care facilities.

Pre-pandemic studies that evaluated the accuracy of various teledentistry methodologies generally found that they were as reliable as in-person clinical examinations across various settings, including patient screening, orthodontic assessment, diagnosis of orofacial diseases, management of dental infections, and indications for oral surgery, although difficulties were noted with the accurate diagnosis of demineralisation of the tooth surface [3]. Some researchers have shown it to be an effective tool for accurately detecting dental caries, comparable to in-person diagnosis [6]. Specialist oral and maxillofacial surgeons reported that teledentistry was effective for diagnosing simple cases but not for more complex issues such as pathology, and they expressed particular concerns about the lack of interventional capacity and the reliability of the technology [7]. The inability to obtain adjunctive diagnostic aids such as radiographs or pulp vitality tests remains a limiting factor.

The technology used is an important factor when assessing the effectiveness and accuracy of teledentistry. Older studies (prior to 2000) raised issues of poor and non-diagnostic image quality, internet connectivity problems, and prohibitive costs associated with information technology setup, which have become less relevant in more recent years [3]. Ongoing advances in information technology and smart devices are likely to improve the accuracy and effectiveness of teledentistry, further increasing acceptability and adoption by both patients and dental practitioners. This is particularly evident in the quality and accessibility of smartphones, enabling the sharing of high-quality images and videos. Nevertheless, limitations remain in the ability to provide high-quality imaging across the entire oral cavity.

11.4 Teledentistry Use During the Pandemic

Once the ability to attend a dental practice was limited during the pandemic, the concepts of access to care took on a completely different meaning. This likely influenced dental practitioners' perceptions of effectiveness. What might previously have been considered unacceptable technology suddenly became viable in the absence of other options.

Since the pandemic affected different parts of the world in various ways, responses from the regulatory and dental professions also differed. The length and type of restrictions on access to dental care likely played a key role in whether teledentistry was considered and used during the pandemic.

A number of studies demonstrate the widespread use of teledentistry during the pandemic across countries including Australia, Canada, China, United States, Japan, Italy, and United Kingdom [8–10]. This uptake and utilisation was generally from a low base. For example, it was reported that in Canada nearly half of all dentists were using teledentistry by December 2021, but only 13% had used it prior to the pandemic [9].

Teledentistry was most commonly used to carry out triage and determine whether the patients' needs were non-urgent or emergent [5, 11]. This enabled urgent cases to be prioritised for care, either through pharmaceutical interventions or through the careful use of in-person treatment.

Some public dental clinics in Australia used teledentistry consultations to triage dental emergencies and manage non-urgent cases during times when physical access to dental services was limited [10]. This typically involved telephone triage conducted by non-clinical staff, followed by a telephone consultation with a dental practitioner. Images were sometimes obtained from the patient, though these were often reported as not very useful. The most commonly recorded diagnoses included irreversible pulpitis, pulpal necrosis, or apical periodontitis; reversible pulpitis and hypersensitivity; periodontal disease; and crown fracture or defective restoration without associated pulpitis.

When comparing teledentistry consultations with subsequent face-to-face consultations, there was high specificity (74.1–99.95%), while sensitivity ranged from 18.8% to 100% [10]. Sensitivity indicates the ability to correctly identify individuals with a disease, whereas specificity refers to correctly identifying those without it. High sensitivity is crucial when the consequences of a disease are serious (for example, cancer), because we do not want to misclassify people as healthy if they actually have the disease. High specificity is essential because misclassifying healthy individuals as having the disease can cause distress and lead to additional (often costly) follow-up procedures to confirm their true health status.

The highest specificity (99.9%) was noted for diagnosing orthodontic concerns, while the lowest (74.1%) was observed for irreversible pulpal diseases [10]. Conversely, sensitivity was low for reversible pulpitis and hypersensitivity (58.8%), periodontal disease (52.2%), and crown fracture or defective restoration (29.2%). This indicates that teledentistry consultations most often overestimate disease severity, recording conditions as irreversible pulpitis, pulpal necrosis, or apical periodontitis when the actual disease is less severe. From a pandemic perspective, this might mean requiring patients to attend an in-person dental appointment, potentially exposing them to the risk of contracting COVID-19.

Across many Southeast Asian countries, teledentistry was used for consultation, diagnosis, monitoring, and education, with diagnosis being the most widely utilised service [12]. The educational aspect enabled dental practitioners to assess oral hygiene and offer advice to children and caregivers or provide smoking cessation counselling to patients.

An evaluation of teledentistry over a one-month period in 2020 at a paediatric dental clinic in the United Kingdom showed a reduction of face-to-face appointments by over one-third [5]. Paediatric dentists were able to offer preventive advice, including prescribing high-strength fluoride toothpaste and dietary guidance, and assess dental development.

11.5 Patient Perspectives

Like dental practitioners, patients also had to navigate the uncertainties of the pandemic. They were keenly aware through media reports that the dental clinic was seen as a high-risk environment for the transmission of COVID-19. Adjusting to new and often unfamiliar technologies to access dental care challenged the idea that dental visits could only be conducted in person.

For many patients, the pandemic was often their first experience of using teledentistry. A study of consumers in the United States in June 2020 found that only 29% had used teledentistry in the previous 12 months, and 68% said they had done so for the first time because of the pandemic [13]. This aligns with the relatively low utilisation reported by Canadian dentists prior to the pandemic [9].

Nonetheless, studies conducted during the pandemic on the implementation and acceptability of teledentistry from the patient perspective generally found that patients were satisfied with the management of their dental issues and the use of teledentistry technology [14–16]. It was considered more acceptable by patients when it led to a resolution of their dental problem or resulted in a referral for treatment [16]. This is important because not all dental problems can be resolved via teledentistry.

It is likely that the widespread acceptance of teledentistry by patients during the pandemic was largely driven by necessity. However, some patients still prefer to visit their dentist in person, which may reflect the inability of teledentistry to address all their dental issues or an ingrained bias favouring in-person dental appointments [14, 16]. Addressing these patient concerns is an important factor to consider in future pandemic planning.

11.6 Limitations

Although the evidence and lived experience support the use of teledentistry, and there is a wide range of use cases for the technology, it is important to recognise that there are limitations from both the patient and dental practitioner perspectives.

For patients, whilst teledentistry can improve access to care and has an important role to play when there are external factors that limit their ability to visit a dental practice, it is important to recognize that it may not be a viable option for all patients. Despite technological improvements and increased affordability, not all patients have access to a smartphone or computer with videoconferencing capability, and internet access, connectivity, and reliability remain variable in many parts of the world.

Even when these technological concerns are addressed, several barriers remain to be overcome, including digital literacy, effective patient communication, working effectively with paediatric patients, a lack of remuneration systems, and some inherent limitations of teledentistry as a tool [12, 17]. Communication can also pose a problem for patients whose native language differs from that of the dental practitioner [7]. Older patients, individuals from socioeconomically disadvantaged backgrounds, or those with physical or learning needs may also face challenges with the technological requirements of teledentistry [7, 15].

Telephone triage, even when complemented with video and still images, can feel restrictive for some clinicians. The inability to perform a visual intra-oral examination using lighting and magnification, take radiographs, or conduct the usual range of clinical tests (for example, periodontal probing or pulp vitality tests) can hinder accurate diagnosis. This limitation was evident in the lower specificity for diagnosing dental conditions such as pulpal disease and the tendency to overestimate the severity of the disease.

The inability to offer definitive treatment beyond a pharmaceutical prescription for patients is also a major limitation for both practitioners and patients. Most dental diseases require physical treatment—for example, restoration, extraction, or endodontic treatment. Antimicrobials are generally not recommended as first-line treatment for dental disease, yet a number of studies suggested that antimicrobial prescriptions either increased or did not decrease to the expected extent due to restricted access to dental care [18–21]. Antimicrobial resistance is a significant global issue, and dental prescribing plays a major role in this problem. It is possible that teledentistry was linked to inappropriate antibiotic prescribing during the pandemic, and this should also be considered in future pandemic planning.

11.7 Conclusion

The pandemic revealed limitations in patients' ability to access dental services and have their oral health properly treated. There is a dependence on in-person visits to diagnose and treat dental issues. Necessity being the mother of invention, when physical access to dental care was halted, practitioners were effectively compelled to choose between using a familiar but underused technology or not seeing patients at all. Similarly, patients also had to navigate the various barriers and challenges that arose.

Nonetheless, although teledentistry was a new concept for many, it appeared to be well accepted. As a result, there was a quick increase in the adoption of virtual technologies to replace or complement traditional dental visits and ensure patients could continue accessing essential dental care. Despite some limitations, evidence indicates that it is acceptable to both patients and dental practitioners. As teledentistry technologies continue to develop, and with the high likelihood of future pandemics, it is important for dental practitioners to become familiar with their use.

References

1. Benzian H, Beltrán-Aguilar E, Mathur MR, Niederman R. Pandemic considerations on essential oral health care. J Dent Res. 2021;100(3):221–5.
2. World Health Organisation (WHO). Consideration for the provision of essential oral health services in the context of COVID-19. Interim guidance. World Health Organisation: Geneva. 2020. Available from: https://www.who.int/publications/i/item/who-2019-nCoV-oral-health-2020.1. Accessed 29 Oct 2025.
3. Irving M, Stewart R, Spallek H, Blinkhorn A. Using teledentistry in clinical practice as an enabler to improve access to clinical care: a qualitative systematic review. J Telemed Telecare. 2017;24(3):129–46.
4. Khan SA, Omar H. Teledentistry in practice: literature review. Telemed J E Health. 2013;19(7):565–7.
5. Wallace CK, Schofield CE, Burbridge LAL, O'Donnell KL. Role of teledentistry in paediatric dentistry. Br Dent J. 2021; https://doi.org/10.1038/s41415-021-3015-y.

6. Casas K, DiPede L, Toema S, Ogwo C. Assessing teledentistry versus in-person examinations to detect dental caries: a systematic review and meta-analysis. JDR Clin Transl Res. 2025:23800844251320974.
7. Lee J, Park JS, Feng B, Wang KN. The utilisation of teledentistry in Australia: a systematic review and meta-analysis. J Dent. 2024;149:105265.
8. Mahdavi A, Atlasi R, Naemi R. Teledentistry during COVID-19 pandemic: scientometric and content analysis approach. BMC Health Serv Res. 2022;22(1):1111.
9. Cheuk R, Adeniyi A, Farmer J, Singhal S, Jessani A. Teledentistry use during the COVID-19 pandemic: perceptions and practices of Ontario dentists. BMC Oral Health. 2023;23(1):72.
10. Mahony T, George A, Kezhekkekara SG, Villarosa A, Friel C, Yaacoub A. The validity of teledentistry examinations during the COVID-19 pandemic in Sydney, Australia. Aust Dent J. 2025;70(2):103–13.
11. Suter N. Teledentistry applications for mitigating risk and balancing the clinical schedule. J Public Health Dent. 2020;80(S2):S126–S31.
12. Jin-Yu ML, Min CW, Si Jin JL, Babar MG, Mahdi SS. Practical applications of teledentistry during the Covid-19 pandemic in ASEAN member states—a systematic review. BMC Oral Health. 2024;24(1):421.
13. O'Malley E, Surdu S, Langelier M. The Impact of Pandemic Concerns on Consumers' Teledentistry Use During the First Months of the COVID-19 Pandemic. Public Health Rep. 2023;138(1_suppl):63S–71S. https://doi.org/10.1177/00333549221133801.
14. Menhadji P, Patel R, Asimakopoulou K, Quinn B, Khoshkhounejad G, Pasha P, et al. Patients' and dentists' perceptions of tele-dentistry at the time of COVID-19. A questionnaire-based study. J Dent. 2021;113:103782.
15. Rahman N, Nathwani S, Kandiah T. Teledentistry from a patient perspective during the coronavirus pandemic. Br Dent J. 2020:1.
16. Watfa MO, Bernfeld NM, Oren D, Shani T, Zigron A, Sela E, et al. Rapid implementation of teledentistry during the Covid-19 lockdown. Adv Oral Maxillofacial Surg. 2021;2:100031.
17. Mahony T, Wang C, Coilparampil A, Kong A, Patterson-Norrie T, Villarosa A, et al. Dental clinicians' perceptions on the use of tele-dentistry consultations during COVID-19 within public dental clinics in Sydney, Australia. Aust Dent J. 2023;68(4):282–93.
18. Kitano T, Brown KA, Daneman N, MacFadden DR, Langford BJ, Leung V, et al. The impact of COVID-19 on outpatient antibiotic prescriptions in Ontario, Canada; an interrupted time series analysis. Open Forum Infect Dis. 2021;8(11):ofab533.
19. Mian M, Teoh L, Hopcraft M. Trends in dental medication prescribing in Australia during the COVID-19 pandemic. JDR Clin Transl Res. 2021;6(2):145–52.
20. Falola A, Demirjian A, Thompson W, Brown CS, Gerver S, Bou-Antoun S. The impact of COVID-19 national restrictions on dental antibiotic dispensing trends and treatment activity in England: January 2016 to July 2021. JAC Antimicrob Resist. 2023;5(4):dlad081.
21. Shah S, Wordley V, Thompson W. How did COVID-19 impact on dental antibiotic prescribing across England? Br Dent J. 2020;229(9):601–4.

Part III

Clinical Manifestations, Management and Prevention of COVID-19

Mechanisms Underlying Severe COVID-19

12

Arjun Bhugra

12.1 Introduction

Coronavirus disease 19 (COVID-19) is a viral pneumonia caused by a novel *Betacoronavirus*, later named as severe acute respiratory syndrome coronavirus 2 (SARS-CoV-2) [1–3]. It belongs to the family Coronaviridae, which also includes other human coronaviruses such as HCoV-NL63, HCoV-229E, HCoV-OC43, and others. These viruses cause endemic infections worldwide throughout the year, usually resulting in a self-limiting disease such as the common cold [4]. Before SARS-Cov-2 triggered the 2020 pandemic, the other two zoonotic coronaviruses deadly outbreaks were severe acute respiratory syndrome (SARS-CoV) and Middle Eastern respiratory syndrome (MERS-CoV) [4]. COVID-19 was declared a global pandemic by the World Health Organisation (WHO) in March 2020 [1, 3, 5, 6].

SARS-CoV-2 is an enveloped, positive-sense, single-stranded RNA virus with 79% genomic sequence similarity to SARS-CoV. It encodes for structural proteins (membrane protein, nucleocapsid protein, envelope protein, and spike glycoprotein) and non-structural proteins (nsp) during replication. The structural proteins, together with the host-derived envelope, form a complete virion that infects new host cells. It gains entry into human host cells by binding its spike (S) glycoprotein to the angiotensin-converting enzyme 2 (ACE2) receptors [4, 7, 8]. These receptors are highly expressed in the ciliated epithelial cells of the respiratory tract (nasopharynx or trachea) and are also found in various other organs, including the heart, kidneys, and intestines [4, 9, 10].

In an immunocompetent host, SARS-Cov-2 infection presents with a wide range of clinical features, from asymptomatic or mild illness to severe and life-threatening critical disease [1, 5]. While most SARS-CoV-2 infections are self-limiting, a

A. Bhugra (✉)
Department of Microbiology and Virology, Queen Elizabeth The Queen Mother Hospital, East Kent Hospitals University NHS Foundation Trust, Margate, UK
e-mail: arjun.bhugra@nhs.net

S. R. Prabhu et al. (eds.), *COVID-19 in Dental Practice*,
https://doi.org/10.1007/978-3-032-26000-0_12

Table 12.1 Predisposing factors leading to severe COVID-19 [5, 8, 12, 13]

Key comorbidities/health conditions implicated in the severity of COVID-19	
Cardiovascular diseases	Coronary artery disease, heart failure
	Hypertension
Other comorbidities	Diabetes mellitus (type 1 and type 2)
Chronic health conditions	Chronic respiratory disease such as COPD, moderate-to-severe asthma
	Chronic kidney disease (CKD)
	Chronic liver disease (CLD)
	Cancer (especially haematological malignancies)

dysregulated, hyperactive immune response in some individuals can lead to a severe hyperinflammatory state, often termed a 'cytokine storm', which can cause acute respiratory distress syndrome (ARDS), multi-organ failure, and death [11]. Severe COVID-19 can often result in significant long-term physical, mental, and organ-specific sequelae [8]. Table 12.1 lists predisposing factors and health conditions associated with an increased risk of severe COVID-19 pneumonia.

12.2 Pathophysiology of Severe COVID-19

The progression from mild to severe COVID-19 is driven primarily by a complex interplay between viral replication and the host immune response [2]. To better understand this, it is important to know how the normal immune response to viral infection occurs.

- *Normal host immune response in viral infections*

During a typical viral respiratory infection, the host's first line of defence is the innate immune system, which plays a prominent role [6]. The immune response to SARS-CoV-2 begins when intracellular pattern recognition receptors (PRRs), such as Toll-like receptors (TLRs) and RIG-I-like receptors (RLRs), recognise SARS-CoV-2 RNA [6, 7].

This initial recognition step is followed by the release of various inflammatory cytokines, interferons (such as type I and III interferons), and chemokines that recruit other immune cells and induce cell death in the infected cell, thereby preventing further infection [6, 7]. The immune cells involved in the primary response to viral proteins are macrophages and neutrophils, although the innate immunity also includes dendritic cells, natural killer (NK) cells, eosinophils, and innate lymphoid cells (ILCs) [6, 14]. Type I and III interferons have an antiviral cytokine-like effect on both the infected and neighbouring cells when upregulated by interferon-stimulated genes (ISGs). Typically, these responses work together to inhibit viral replication and activate the adaptive immune response to eliminate the viral infection from the host [6].

These sequential steps eliminate the virus while minimising tissue damage in the host [6, 7]. In cases where this normal immune response becomes dysregulated—potentially due to viral evasion strategies like genetic mutations that adapt to immune pressure—there is uncontrolled production of inflammatory cytokines such as tumour necrosis factor (TNF) and interferons, which leads to a cytokine storm and promotes PANoptosis.

- *Mechanisms of dysregulated immune response in severe COVID-19*

One of the main reasons for the development of severe COVID-19 is profound dysregulation of the normal immune response to viral infection. Several mechanisms have been described for this, among which the most important are as follows [2, 6–8, 11, 14, 15]:

- Impaired Interferon Response: This can be attributed to SARS-CoV-2's ability to evade the normal immune response due to mutations and genome variations. When this occurs, the delay in IFN-I and IFN-III responses is caused by several factors [4]:
  - *Viral factors*:
    - Antagonistic actions of several viral proteins, including nsp1, nsp3, ORF6, and the N protein, lead to uncontrolled viral replication during the early phase of infection. High-level viraemia has been associated with the severity of the disease [16].
  - *Host factors*:
    - Autoantibodies to interferons.
    - Inborn defects to interferon signalling leading to low induction of local and systemic response.
- *Hyperinflammation and Cytokine Storm*: The impaired early innate immune response to viral infection results in an exaggerated and dysregulated inflammatory reaction. A high viral load in the host triggers a massive influx of neutrophils and macrophages into the lungs, leading to the release of large quantities of pro-inflammatory cytokines (e.g., IL-1β, IL-6, TNF-α) and chemokines (e.g., CXCL8, CXCL10). This phenomenon is known as cytokine release syndrome (CRS) or cytokine storm. Among these, IL-6 plays the most critical role and can be used independently to predict disease severity. The cytokine storm operates via a positive feedback loop: increased inflammatory mediators induce cell death (PANoptosis), which in turn releases more cytokines. This systemic hyperinflammation, particularly high levels of IL-6, causes extensive immunopathological damage to pulmonary tissue, leading to acute respiratory distress syndrome (ARDS) and multi-organ failure, which can result in death. Other biochemical parameters that can be assessed alongside IL-6 include known acute phase reactants and markers of tissue damage, such as C-reactive protein (CRP), ferritin, D-dimer, alanine aminotransferase (ALT), and lactate dehydrogenase (LDH).

- *Lymphopenia*: This is a hallmark of severe COVID-19 characterised by a significant reduction in circulating lymphocytes, especially CD4+ and CD8+ T-cells. Contributing factors include suppressive effects of high cytokine levels (TNF-α and IL-6), direct viral effects, and the sequestration of T-cells in the inflamed lungs. This results in T-cell depletion or T-cell exhaustion, which further hampers the host's ability to clear the virus from the body.
- *Endotheliitis and Coagulopathies*: Due to the presence of ACE2 receptors, endothelial cells can be directly infected and adversely affected by SARS-CoV-2. Infection leads to widespread endothelial inflammation, known as endotheliitis. Published studies, including autopsy reports of patients who succumbed to severe COVID-19, have demonstrated a significantly higher burden of microthrombi in the pulmonary capillaries compared with classic ARDS, contributing to organ damage and increased mortality. The lung injury caused by severe COVID-19 is also called diffuse alveolar damage (DAD). DAD results in cellular exudation, leading to interstitial fibrosis [4]. This fibrosis is a direct result of the host's attempt to repair the damage caused by SARS-CoV-2 infection and immunopathological insult to the pulmonary parenchyma [4, 14]. Histological examination after death shows features such as AT2 cell hyperplasia, dying pneumocytes, microvascular thrombi, and hyaline membranes (with increased D-dimers) [4]. In severe cases, damage to endothelial cells causes a hypercoagulable state through activation of the coagulation cascade and platelets. This mainly results from an imbalance between coagulation and fibrinolysis during the exudative phase of DAD. Although it is not fully understood, published studies suggest that hypoxia, chemokines, and disruption of alveolar epithelium are probable causes of this imbalance [4, 17]. Activation of platelets for clotting can also lead to thrombocytopenia in the acute phase of severe disease.

12.3 Is Severe COVID-19 a Systemic Disease?

Although primarily a pulmonary disease, severe COVID-19 can lead to systemic sequelae, making it a multi-organ disease [9, 14]. Systemic inflammation and coagulopathy contribute to indirect tissue damage throughout the body, particularly in organs that express ACE2 receptors. Furthermore, the virus can directly infect and harm cells in multiple organs through immunopathological mechanisms as described earlier in the chapter [8, 9]. As a result, severe COVID-19 can cause long-term complications affecting various organ systems, presenting with a wide range of systemic symptoms.

- *Cardiovascular system*: Common complications include heart failure, arrhythmias, myocardial damage, myocarditis (inflammation of the heart muscle), and thromboembolic events such as stroke and pulmonary embolism [7, 9].
- *Renal System*: Acute kidney injury (AKI), a common complication associated with high mortality rates, frequently occurs in critically ill COVID-19 patients [5, 14].

Table 12.2 This table provides a brief list of immune-related disorders reported in COVID-19

Immune-related disorders reported in COVID-19	
Systemic immune-related manifestations such as SLE-related symptoms, sarcoidosis, antiphospholipid antibodies, and multisystem inflammatory syndrome in the paediatric age group	
Vasculitis	Kawasaki disease in children and adults
	CNS vasculitis
	Retinal vasculitis
	IgA vasculitis
Myositis	Acute myalgia, rhabdomyolysis
	Autoimmune inflammatory myopathy
Arthritis	Acute arthralgias
	Symmetric polyarthritis
	Asymmetric oligoarthritis
	Monoarthritis
Organ-specific immune-related manifestations (brief list)	Oral ulcers, chilblain lesions, erythema nodosum, uveitis, conjunctivitis, and periorbital erythema

CNS central nervous system, *IgA* immunoglobulin A

- *Nervous System*: Common neurological symptoms include loss of taste and smell, while more serious issues include seizures, stroke, and encephalopathy [7, 9]. 'Brain fog', a chronic cognitive impairment, is a well-established long-term consequence [7].
- *Hepatic System*: Liver injury, indicated by elevated liver enzymes, is common in hospitalised patients, particularly those with severe disease [10, 14].
- *Gastrointestinal System*: Symptoms such as diarrhoea, nausea, and vomiting can occur due to direct viral infection of the gut epithelium [9].

The systemic nature of COVID-19 is particularly important for dental patients and practitioners [15]. The oral cavity can be a site for viral replication, and dental procedures that generate aerosols can significantly increase the risk of SARS-CoV-2 transmission [15]. Table 12.2 enumerates various immune-related disorders reported in patients with severe COVID-19 [18]

12.4 Conclusion

Although COVID-19 often presents as a primary lung disease, its development reveals a complex condition capable of causing severe systemic illness. Consequently, it is essential for dentists and oral hygienists to take proper precautions when treating known or susceptible cases of the virus. The infection's nature can lead to multisystem involvement. Therefore, patient management must be holistic and multidisciplinary, involving a comprehensive review of medical history, including any previous COVID-19 infections, and close collaboration with other healthcare professionals to reduce risks and ensure the best outcomes for vulnerable patients.

References

1. Yip JQ, Oo A, Ng YL, Chin KL, Tan KK, Chu JJH, et al. The role of inflammatory gene polymorphisms in severe COVID-19: a review. Virol J [Internet]. 2024;21(1):327. Available from: https://virologyj.biomedcentral.com/articles/10.1186/s12985-024-02597-3
2. Rovito R, Augello M, Ben-Haim A, Bono V, d'Arminio Monforte A, Marchetti G. Hallmarks of severe COVID-19 pathogenesis: a pas de Deux between viral and host factors. Front Immunol [Internet] 2022 13;912336. Available from: https://www.frontiersin.org/articles/10.3389/fimmu.2022.912336/full.
3. Jin Y, Yang H, Ji W, Wu W, Chen S, Zhang W, et al. Virology, epidemiology, pathogenesis, and control of COVID-19. Viruses [Internet]. 2020;12(4):372. Available from: https://www.mdpi.com/1999-4915/12/4/372.
4. Lamers MM, Haagmans BL. SARS-CoV-2 pathogenesis. Nat Rev Microbiol [Internet]. 2022;20(5):270–84. Available from: https://www.nature.com/articles/s41579-022-00713-0.
5. Sim BLH, Chidambaram SK, Wong XC, Pathmanathan MD, Peariasamy KM, Hor CP, et al. Clinical characteristics and risk factors for severe COVID-19 infections in Malaysia: a nationwide observational study. Lancet Reg Health West Pac [Internet]. 2020;4:100055. Available from: https://linkinghub.elsevier.com/retrieve/pii/S2666606520300559.
6. Malireddi RKS, Sharma BR, Kanneganti TD. Innate immunity in protection and pathogenesis during coronavirus infections and COVID-19. Annu Rev Immunol [Internet]. 2024;42(1):615–45. Available from: https://www.annualreviews.org/content/journals/10.1146/annurev-immunol-083122-043545.
7. Torres Acosta MA, Singer BD. Pathogenesis of COVID-19-induced ARDS: implications for an ageing population. Eur Respir J [Internet]. 2020;56(3):2002049. Available from: https://publications.ersnet.org/lookup/doi/10.1183/13993003.02049-2020.
8. Attaway AH, Scheraga RG, Bhimraj A, Biehl M, Hatipoğlu U. Severe covid-19 pneumonia: pathogenesis and clinical management. BMJ [Internet]. 2021;372:n436. Available from: https://www.bmj.com/lookup/doi/10.1136/bmj.n436.
9. Yuki K, Fujiogi M, Koutsogiannaki S. COVID-19 pathophysiology: a review. Clin Immunol [Internet]. 2020;215:108427. Available from: https://linkinghub.elsevier.com/retrieve/pii/S152166162030262X.
10. Shao HH, Yin RX. Pathogenic mechanisms of cardiovascular damage in COVID-19. Mol Med [Internet]. 2024;30(1):92. Available from: https://molmed.biomedcentral.com/articles/10.1186/s10020-024-00855-2.
11. Nile SH, Nile A, Qiu J, Li L, Jia X, Kai G. COVID-19: pathogenesis, cytokine storm and therapeutic potential of interferons. Cytokine Growth Factor Rev [Internet]. 2020;53:66–70. Available from: https://linkinghub.elsevier.com/retrieve/pii/S1359610120300708.
12. Carreira H, Strongman H, Peppa M, McDonald HI, dos-Santos-Silva I, Stanway S, et al. Prevalence of COVID-19-related risk factors and risk of severe influenza outcomes in cancer survivors: a matched cohort study using linked English electronic health records data. EClinicalMedicine [Internet]. 2020;29–30:100656. Available from: https://linkinghub.elsevier.com/retrieve/pii/S2589537020304004.
13. Clark A, Jit M, Warren-Gash C, Guthrie B, Wang HHX, Mercer SW, et al. Global, regional, and national estimates of the population at increased risk of severe COVID-19 due to underlying health conditions in 2020: a modelling study. Lancet Glob Health [Internet]. 2020;8(8):e1003–17. Available from: https://linkinghub.elsevier.com/retrieve/pii/S2214109X20302643.
14. Li C, He Q, Qian H, Liu J. Overview of the pathogenesis of COVID-19 (review). Exp Ther Med [Internet]. 2021;22(3):1011. Available from: http://www.spandidos-publications.com/10.3892/etm.2021.10444.
15. Parasher A. COVID-19: current understanding of its pathophysiology, clinical presentation and treatment. Postgrad Med J [Internet]. 2021;97(1147):312–20. Available from: https://academic.oup.com/pmj/article/97/1147/312/6969661.

16. Ringlander J, Martner A, Huiqi L, Gisslén M, Lindh M, Westin J, et al. Influence of viral load on severity and mortality in COVID-19. Infect Dis. 2025;57(9):811–8.
17. Millar FR, Summers C, Griffiths MJ, Toshner MR, Proudfoot AG. The pulmonary endothelium in acute respiratory distress syndrome: insights and therapeutic opportunities. Thorax [Internet]. 2016;71(5):462–73. Available from: https://thorax.bmj.com/lookup/doi/10.1136/thoraxjnl-2015-207461.
18. Ramos-Casals M, Brito-Zerón P, Mariette X. Systemic and organ-specific immune-related manifestations of COVID-19. Nat Rev Rheumatol [Internet]. 2021;17(6):315–32. Available from: https://www.nature.com/articles/s41584-021-00608-z.

Signs and Symptoms of Severe COVID-19 with Predisposing Risk Factors

13

Arjun Bhugra

13.1 Introduction

In December 2019, a cluster of atypical respiratory diseases emerged in Wuhan, China [1–3], leading to the discovery of a novel coronavirus named as severe acute respiratory syndrome coronavirus 2 (SARS-CoV-2). The name was assigned due to its genetic similarity to the SARS-CoV that caused the 2002–2003 outbreak [1, 2, 4]. The disease caused by SARS-Cov-2 was named Coronavirus Disease 2019 (COVID-19). It is an enveloped, positive-sense, single-stranded RNA, virus belonging to the *Betacoronavirus* genus, with a genome size of approximately 30 kb [1, 2, 5]. Its structural proteins, particularly the spike (S) protein, are vital for its lifecycle. The S protein binds to the host cell receptor, angiotensin-converting enzyme 2 (ACE2), to initiate viral entry [1, 2]. Subsequently, the S protein is cleaved by host proteases such as TMPRSS2, cathepsin L, and furin, which are essential for the virus to fuse with the host cell membrane and release its genetic material into the cytoplasm. This process, which can occur in a wide range of cells expressing ACE2—including those in the respiratory tract, heart, kidneys, and gastrointestinal tract—explains the virus's multiorgan tropism [1, 2, 6, 7]. COVID-19 can be divided into distinct phases: the viral response phase, the pulmonary phase, and the inflammatory phase [8].

- *Viral response phase*: During the early stage of infection, the virus replicates locally in the upper respiratory tract [2]. For most patients, the immune system can contain the infection, resulting in a self-limiting illness with mild constitutional symptoms [1, 2, 9]. Initial symptoms often include fever, dry cough, and fatigue, but some cases can be entirely asymptomatic [1, 2].

A. Bhugra (✉)
Department of Microbiology and Virology, Queen Elizabeth The Queen Mother Hospital, East Kent Hospitals University NHS Foundation Trust, Margate, UK
e-mail: arjun.bhugra@nhs.net

S. R. Prabhu et al. (eds.), *COVID-19 in Dental Practice*,
https://doi.org/10.1007/978-3-032-26000-0_13

- *Pulmonary phase*: In some individuals, the disease progresses to a pulmonary phase characterised by dyspnoea and lung infiltrates [8].
- *Inflammatory phase*: This follows the pulmonary infiltration and is responsible for most of the morbidity and mortality. This phase is marked by a dysregulated immune response and a hypercoagulable state that can lead to multi-system organ failure and acute respiratory distress syndrome (ARDS) [6, 8].

As explained, COVID-19 presents with a wide spectrum of symptoms, from mild and constitutional to severe and life-threatening [6]. Table 13.2 provides an overview of factors that may contribute to severe COVID-19.

13.2 Signs and Symptoms of COVID-19

Table 13.1 summarises and compares the presentations and manifestations of COVID-19 in paediatric and adult patients.

- *Paediatric Presentation and Multisystem Inflammatory Syndrome in children (MIS-C)*: The paediatric population usually experiences a mild or asymptomatic acute phase, often presenting with simple fever (71.9%), cough, or rhinorrhoea. Severe COVID-19 in children predominantly presents as multisystem inflammatory syndrome in children (MIS-C). Risk factors that primarily increase the risk of severe infection in children include age, viral load, and chronic comorbidities [3]. Babies younger than one year are at higher risk of developing severe COVID-19, which shifts after one year of age, with the youngest children experiencing asymptomatic or milder disease [3]. Unlike adults, who typically present with acute viral pneumonia, MIS-C typically presents 2–6 weeks after the initial infection [3, 10]. These children often present with hyperinflammatory

Table 13.1 A summary of the important differences in presentation of COVID-19 in the paediatric age group and adults

Feature	Paediatric age group	Adult age group
Primary disease in the age group	MIS-C (multisystem inflammatory syndrome)	ARDS (acute respiratory distress syndrome)
Most common timing for severity	Post-infectious (2–6 weeks after onset)	Acute phase (during active infection)
Most common symptom of infection	Persistent fever and GI distress (pain/vomiting)	Dyspnoea and dry cough
Primary organ failure	Cardiovascular (shock/myocarditis)	Pulmonary (respiratory failure)
Typical biomarkers to predict the severity of COVID-19	Very high CRP, procalcitonin, and troponins	Elevated D-dimer & IL-6; moderate CRP
Unique findings	Kawasaki-like signs (rash, conjunctivitis)	Anosmia (loss of smell) and ageusia
Common comorbidities	Often previously healthy	Chronic disease such as obesity, hypertension, diabetes mellitus

shock requiring high inotropic support (100% in paediatric ICU cohorts). MIS-C clinically resembles conditions such as Kawasaki disease and toxic shock syndrome, characterised by persistent fever, gastrointestinal symptoms like abdominal pain and diarrhoea, and mucocutaneous signs such as rash or conjunctivitis. A key feature of the severe paediatric form is cardiac dysfunction, evidenced by significantly elevated NT-proBNP and troponins. While respiratory support may sometimes be necessary, it is often due to haemodynamic instability rather than primary lung parenchymal damage [3, 10].

- *Presentation in Adults and Acute Respiratory Distress Syndrome (ARDS)*: Unlike paediatric patients, while fever and cough are common in adults, they more frequently report fatigue (80.7%), anosmia (70.3%), and shortness of breath. In contrast, severe disease is characterised by acute respiratory distress syndrome (ARDS) [3]. ICU admissions in adults are primarily due to respiratory failure, requiring high positive end-expiratory pressure (PEEP) and prone positioning. Although other parameters are compared, C-reactive protein (CRP) and procalcitonin are often lower than those seen in paediatric MIS-C, suggesting that adult pathology is more localised to the pulmonary system rather than involving a widespread multisystem storm [3, 10]. The higher incidence of healthcare-associated infections and thrombotic complications is often linked to prolonged immobilisation and a hypercoagulable state.

13.3 Clinical Features of Long COVID-19

WHO defines post-COVID condition (PCC) as a range of symptoms that usually begin within 3 months of the initial COVID-19 illness and persist for at least 2 months, without an alternative explanation. PCC can impair a person's ability to carry out daily activities such as work or household chores and limit social participation. The following are some of the key clinical features that define long COVID-19 or PCC [11–13]:

- General and Systemic features.
  - Fatigue.
  - Post-exertional malaise (PEM).
  - Sleep disturbances.
- Neurological and psychological features also known as 'brain fog'.
  - Cognitive Impairment: It is characterised by loss of concentration, memory issues, and 'slowness of thought'.
  - Psychological Impact: This includes anxiety, depression, and mood swings, particularly in children whose social development and schooling are disrupted.
  - Sensory Changes: Altered or lost sense of smell (anosmia) and taste (ageusia), more common in adults.
- Organ-specific manifestations.

- *Cardiovascular manifestations*: patients of PCC may end up having palpitations, chest pain, and postural orthostatic tachycardia syndrome (POTS), etc.
- *Respiratory manifestations*: persistent dry cough and shortness of breath (dyspnoea), even in patients with normal lung function tests.
- *Gastrointestinal manifestations*: they may be abdominal pain, nausea, and diarrhoea. In children, persistent gut symptoms may be linked to viral fragments remaining in the intestinal lining.

13.4 Predisposing Risk Factors of Severe COVID-19

Severe COVID-19 is associated with a number of host, viral, and environmental factors [14, 15]. Table 13.2 summarises the factors that influence and contribute to severe COVID-19 as predisposing risk factors.

13.4.1 Human/Host Factors

- *Age*: Age is a significant factor reported since 2020 that influences disease severity. Older age consistently emerges as the most important risk factor for severe disease and high mortality [1, 8, 16]. This has been confirmed by several meta-analyses. In addition to higher mortality, older patients are also known to experience prolonged illness (long COVID-19) and longer hospital stays. They are more likely to progress to respiratory failure requiring level three care in the intensive care unit with mechanical ventilation [15, 17–19]. This also increases the healthcare system's costs. Patients with advanced age suffer from chronic low-grade inflammation that can worsen cytokine storms (as explained in Chap. 14) [20, 21]. The other end of the age spectrum, i.e., children, are least affected due to their lack of comorbidities and robust immune response.
- *Biological Sex*: According to the published literature, males face a significantly higher risk of severe COVID-19 as compared to females, where a predominance

Table 13.2 Overview of the predisposing risk factors resulting in severe COVID-19

Factors affecting the severity of COVID-19	
Host factors	Age—usually older population is at higher risk
	Biological sex—male >> females; can be different in pregnancy
	Genetic variations and mutations
	Underlying health conditions and comorbidities
	Immune-mediated diseases
	Other infections—co-infections, superinfections, lifestyle factors such as smoking, substance use, and malnutrition put the patients at more risk of developing severe COVID-19
Viral factors	Viral genetic variations and infective dose of the virus
Social factors	Socioeconomic status and air pollution

is seen in other viral-induced ARDS [8, 14]. This sex-based difference may be linked to variations in immune responses regulated by hormonal influence (oestrogen) and the expression of the ACE2 receptor [6, 14, 15]. Additionally, females tend to have better viral clearance than males [15]. However, this shift occurs during pregnancy, when females are also more likely to develop severe COVID-19 [15, 22, 23]. Pregnant women infected with SARS-CoV-2 may also face higher risks of pre-eclampsia and preterm labour due to placental inflammation [15].

- *Host Genetic Variation*: Key genetic variations implicated in severe COVID-19 include polymorphisms in the ACE2 and TMPRSS2 genes, which facilitate the virus's entry into host cells [24, 25]. Variations in inflammatory genes can substantially influence disease severity. For example, polymorphisms in the genes for IL-6 and IL-8 are associated with a higher risk of severe COVID-19 [26]. Other significant genetic factors affecting disease severity, though beyond the scope of this book's discussion, include loss-of-function mutations in the TLR7 gene and a genetic cluster on chromosome 3 (3p21.31), identified as a major risk locus.
- *Underlying Health Conditions and Comorbidities*: A wide range of comorbidities are linked to an increased risk of severe COVID-19. These include hypertension, diabetes, cardiovascular disease, chronic kidney disease, chronic obstructive pulmonary disease (COPD), and cancer [14, 15, 27–30]. Patients with multiple comorbidities (multimorbidity) have a doubled mortality rate compared to those without [31].
- *Immune-Mediated Diseases*: Patients with immune-mediated inflammatory diseases (IMIDs) and those taking immunomodulatory medications (IMMs) also face a higher risk of severe outcomes. Although the specific IMID or IMM is less significant than age or comorbidities, diseases such as rheumatoid arthritis (RA) and multiple sclerosis (MS) have been linked to poorer outcomes [32]. Conversely, some conditions like asthma, psoriasis, and spondyloarthritis may be linked to a lower risk of severe COVID-19 [32].
- *Superinfections and Previous Infections*: Bacterial superinfections caused by pathogens such as *Staphylococcus aureus* or *Klebsiella pneumoniae* worsen the prognosis of COVID-19 [15, 30, 33]. Prior infection with seasonal coronaviruses may provide some cross-reactive T-cell immunity to SARS-CoV-2 [15], which is more common in children and could explain their milder symptoms [6]. Conversely, HIV infection is an independent risk factor for both severe COVID-19 at admission and in-hospital mortality [34].

13.5 Viral Factors

- Viral genetic mutations and infection of the virus due to its mode of transmission causes propagated outbreaks in the community. This kind of spread, along with the rapid development of vaccines and antivirals against severe disease, puts immune pressure on the virus, leading to rapid evolution of the viral genome over a short period of time. WHO has classified these variants into variants of concern (VOCs) and variants of interest (VoIs). Early VOCs, such as the alpha and delta variants of SARS-CoV-2, were highly transmissible and virulent [35, 36]. They have been associated with increased mortality and longer hospital stays. Additionally, a higher initial infectious dose (inoculum) is believed to cause more severe disease by overwhelming early innate defences. This highlights the importance of public health measures like masking to reduce viral load during exposure.

13.6 Summary

The development of severe COVID-19, characterised by a hyperinflammatory and hypercoagulable state, poses distinct challenges and risks for dental patients, especially those requiring surgical procedures. Dental patients with existing conditions such as hypertension, diabetes, or cardiovascular disease are already more vulnerable to severe COVID-19 outcomes [7]. For these individuals, an acute SARS-CoV-2 infection could provoke an amplified inflammatory response that worsens their underlying health issues, potentially resulting in cardiac events or stroke.

The management of dental patients must therefore consider the possibility of both active and past COVID-19 infections. For patients who are actively infected or recovering, elective dental procedures, especially aerosol-generating ones, should be delayed. Before surgery, a comprehensive medical history should be taken to identify any risk factors for severe COVID-19. In emergency dental procedures, clinicians must wear suitable personal protective equipment (PPE) and reduce aerosol production to prevent viral transmission.

Furthermore, a patient's post-COVID-19 status should be a considered. The long-term effects of COVID-19 can include persistent symptoms such as fatigue and hypoxia. These ongoing health issues may affect a patient's ability to tolerate a dental procedure and could increase the risk of complications. Therefore, a comprehensive and collaborative approach, involving consultation with the patient's primary care physician, is crucial to ensure patient safety and to mitigate the risks associated with dental procedures in this vulnerable population.

References

1. Yuki K, Fujiogi M, Koutsogiannaki S. COVID-19 pathophysiology: a review. Clin Immunol [Internet]. 2020;215:108427. Available from: https://linkinghub.elsevier.com/retrieve/pii/S152166162030262X.
2. Parasher A. COVID-19: current understanding of its pathophysiology, clinical presentation and treatment. Postgrad Med J [Internet]. 2021;97(1147):312–20. Available from: https://academic.oup.com/pmj/article/97/1147/312/6969661.
3. Jiang L, Tang K, Levin M, Irfan O, Morris SK, Wilson K, et al. COVID-19 and multisystem inflammatory syndrome in children and adolescents. Lancet Infect Dis [Internet]. 2020;20(11):e276–88. Available from: https://linkinghub.elsevier.com/retrieve/pii/S1473309920306514.

4. Tomokazu Tamura, Jumpei Ito, Keiya Uriu, Jiri Zahradnik, Izumi Kida, Hesham Nasser, et al. Virological characteristics of the SARS-CoV-2 XBB variant derived from recombination of two omicron subvariants. bioRxiv [Internet]. 2023:1–43. Available from: https://doi.org/10.1101/2022.12.27.521986.
5. Xu X, Chen P, Wang J, Feng J, Zhou H, Li X, et al. Evolution of the novel coronavirus from the ongoing Wuhan outbreak and modeling of its spike protein for risk of human transmission. Sci China Life Sci. 2020;63(3):457–60.
6. Rovito R, Augello M, Ben-Haim A, Bono V, d'Arminio Monforte A, Marchetti G. Hallmarks of severe COVID-19 pathogenesis: a pas de Deux between viral and host factors. Front Immunol [Internet]. 2022;13. Available from: https://www.frontiersin.org/articles/10.3389/fimmu.2022.912336/full.
7. Shao HH, Yin RX. Pathogenic mechanisms of cardiovascular damage in COVID-19. Mol Med [Internet]. 2024;30(1):92. Available from: https://molmed.biomedcentral.com/articles/10.1186/s10020-024-00855-2.
8. Torres Acosta MA, Singer BD. Pathogenesis of COVID-19-induced ARDS: implications for an ageing population. Eur Respir J [Internet]. 2020;56(3):2002049. Available from: https://publications.ersnet.org/lookup/doi/10.1183/13993003.02049-2020.
9. Nile SH, Nile A, Qiu J, Li L, Jia X, Kai G. COVID-19: pathogenesis, cytokine storm and therapeutic potential of interferons. Cytokine Growth Factor Rev [Internet]. 2020;53:66–70. Available from: https://linkinghub.elsevier.com/retrieve/pii/S1359610120300708.
10. Girona-Alarcon M, Bobillo-Perez S, Sole-Ribalta A, Hernandez L, Guitart C, Suarez R, et al. The different manifestations of COVID-19 in adults and children: a cohort study in an intensive care unit. BMC Infect Dis [Internet]. 2021;21(1):87. Available from: https://bmcinfectdis.biomedcentral.com/articles/10.1186/s12879-021-05786-5.
11. Davis HE, McCorkell L, Vogel JM, Topol EJ. Long COVID: major findings, mechanisms and recommendations. Nat Rev Microbiol [Internet]. 2023;21(3):133–46. Available from: https://www.nature.com/articles/s41579-022-00846-2
12. Ely EW, Brown LM, Fineberg HV. Long Covid defined. N Engl J Med [Internet]. 2024;391(18):1746–53. Available from: http://www.nejm.org/doi/10.1056/NEJMsb2408466.
13. Greenhalgh T, Sivan M, Perlowski A, Nikolich JŽ. Long COVID: a clinical update. The Lancet [Internet]. 2024;404(10453):707–24. Available from: https://linkinghub.elsevier.com/retrieve/pii/S014067362401136X.
14. Attaway AH, Scheraga RG, Bhimraj A, Biehl M, Hatipoğlu U. Severe covid-19 pneumonia: pathogenesis and clinical management. BMJ [Internet]. 2021;372:n436. Available from: https://www.bmj.com/lookup/doi/10.1136/bmj.n436.
15. Zsichla L, Müller V. Risk factors of severe COVID-19: a review of host, viral and environmental factors. Viruses [Internet]. 2023;15(1):175. Available from: https://www.mdpi.com/1999-4915/15/1/175.
16. Fang X, Li S, Yu H, Wang P, Zhang Y, Chen Z, et al. Epidemiological, comorbidity factors with severity and prognosis of COVID-19: a systematic review and meta-analysis. Aging. 2020;12(13):12493–503.
17. Pijls BG, Jolani S, Atherley A, Derckx RT, JIR D, GHL F, et al. Demographic risk factors for COVID-19 infection, severity, ICU admission and death: a meta-analysis of 59 studies. BMJ Open [Internet]. 2021;11(1):e044640. Available from: https://bmjopen.bmj.com/lookup/doi/10.1136/bmjopen-2020-044640.
18. Du P, Li D, Wang A, Shen S, Ma Z, Li X. A systematic review and meta-analysis of risk factors associated with severity and death in COVID-19 patients. Uhanova J, editor. Can J Infect Dis Med Microbiol [Internet]. 2021;2021:1–12. Available from: https://www.hindawi.com/journals/cjidmm/2021/6660930/.
19. Booth A, Reed AB, Ponzo S, Yassaee A, Aral M, Plans D, et al. Population risk factors for severe disease and mortality in COVID-19: a global systematic review and meta-analysis. Madeddu G, editor. PLoS One [Internet]. 2021;16(3):e0247461. Available from: https://dx.plos.org/10.1371/journal.pone.0247461.

20. Schmitt CA, Tchkonia T, Niedernhofer LJ, Robbins PD, Kirkland JL, Lee S. COVID-19 and cellular senescence. Nat Rev Immunol [Internet]. 2023;23(4):251–63. Available from: https://www.nature.com/articles/s41577-022-00785-2.
21. Bartleson JM, Radenkovic D, Covarrubias AJ, Furman D, Winer DA, Verdin E. SARS-CoV-2, COVID-19 and the aging immune system. Nat Aging [Internet]. 2021;1(9):769–82. Available from: https://www.nature.com/articles/s43587-021-00114-7.
22. Di Toro F, Gjoka M, Di Lorenzo G, De Santo D, De Seta F, Maso G, et al. Impact of COVID-19 on maternal and neonatal outcomes: a systematic review and meta-analysis. Clin Microbiol Infect. Elsevier B.V. 2021;27:36–46.
23. Martinez-Portilla RJ, Sotiriadis A, Chatzakis C, Torres-Torres J, Espino y Sosa S, Sandoval-Mandujano K, et al. Pregnant women with SARS-CoV-2 infection are at higher risk of death and pneumonia: propensity score matched analysis of a nationwide prospective cohor. Ultrasound Obstetr Gynecol [Internet]. 2021;57(2):224–31. Available from: https://obgyn.onlinelibrary.wiley.com/doi/10.1002/uog.23575.
24. Kurki SN, Kantonen J, Kaivola K, Hokkanen L, Mäyränpää MI, Puttonen H, et al. APOE ε4 associates with increased risk of severe COVID-19, cerebral microhaemorrhages and post-COVID mental fatigue: a Finnish biobank, autopsy and clinical study. Acta Neuropathol Commun [Internet]. 2021;9(1):199. Available from: https://actaneurocomms.biomedcentral.com/articles/10.1186/s40478-021-01302-7.
25. Hernández Cordero AI, Li X, Milne S, Yang CX, Bossé Y, Joubert P, et al. Multi-omics highlights ABO plasma protein as a causal risk factor for COVID-19. Hum Genet [Internet]. 2021;140(6):969–79. Available from: https://link.springer.com/10.1007/s00439-021-02264-5.
26. Yip JQ, Oo A, Ng YL, Chin KL, Tan KK, Chu JJH, et al. The role of inflammatory gene polymorphisms in severe COVID-19: a review. Virol J [Internet]. 2024;21(1):327. Available from: https://virologyj.biomedcentral.com/articles/10.1186/s12985-024-02597-3.
27. Pardhan S, Wood S, Vaughan M, Trott M. The risk of COVID-19 related hospitalsation, intensive care unit admission and mortality in people with underlying asthma or COPD: a systematic review and meta-analysis. Front Med (Lausanne) [Internet]. 2021;8. Available from: https://www.frontiersin.org/articles/10.3389/fmed.2021.668808/full.
28. Vegivinti CTR, Evanson KW, Lyons H, Akosman I, Barrett A, Hardy N, et al. Efficacy of antiviral therapies for COVID-19: a systematic review of randomized controlled trials. BMC Infect Dis [Internet]. 2022;22(1):107. Available from: https://bmcinfectdis.biomedcentral.com/articles/10.1186/s12879-022-07068-0.
29. Barnes PJ. Inflammatory mechanisms in patients with chronic obstructive pulmonary disease. J Allergy Clin Immunol [Internet]. 2016;138(1):16–27. Available from: https://linkinghub.elsevier.com/retrieve/pii/S0091674916303621.
30. Filardo TD, Khan MR, Krawczyk N, Galitzer H, Karmen-Tuohy S, Coffee M, et al. Comorbidity and clinical factors associated with COVID-19 critical illness and mortality at a large public hospital in New York City in the early phase of the pandemic (March–April 2020). Cheungpasitporn W, editor. PLoS One [Internet]. 2020;15(11):e0242760. Available from: https://dx.plos.org/10.1371/journal.pone.0242760.
31. Chung YS, Lam CY, Tan PH, Tsang HF, Wong SCC. Comprehensive review of COVID-19: epidemiology, pathogenesis, advancement in diagnostic and detection techniques, and post-pandemic treatment strategies. Int J Mol Sci [Internet]. 2024;25(15):8155. Available from: https://www.mdpi.com/1422-0067/25/15/8155.
32. Jin Y, Yang H, Ji W, Wu W, Chen S, Zhang W, et al. Virology, epidemiology, pathogenesis, and control of COVID-19. Viruses [Internet]. 2020;12(4):372. Available from: https://www.mdpi.com/1999-4915/12/4/372.
33. Feldman C, Anderson R. The role of co-infections and secondary infections in patients with COVID-19. Pneumonia [Internet]. 2021;13(1):5. Available from: https://pneumonia.biomedcentral.com/articles/10.1186/s41479-021-00083-w.
34. Bertagnolio S, Thwin SS, Silva R, Nagarajan S, Jassat W, Fowler R, et al. Clinical features of, and risk factors for, severe or fatal COVID-19 among people living with HIV admitted

to hospital: analysis of data from the WHO Global Clinical Platform of COVID-19. Lancet HIV. 2022;9(7):e486–95.
35. Davies NG, Jarvis CI, Edmunds WJ, Jewell NP, Diaz-Ordaz K, Keogh RH. Increased mortality in community-tested cases of SARS-CoV-2 lineage B.1.1.7. Nature [Internet]. 2021;593(7858):270–4. Available from: https://www.nature.com/articles/s41586-021-03426-1.
36. Challen R, Brooks-Pollock E, Read JM, Dyson L, Tsaneva-Atanasova K, Danon L. Risk of mortality in patients infected with SARS-CoV-2 variant of concern 202012/1: matched cohort study. BMJ [Internet]. 2021;372:n579. Available from: https://www.bmj.com/lookup/doi/10.1136/bmj.n579.

COVID-19 Complications

14

M. A. Ashwini

14.1 Introduction

Coronavirus disease 2019 (COVID-19), caused by severe acute respiratory syndrome coronavirus 2 (SARS-CoV-2), rapidly evolved from a predominantly respiratory illness into a multisystem disease since its emergence in late 2019, profoundly disrupting global health systems and revealing extensive organ complications beyond the lungs [1–3]. While severe pneumonia and acute respiratory distress syndrome (ARDS) remain hallmarks of critical cases, COVID-19 triggers widespread vascular, thrombotic, neurological, cardiac, renal, and even oral manifestations through dysregulated immune responses, endothelial injury, and immunothrombosis—processes that collectively explain its high morbidity and mortality [4–9].

This chapter deals with essential knowledge of COVID-19 immunopathogenesis, acute/subacute/long-term complications across organ systems, variant-specific patterns (delta vs. omicron), and management strategies to ensure safe practice, facilitate patient referrals, and contribute to interdisciplinary recovery efforts amid persistent post-acute sequelae.

14.2 Immunopathogenesis

Severe complications of COVID-19 result from an abnormal immune response that links excessive inflammation, blood vessel injury, and abnormal clot formation, ultimately leading to damage of multiple organs [4–6].

M. A. Ashwini (✉)
Department of Neurovirology, National Institute of Mental Health and Neurosciences, Bengaluru, Karnataka, India

S. R. Prabhu et al. (eds.), *COVID-19 in Dental Practice*,
https://doi.org/10.1007/978-3-032-26000-0_14

Cytokine Storm and Immune Cell Dysfunction SARS-CoV-2 infection can trigger an exaggerated immune response known as a cytokine storm, with increased levels of inflammatory mediators such as interleukin (IL)-6, tumor necrotic factor (TNF)-α, IL-1β, and interferon (IFN)-γ. These elevated cytokines are associated with high C-reactive protein (CRP) and D-dimer levels and worse clinical outcomes. Persistent inflammation leads to a reduction and functional exhaustion of protective immune cells, including T lymphocytes and natural killer (NK) cells, weakening viral clearance while sustaining inflammation [5, 6].

Endothelial Injury, Oxidative Stress, and Complement Activation Inflammatory cytokines and direct viral infection damage endothelial cells lining blood vessels. This damage causes oxidative stress, loss of barrier function, and reduced anticoagulant activity, making blood vessels more prone to inflammation and clot formation. Activation of the complement system further amplifies vascular inflammation and tissue injury [4, 6, 9, 10].

Immunothrombosis and Organ Damage Endothelial dysfunction, platelet activation, and release of clot-promoting factors lead to immunothrombosis, a process in which immune responses and coagulation pathways interact to form micro-clots within blood vessels. These microthrombi impair blood flow, contributing to acute respiratory distress syndrome (ARDS), shock, and injury to organs such as the lungs, heart, kidneys, and brain [5, 6].

Multisystem Inflammatory Syndrome in Children (MIS-C) and Multisystem Involvement In some children, SARS-CoV-2 infection can cause MIS-C, characterized by widespread inflammation, blood vessel involvement, and immune cell activation. This condition can resemble vasculitis and affects multiple organs, including the heart [4, 5, 11, 12].

14.3 Classification of COVID-19 Complications

COVID-19 complications can be broadly categorized into:

1. Acute complications (during infection).
2. Subacute complications (within 4–12 weeks).
3. Long-term complications or post-acute sequelae of SARS-CoV-2 infection (>12 weeks).

Complications of COVID-19 can also be classified according to the organ or body system involved, including respiratory, cardiovascular, neuropsychiatric, renal, hematological, gastrointestinal, dermatological, endocrine, and metabolic systems [3, 13–15] (Fig. 14.1). The following section outlines the effects of COVID-19 on each of these systems, along with the probable pathogenic mechanisms and corresponding therapeutic strategies [16–18] (Table 14.1).

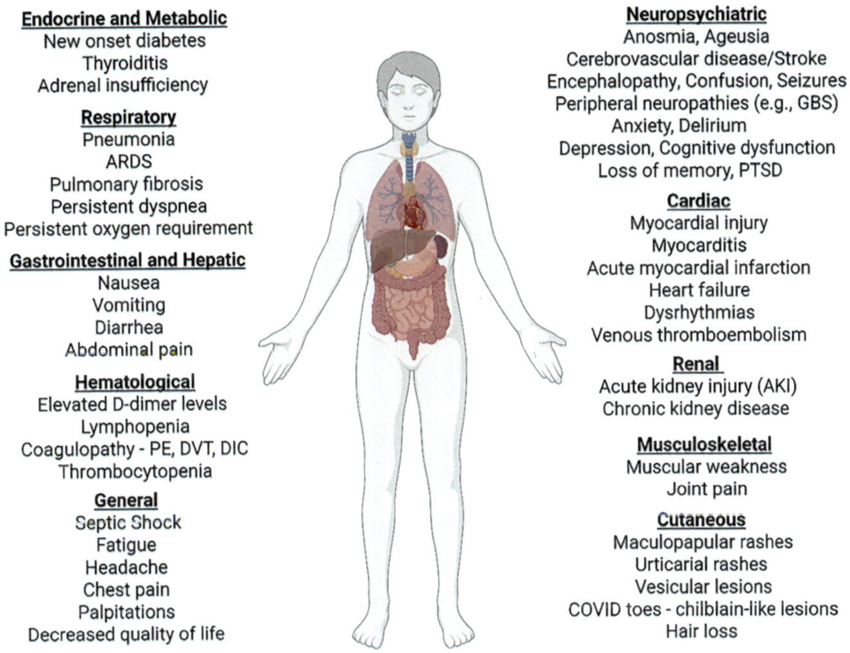

Fig. 14.1 Complications of COVID-19 (Created in https://BioRender.com). ARDS Acute Respiratory Distress Syndrome, PE Pulmonary Embolism, DVT Deep Vein Thrombosis, DIC Disseminated Intravascular Coagulopathy, GBS Guillain-Barré syndrome, PTSD Posttraumatic stress disorder

Respiratory Complications The respiratory system is the primary target of SARS-CoV-2 infection, with disease severity ranging from mild upper respiratory tract involvement to severe pneumonia and acute respiratory distress syndrome (ARDS). The virus primarily enters host cells through angiotensin-converting enzyme 2 (ACE2) receptors expressed on airway epithelial cells and alveolar pneumocytes, leading to direct cytopathic effects and immune-mediated injury [19].

Common respiratory manifestations include fever, persistent cough (often lasting beyond 8 weeks), dyspnea, and hypoxemia. Pneumonia is the most frequent complication observed in moderate to severe cases and is characterized by radiological findings such as bilateral ground-glass opacities and infiltrates. Severe cases may progress to ARDS, marked by diffuse alveolar damage, pulmonary edema, and reduced lung compliance, often necessitating oxygen supplementation or mechanical ventilation [20].

Table 14.1 COVID-19 complications: clinical manifestations, risk factors, probable pathogenesis, and clinical management

COVID-19 complications	Clinical manifestations	Risk factors	Probable pathogenesis	Clinical management
Respiratory	Fever, persistent cough, dyspnea (breathlessness), hypoxia, chest pain, pneumonia, ARDS, chronic pulmonary sequelae (pulmonary fibrosis and persistent dyspnea)	Elder age (>60 years), Male gender, pulmonary consolidation. Comorbidities—Hypertension, obesity, diabetes, chronic obstructive lung disease/chronic lung disease	Virus attaches to ACE2 receptors on airway epithelial cells and alveolar pneumocytes, leading to direct cytopathic effects, vascular thrombosis, immune-mediated injury and fibrosis	CT scan-ground glass opacities; supportive care, oxygen therapy, corticosteroids, antiviral agents, and immunomodulators, long-term pulmonary rehabilitation
Cardiac	Chest pain, palpitations, dyspnea, myocardial injury, myocarditis, acute myocardial infarction, ventricular dysfunction, acute/decompensated heart failure, acute coronary syndrome, arrhythmias/dysrhythmias, venous thromboembolism, sudden cardiac arrest	Older age; Comorbidities—Diabetes, cardiovascular, lung, and renal diseases; Systemic inflammation; Coagulation abnormalities; Severe illness; multiorgan dysfunction; immobility; medication interactions-remdesivir, ribavirin, chloroquine, corticosteroid etc.	Direct viral invasion, downregulation of ACE2, inflammation and immunologic response affecting structural integrity of myocardium, pericardium, and conduction system. Myocardial fibrosis or scarring lead to arrythmias	Serial clinical and imaging evaluation with ECG and echocardiography at 4–12 weeks. Advanced cardiac imaging considered on case- by-case basis. COVID-19 patients with cardiovascular disease experience poorer outcomes
Neurological	*Mild symptoms*: Headache, myalgia, weakness, vertigo, chemosensory dysfunction (anosmia/ageusia) *Serious complications*: Seizures, hypoxic encephalopathy, and cerebrovascular disease (stroke). Cognitive function impairment—Confusion, short-term memory loss, dizziness, inability to concentrate/attention deficits Encephalopathy, meningoencephalitis, GBS, peripheral neuropathy, myasthenia gravis, myositis, relapse of MS, corticospinal tract signs, autonomic dysfunction (POTS)	Advanced age, comorbidities—Hypertension, diabetes, cardiovascular disease, neurodegenerative disease (Alzheimer, Parkinson), severe COVID-19, prolonged ICU stay, mechanical ventilation	Direct virus invasion through ACE2 and TMPRSS2 receptors, hyper-inflammatory reactions, multi-system failure, prothrombotic states and immune-mediated processes (cytokine storm), hypoxia and mitochondrial dysfunction lead to microstructural damage	Multidisciplinary approach integrating neurology, infectious disease, critical care, and rehabilitation expertise. Early identification and evaluation: Detailed neurological examination, neuroimaging (CT/MRI), and, when indicated, CSF analysis and EEG. Supportive care and symptomatic treatment. Targeted management for syndromes

Psychiatric	*Acute phase (4 weeks)*: anxiety, delirium *Mid-term (4–12 weeks)*: anxiety, depression, sleep disturbances *Long-term (>12 weeks)*: chronic sleep disturbances, persistent depression, PTSD, chronic anxiety	Older age, female, diabetes, hypertension, smoking, obesity, genetic predisposition, severe COVID-19 requiring oxygen support or mechanical ventilation, social isolation, economic stress, special populations—Preexisting psychiatric disorders (mood disorders, schizophrenia, alcohol use disorder); children and adolescents; health care workers; pregnant women and infants	Neuroinvasive properties; cytokine storm and microglia activation; inflammation and neurotransmitter systems; prothrombotic state and formation of microthrombi	Psychological counseling, antidepressants, and anti-anxiety medications Physical exercise, dietary supplements with antioxidant, anti-inflammatory, and neuroprotective properties such as vitamins A, C, D, E, B12, omega-3 fatty acids, zinc, or selenium Cognitive behavioral therapy Long-term follow-up
Gastrointestinal and hepatic	Nausea, vomiting, diarrhea, abdominal pain, and liver involvement	Prolonged viral shedding, COVID-19 therapies—Chloroquine and hydroxychloroquine (hepatotoxicity); lopinavir/ritonavir (diarrhea and acute liver failure); favipiravir and remdesivir (mild to moderate hepatic effects)	Viral invasion of gastrointestinal mucosa, systemic inflammation, or drug toxicity Liver—Viral replication, cytokine-mediated damage, or hepatotoxic drugs	Routine monitoring of GI symptoms and liver function in patients receiving hepatotoxic treatments. Early recognition and supportive management
Renal	Severe acute kidney injury (AKI), chronic kidney disease	Hospitalized patients, critically ill patients with acute COVID-19, severe infections requiring mechanical ventilation APOL1 risk alleles	Virus infects renal tissue, causing acute tubular necrosis and COVID-19-associated nephropathy (COVAN), Thrombotic microangiopathy	Early follow-up with nephrologists after discharge for patients with COVID-19 and AKI
Endocrine and metabolic	New-onset diabetes or worsen glycemic control in patients with preexisting diabetes Subacute thyroiditis, adrenal insufficiency, and hypothalamic-pituitary axis dysfunction	Preexisting diabetes, obesity, and metabolic syndromes; corticosteroid therapy, critical illness, prolonged ICU stay	Direct viral damage to pancreatic β-cells, systemic inflammation, and immune-mediated injury	Targeted laboratory evaluation and further managed in endocrinology. Early recognition and long-term monitoring
Cutaneous	Maculopapular, urticarial, vesicular, and pseudo-chilblain or "COVID toes" lesions, hair loss	Preexisting dermatoses, drug-related eruptions	Immune and vascular involvement	Nailfold capillaroscopy, symptomatic therapy

Abbreviations: *COVID-19* Coronavirus Disease 2019, *ARDS* Acute Respiratory Distress Syndrome, *ACE2* angiotensin-converting enzyme 2, *CT* Computed Tomography, *ECG* Electrocardiography, *ICU* Intensive care unit, *TMPRSS2* Transmembrane protease, serine 2, *GBS* Guillain-Barré syndrome, *MS* Multiple sclerosis, *MRI* Magnetic Resonance Imaging, *CSF* Cerebrospinal fluid, *EEG* Electroencephalography, *PTDS* Posttraumatic stress disorder

Chronic pulmonary sequelae, including pulmonary fibrosis and persistent dyspnea, have been documented among recovered patients. Advanced age (over 60 years) and the presence of pulmonary consolidations on imaging are associated with a higher risk of post-COVID-19 pulmonary complications [16–20].

Management primarily focuses on supportive care, oxygen therapy, corticosteroids, antiviral agents, and immunomodulators to mitigate lung injury and improve oxygenation. Long-term pulmonary rehabilitation plays a crucial role in enhancing functional recovery and quality of life among survivors with chronic respiratory impairment [3, 20].

Cardiovascular Complications COVID-19 is associated with a wide range of cardiovascular complications, including myocardial injury and myocarditis, acute myocardial infarction (AMI), heart failure, dysrhythmias, and venous thromboembolic events (VTE). The underlying mechanisms involve direct viral invasion via ACE2 receptors on cardiac tissue, systemic inflammation, cytokine-mediated injury, immune dysregulation, and hypercoagulability. Preexisting cardiovascular disease (CVD) increases susceptibility to severe infection and mortality [21].

Myocardial injury, reflected by elevated troponin levels, occurs in 7–17% of hospitalized patients and up to 30% in ICU settings. Myocarditis presents with chest pain, dyspnea, arrhythmia, and left ventricular dysfunction, often mimicking acute coronary syndrome (ACS). ECG findings include nonspecific ST–T changes, while echocardiography may reveal global or focal wall motion abnormalities. Acute heart failure and cardiogenic shock may develop in critically ill patients [21, 22].

AMI can result from plaque rupture or microthrombi due to systemic inflammation and endothelial injury. Dysrhythmias, particularly sinus tachycardia and atrial fibrillation, are common and linked to hypoxia, fever, or metabolic stress. VTE, including pulmonary embolism, arises from COVID-19–associated hypercoagulability and prolonged immobilization [21, 22].

Neurological Complications COVID-19 has been associated with a wide spectrum of neurological manifestations involving both the central and peripheral nervous systems. Common symptoms include anosmia (loss of smell) and ageusia (loss of taste), often occurring early or even in isolation. Central nervous system (CNS) complications comprise encephalopathy, encephalitis, seizures, stroke, and acute disseminated encephalomyelitis (ADEM). Peripheral nervous system (PNS) involvement includes Guillain-Barré syndrome (GBS) and other acute neuropathies [23].

The mechanisms underlying these manifestations include direct viral invasion via ACE2 receptors, immune-mediated inflammation, cytokine storm, and systemic complications such as hypoxia, metabolic derangements, and coagulopathy. In large cohort studies, up to 31% of hospitalized patients exhibited neurological symptoms, including encephalopathy, psychiatric disturbances, and cerebrovascular events. Ischemic stroke is particularly notable, sometimes occurring in young individuals without traditional risk factors, likely due to COVID-19 associated hypercoagulability and endothelial injury [23].

Encephalitis and encephalopathy may present with altered mental status, confusion, or seizures. CSF findings are often nonspecific, and MRI may reveal focal or diffuse abnormalities. GBS typically develops within weeks of infection, suggesting a post-infectious immune-mediated mechanism, with most cases responding to intravenous immunoglobulin or corticosteroids [23, 24].

Long-term sequelae include cognitive dysfunction, mood disturbances, and post-COVID fatigue, collectively termed neuro-COVID. Early recognition and multidisciplinary management are essential to prevent permanent deficits. Ongoing research aims to clarify the pathophysiological basis of these complications and guide targeted neuroprotective therapies [24].

Psychiatric Complications The COVID-19 pandemic has significantly affected mental health, aggravating preexisting psychiatric disorders and triggering new-onset conditions in both infected individuals and the general population. Psychiatric manifestations evolve through acute (0–4 weeks: anxiety, stress reactions, delirium), mid-term (4–12 weeks: depression, sleep disturbances, cognitive dysfunction), and long-term (>12 weeks: post-traumatic stress disorder, fatigue) phases.

Vulnerable groups such as healthcare workers, children, adolescents, and pregnant women face unique psychosocial and biological stressors. Psychosocial factors including social isolation, lockdowns, financial instability, and fear of infection have led to widespread anxiety, depression, and burnout. In children and the elderly, disrupted routines and confinement have worsened behavioral and cognitive symptoms.

Biologically, SARS-CoV-2 may exert neuroinvasive effects through neuroinflammation and cytokine-mediated pathways, leading to neurotransmitter dysregulation and vascular injury. Elevated cytokines such as IL-6 and TNF-α, along with genetic predispositions and comorbidities like obesity and diabetes, may heighten vulnerability to psychiatric and neurological complications.

Management includes psychological therapies, antidepressants, and anxiolytics, complemented by exercise, nutritional supplementation, and cognitive behavioral therapy, which have shown benefit in reducing fatigue and distress. Long-term mental health surveillance and integrative care are essential to mitigate the enduring psychiatric impact of COVID-19 [25].

Gastrointestinal and Hepatic Complications Gastrointestinal and hepatic manifestations are frequent in COVID-19, affecting around 10% of patients. Common symptoms include nausea, vomiting, diarrhea, and abdominal pain, attributed to viral invasion of the gastrointestinal mucosa, systemic inflammation, or drug toxicity. Liver involvement, seen in approximately 15% of cases, is marked by elevated aspartate and alanine transaminases due to viral replication, cytokine-mediated damage, or hepatotoxic drugs [18, 26].

COVID-19 therapies can exacerbate these effects—chloroquine and hydroxychloroquine occasionally cause hepatotoxicity; lopinavir/ritonavir induces dose-dependent diarrhea and, rarely, acute liver failure; favipiravir and remdesivir have mild to moderate hepatic effects. Several agents also interact with CYP enzymes and transport proteins, influencing drug metabolism. Routine monitoring of gastrointestinal symptoms and liver function is essential, especially in patients receiving potentially hepatotoxic treatments. Early recognition and supportive management of these complications are crucial to prevent disease progression and improve clinical outcomes [26].

Renal Complications Renal complications in COVID-19 are common, with severe acute kidney injury (AKI) requiring renal replacement therapy (RRT) in up to 31% of critically ill patients. Among those needing RRT, 27–64% recover dialysis independence within 28 days, though mortality remains high. At 6 months, 35% show reduced estimated glomerular filtration rate (eGFR), and 13% develop new-onset renal impairment. SARS-CoV-2 can infect renal tissue, causing acute tubular necrosis and COVID-19-associated nephropathy (COVAN), often linked to APOL1 risk alleles. Thrombotic microangiopathy may worsen injury. Persistent dysfunction warrants long-term nephrology follow-up for early intervention and improved renal outcomes [27].

Hematological Complications COVID-19 is frequently associated with hematological abnormalities that reflect disease severity and prognosis. Elevated D-dimer levels are strongly correlated with increased risk of thrombosis, severe disease, and mortality. Critically ill patients may develop disseminated intravascular coagulation (DIC), reflecting widespread endothelial injury and hypercoagulability. Lymphopenia is a characteristic laboratory finding, indicating immune dysregulation and poor outcomes. Post-acute COVID-19 phases may still exhibit thromboembolic events, though typically <5% in retrospective studies. The duration of the infection-induced hyperinflammatory and prothrombotic state remains uncertain. Extended thromboprophylaxis using direct oral anticoagulants or low-molecular-weight heparin can be considered in high-risk individuals, especially those with immobility, active malignancy, or persistently elevated D-dimer levels (>2× upper limit of normal). Close monitoring and individualized management of coagulation parameters are crucial to prevent thrombotic complications and improve recovery in COVID-19 patients [13, 15].

Endocrine and Metabolic Complications COVID-19 has significant effects on the endocrine and metabolic systems. It may induce new-onset diabetes or worsen glycemic control in patients with preexisting diabetes, likely due to direct viral damage to pancreatic β-cells, systemic inflammation, and corticosteroid therapy. Cases of subacute thyroiditis, adrenal insufficiency, and hypothalamic-pituitary axis dysfunction have been reported, reflecting viral or immune-mediated injury. Post-infection endocrine sequelae such as persistent hyperglycemia, thyroid dysfunction, and bone demineralization may also occur. Patients presenting with new-onset diabetes without traditional risk factors, unexplained thyroid symptoms, or suspected adrenal suppression should undergo targeted laboratory evaluation and be referred to endocrinology for further management. Early recognition and long-term monitoring of endocrine complications are essential for optimal recovery and metabolic control in COVID-19 survivors [13].

Dermatological Complications Dermatological manifestations are increasingly recognized in COVID-19, reflecting immune and vascular involvement. Common findings include maculopapular (47%), urticarial (19%), vesicular (9%), and pseudo-chilblain or "COVID toes" (19%) lesions, while livedo or necrosis (6%) occurs in severe cases. Vesicular eruptions often appear early, whereas pseudo-chilblain lesions emerge later. Hair loss, seen in about 20% of survivors, typically represents post-infectious telogen effluvium. These cutaneous signs may correlate with disease severity—acral lesions with milder illness and necrotic patterns with severe disease. Reported COVID-19-related skin findings also include morbilliform rashes, urticarial eruptions, and papulo-squamous lesions. Urticarial and morbilliform rashes are usually short-lived, whereas pernio (6.8%) and livedo reticularis can persist beyond 60 days. Altered peripheral microangiopathy may underlie chilblain-like lesions in long COVID-19, and nailfold capillaroscopy has been suggested to assess microvascular hemodynamics. Drug-related eruptions and exacerbation of pre-existing dermatoses should also be considered during evaluation [13, 15, 18].

Multisystem Inflammatory Syndrome in Children (MIS-C) It is also known as pediatric inflammatory multisystem syndrome temporally associated with SARS-CoV-2 (PIMS-TS) and occurs in children and adolescents (0–19 years), presenting with fever (≥3 days), elevated inflammatory markers, and multisystem involvement, along with evidence of current or recent COVID 19 infection or exposure. Common manifestations include rash, non-purulent conjunctivitis, mucocutaneous inflammation, hypotension or shock, myocardial dysfunction, coronary artery aneurysms, coagulopathy, and gastrointestinal symptoms. MIS-C usually appears 2–6 weeks after SARS-CoV-2 infection and is more frequent among children of African, Afro-Caribbean, or Hispanic origin. Neurological features such as headache, encephalopathy, seizures, and stroke may also occur. The condition likely reflects a post-infectious immune dysregulation involving cytokine storm, immune complex formation, complement activation, and superantigen-mediated T-cell activation. Management includes intravenous immunoglobulin, corticosteroids, and low-dose aspirin, with anticoagulation for those with significant cardiac involvement. Serial echocardiography and cardiac MRI are advised to monitor coronary and ventricular function [11–13, 15].

Mucormycosis and COVID-19 Mucormycosis, an opportunistic fungal infection caused by *Mucorales* species, emerged as a serious complication during the COVID-19 pandemic, particularly in India. It predominantly affects patients with uncontrolled diabetes, prolonged corticosteroid use, or immunosuppression. COVID-19-associated immune dysregulation, hypoxia, acidosis, and elevated serum iron create a favorable environment for fungal proliferation. The infection commonly involves the rhino-orbital-cerebral region, but pulmonary and disseminated forms may also occur. Clinical features include facial pain, nasal congestion with black discharge, visual disturbances, and neurological deficits. Early diagnosis, prompt antifungal therapy (amphotericin B), strict glycemic control, and surgical debridement are crucial for improving survival outcomes [28].

14.4 Impact of SARS-CoV-2 Variants: Differential Complication Patterns (Delta vs. Omicron)

The emergence of successive SARS-CoV-2 variants has reshaped the spectrum of COVID-19 complications, with the delta and omicron lineages showing distinct virological and clinical profiles [29, 30]. Early comparative data consistently demonstrated that infection with the delta variant was associated with a substantially higher risk of hospitalization, need for advanced respiratory support, and death than infection with omicron, particularly in unvaccinated or minimally immunized populations, reflecting greater intrinsic virulence and a stronger propensity for severe lower-respiratory tract disease [29, 31, 32]. In contrast, omicron and its subvariants, which rapidly displaced delta and have remained the globally dominant lineages since late 2021, are characterized by markedly increased transmissibility and substantial immune escape but, on average, lower risks of progression to hypoxemic respiratory failure and critical illness [29, 32].

14.5 Conclusion

- COVID-19 is a multisystem disease, with complications driven by interconnected hyperinflammation, endothelial injury, and immunothrombosis, leading to acute and long-term organ damage.
- Comprehensive understanding of its pathophysiology and organ-specific effects is crucial for timely diagnosis, effective management, and prevention of long-term sequelae.
- Disease severity and complication patterns vary by viral variant, with the delta variant associated with higher virulence and the omicron variant characterized by immune evasion, influenced by evolving population immunity.
- Early identification and appropriate referral of patients with persistent post-COVID symptoms, such as chronic fatigue or pulmonary fibrosis, can improve outcomes.
- Multidisciplinary care, vaccination, and structured rehabilitation play vital roles in reducing long-term morbidity and improving quality of life among COVID-19 survivors.

References

1. Hu B, Guo H, Zhou P, Shi ZL. Characteristics of SARS-CoV-2 and COVID-19. Nat Rev Microbiol. 2021;19(3):141–54. https://doi.org/10.1038/s41579-020-00459-7. Epub 2020 Oct 6. Erratum in: Nat Rev Microbiol. 2022 May;20(5):315. 10.1038/s41579-022-00711-2. PMID: 33024307; PMCID: PMC7537588.
2. Lai CC, Shih TP, Ko WC, Tang HJ, Hsueh PR. Severe acute respiratory syndrome coronavirus 2 (SARS-CoV-2) and coronavirus disease-2019 (COVID-19): the epidemic and the challenges. Int J Antimicrob Agents. 2020;55(3):105924. https://doi.org/10.1016/j.ijantimicag.2020.105924. Epub 2020 Feb 17. PMID: 32081636; PMCID: PMC7127800.
3. World Health Organization (WHO). Clinical management of COVID-19: living guideline, 13 January 2023. Geneva: World Health Organization; 2023. (WHO/2019-nCoV/clinical/2023.1).
4. Chang R, Mamun A, Dominic A, Le NT. SARS-CoV-2 mediated endothelial dysfunction: the potential role of chronic oxidative stress. Front Physiol. 2021;11:605908. https://doi.org/10.3389/fphys.2020.605908. PMID: 33519510; PMCID: PMC7844210.
5. Bonaventura A, Vecchié A, Dagna L, Martinod K, Dixon DL, Van Tassell BW, Dentali F, Montecucco F, Massberg S, Levi M, Abbate A. Endothelial dysfunction and immunothrombosis as key pathogenic mechanisms in COVID-19. Nat Rev Immunol. 2021;21(5):319–29. https://doi.org/10.1038/s41577-021-00536-9. Epub 2021 Apr 6. PMID: 33824483; PMCID: PMC8023349.
6. Fujimura Y, Holland LZ. COVID-19 microthrombosis: unusually large VWF multimers are a platform for activation of the alternative complement pathway under cytokine storm. Int J Hematol. 2022;115(4):457–69. https://doi.org/10.1007/s12185-022-03324-w. Epub 2022 Mar 22. PMID: 35316498; PMCID: PMC8938647.
7. Georgieva E, Ananiev J, Yovchev Y, Arabadzhiev G, Abrashev H, Abrasheva D, Atanasov V, Kostandieva R, Mitev M, Petkova-Parlapanska K, Karamalakova Y, Koleva-Korkelia I, Tsoneva V, Nikolova G. COVID-19 complications: oxidative stress, inflammation, and mitochondrial and endothelial dysfunction. Int J Mol Sci. 2023;24(19):14876. https://doi.org/10.3390/ijms241914876. PMID: 37834324; PMCID: PMC10573237.
8. Shahgolzari M, Yavari A, Arjeini Y, Miri SM, Darabi A, Mozaffari Nejad AS, Keshavarz M. Immunopathology and Immunopathogenesis of COVID-19, what we know and what we should learn. Gene Rep. 2021;25:101417. https://doi.org/10.1016/j.genrep.2021.101417. Epub 2021 Nov 5. PMID: 34778602; PMCID: PMC8570409.
9. Berber NK, Kurt O, Altıntop Geçkil A, Erdem M, Kıran TR, Otlu Ö, Ecin SM, İn E. Evaluation of oxidative stress and endothelial dysfunction in COVID-19 patients. Medicina (Kaunas). 2024;60(7):1041. https://doi.org/10.3390/medicina60071041. PMID: 39064471; PMCID: PMC11279166.
10. Wu J, Xu S, Li Z, Cong B, Yang Z, Yang Z, Gao W, Liu S, Yu Z, Xu S, Li N, Hou J, Wang G, Cao X, Liu S. SARS-CoV-2 enhances complement-mediated endothelial injury via the suppression of membrane complement regulatory proteins. Emerg Microbes Infect. 2025;14(1):2467781. https://doi.org/10.1080/22221751.2025.2467781. Epub 2025 Feb 28. PMID: 39945674; PMCID: PMC11873982.
11. Kouo T, Chaisawangwong W. SARS-CoV-2 as a superantigen in multisystem inflammatory syndrome in children. J Clin Invest. 2021;131(10):e149327. https://doi.org/10.1172/JCI149327. PMID: 33844652; PMCID: PMC8121522.
12. Lam KP, Chiñas M, Julé AM, Taylor M, Ohashi M, Benamar M, Crestani E, Son MBF, Chou J, Gebhart C, Chatila T, Newburger J, Randolph A, Gutierrez-Arcelus M, Henderson LA. SARS-CoV-2-specific T cell responses in patients with multisystem inflammatory syndrome in children. Clin Immunol. 2022;243:109106. https://doi.org/10.1016/j.clim.2022.109106. Epub 2022 Aug 30. PMID: 36049601; PMCID: PMC9423880.
13. Nalbandian A, Sehgal K, Gupta A, Madhavan MV, McGroder C, Gupta A, et al. Post-acute COVID-19 syndrome. Nat Med. 2021;27:601–15. https://doi.org/10.1038/s41591-021-01283-z.

14. Greenhalgh T, Knight M, A'Court C, Buxton M, Husain L. Management of post-acute covid-19 in primary care. BMJ. 2020;370:m3026. https://doi.org/10.1136/bmj.m3026. PMID: 32784198.
15. Mallah SI, Ghorab OK, Al-Salmi S, Abdellatif OS, Tharmaratnam T, Iskandar MA, et al. COVID-19: breaking down a global health crisis. Ann Clin Microbiol Antimicrob. 2021;20(1):35. https://doi.org/10.1186/s12941-021-00438-7. PMID: 34006330; PMCID: PMC8129964.
16. Zhang JJ, Dong X, Liu GH, Gao YD. Risk and protective factors for COVID-19 morbidity, severity, and mortality. Clin Rev Allergy Immunol. 2023;64(1):90–107. https://doi.org/10.1007/s12016-022-08921-5. Epub 2022 Jan 19. PMID: 35044620; PMCID: PMC8767775.
17. Chams N, Chams S, Badran R, Shams A, Araji A, Raad M, et al. COVID-19: a multidisciplinary review. Front Public Health. 2020;8:383. https://doi.org/10.3389/fpubh.2020.00383. PMID: 32850602; PMCID: PMC7403483.
18. Garg M, Maralakunte M, Garg S, Dhooria S, Sehgal I, Bhalla AS, et al. The conundrum of 'Long-COVID-19': a narrative review. Int J Gen Med. 2021;14:2491–506. https://doi.org/10.2147/IJGM.S316708. PMID: 34163217; PMCID: PMC8214209.
19. Huang C, Wang Y, Li X, Ren L, Zhao J, Hu Y, et al. Clinical features of patients infected with 2019 novel coronavirus in Wuhan, China. Lancet. 2020;395(10223):497–506. https://doi.org/10.1016/S0140-6736(20)30183-5. Epub 2020 Jan 24. Erratum in: Lancet. 2020 Feb 15;395(10223):496. 10.1016/S0140-6736(20)30252-X. PMID: 31986264; PMCID: PMC7159299.
20. Seyoum AB, Tegegnework SS, Mengistu MM, Mekonnen TD, Asabel AM, Dagnaw AG, et al. Post-COVID-19 pulmonary complications among recovered COVID-19 patients: a cross-sectional study from Addis Ababa, Ethiopia. BMC Pulm Med. 2023;23(1):409. https://doi.org/10.1186/s12890-023-02731-x. PMID: 37891593; PMCID: PMC10612275.
21. Long B, Brady WJ, Koyfman A, Gottlieb M. Cardiovascular complications in COVID-19. Am J Emerg Med. 2020;38(7):1504–7. https://doi.org/10.1016/j.ajem.2020.04.048. Epub 2020 Apr 18. PMID: 32317203; PMCID: PMC7165109.
22. Louis DW, Saad M, Vijayakumar S, Ilyas S, Kokkirala A, Aronow HD. The cardiovascular manifestations of COVID-19. Heart Fail Clin. 2023;19(2):153–61. https://doi.org/10.1016/j.hfc.2022.08.001. PMID: 36863807; PMCID: PMC9973545.
23. Ellul MA, Benjamin L, Singh B, Lant S, Michael BD, Easton A, et al. Neurological associations of COVID-19. Lancet Neurol. 2020;19(9):767–83. https://doi.org/10.1016/S1474-4422(20)30221-0. Epub 2020 Jul 2. PMID: 32622375; PMCID: PMC7332267.
24. Valderas C, Méndez G, Echeverría A, Suarez N, Julio K, Sandoval F. COVID-19 and neurologic manifestations: a synthesis from the child neurologist's corner. World J Pediatr. 2022;18(6):373–82. https://doi.org/10.1007/s12519-022-00550-4. Epub 2022. PMID: 35476245; PMCID: PMC9044375.
25. Ahmed GK, Ramadan HKA, Khedr EM. Short- and long-term psychiatric complications of COVID-19. Egypt J Neurol Psychiatry Neurosurg. 2025;61:40. https://doi.org/10.1186/s41983-025-00972-7.
26. Sultan S, Altayar O, Siddique SM, Davitkov P, Feuerstein JD, Lim JK, et al. AGA institute rapid review of the gastrointestinal and liver manifestations of COVID-19, meta-analysis of international data, and recommendations for the consultative management of patients with COVID-19. Gastroenterology. 2020;159(1):320–334.e27. https://doi.org/10.1053/j.gastro.2020.05.001. Epub 2020. PMID: 32407808; PMCID: PMC7212965.
27. Cheng Y, Luo R, Wang K, Zhang M, Wang Z, Dong L, et al. Kidney disease is associated with in-hospital death of patients with COVID-19. Kidney Int. 2020;97(5):829–38. https://doi.org/10.1016/j.kint.2020.03.005. Epub 2020. PMID: 32247631; PMCID: PMC7110296.
28. Sen M, Honavar SG, Bansal R, Sengupta S, Rao R, Kim U, et al., members of the Collaborative OPAI-IJO Study on Mucormycosis in COVID-19 (COSMIC) Study Group. Epidemiology, clinical profile, management, and outcome of COVID-19-associated rhino-orbital-cerebral mucormycosis in 2826 patients in India - Collaborative OPAI-IJO Study on Mucormycosis

in COVID-19 (COSMIC), Report 1. Indian J Ophthalmol. 2021;69(7):1670–92. https://doi.org/10.4103/ijo.IJO_1565_21. PMID: 34156034; PMCID: PMC8374756.

29. Relan P, Motaze NV, Kothari K, Askie L, Le Polain O, Van Kerkhove MD, Diaz J, Tirupakuzhi Vijayaraghavan BK. Severity and outcomes of Omicron variant of SARS-CoV-2 compared to Delta variant and severity of Omicron sublineages: a systematic review and metanalysis. BMJ Glob Health. 2023;8(7):e012328. https://doi.org/10.1136/bmjgh-2023-012328. PMID: 37419502; PMCID: PMC10347449.
30. Andre M, Lau LS, Pokharel MD, Ramelow J, Owens F, Souchak J, Akkaoui J, Ales E, Brown H, Shil R, Nazaire V, Manevski M, Paul NP, Esteban-Lopez M, Ceyhan Y, El-Hage N. From alpha to omicron: how different variants of concern of the SARS-coronavirus-2 impacted the world. Biology (Basel). 2023;12(9):1267. https://doi.org/10.3390/biology12091267. PMID: 37759666; PMCID: PMC10525159.
31. Meesoontorn S, Pakdee W, Cheranakhorn C, Sangkaew S. Understanding the change of in-hospital mortality and respiratory failure between Delta and Omicron waves from a tertiary hospital in Southern Thailand: a retrospective cohort study. IJID Reg. 2024;13:100446. https://doi.org/10.1016/j.ijregi.2024.100446. PMID: 39430602; PMCID: PMC11490909.
32. Thi Hong Nguyen N, Ou TY, Huy LD, Shih CL, Chang YM, Phan TP, Huang CC. A global analysis of COVID-19 infection fatality rate and its associated factors during the Delta and Omicron variant periods: an ecological study. Front Public Health. 2023;11:1145138. https://doi.org/10.3389/fpubh.2023.1145138. PMID: 37333556; PMCID: PMC10274323.

Management of COVID-19 Patients 15

Shivdas Rajaram Naik

15.1 Introduction

The treatment for COVID-19 has evolved since the beginning of the pandemic and now mainly consists of antivirals, immunomodulatory agents, oxygen therapy, supportive care, and prevention and management of complications [1, 2]. The treatment varies depending on the phase and severity of the illness. Antivirals are most effective in the early phase of disease, when there is active viral replication, whereas in the inflammatory or cytokine-storm phase, immunomodulatory agents take the lead. Certain principles can guide optimal therapy for patients with COVID-19 (Box 15.1).

Box 15.1: General Principles in the Management of COVID-19 Patients

1. Appropriate patient stratification based on severity and need for admission.
2. Timely antiviral therapy.
3. Appropriate anti-inflammatory therapy.
4. Antithrombotic prophylaxis.
5. Oxygen therapy.
6. Supportive care.

S. R. Naik (✉)
Department of Infectious Diseases, Kasturba Medical College, MAHE, Manipal, India
e-mail: shivdas.naik@manipal.edu

S. R. Prabhu et al. (eds.), *COVID-19 in Dental Practice*,
https://doi.org/10.1007/978-3-032-26000-0_15

15.2 Patient Stratification

Not all patients with COVID-19 will require hospitalisation or treatment. Disease severity guides the need for treatment or hospitalisation, as well as whether the patient is at higher risk for severe disease. Conditions at risk of developing severe disease are listed in Box 15.2.

Box 15.2: Conditions at Risk of Developing Severe Disease [4, 5]

- *Underlying structural or functional lung disease*
  Bronchial asthma, bronchiectasis, chronic obstructive airway disease and interstitial lung disease.
- *Liver disease*
  Cirrhosis, non-alcoholic fatty liver disease, alcoholic liver disease and autoimmune hepatitis.
- *Heart diseases*
  Coronary artery disease, cardiomyopathies and heart failure.
- *Other*
  Cystic fibrosis, diabetes, obesity and pregnancy.
- *Immunocompromised states*
  HIV, solid or haematopoietic stem cell transplant patients and those on corticosteroids or other immunosuppressants.

Once the diagnosis is confirmed, stratify patients into asymptomatic/mild, moderate and severe disease.

- The patients with mild disease, without the risk for severe disease or mortality, are usually managed on an OPD basis, with advice for home isolation and self-monitoring [1, 3].
- Patients with mild illness but at risk of severe disease are to be admitted to the dedicated COVID-19 wards in the hospital.
- Patients with moderate to severe disease are admitted to a hospital ward that provides a level of care (HDU and intensive care unit (ICU)) based on the severity of the disease.
- If the patients with mild disease are hospitalised for other reasons and do not require supplemental oxygen, then they should be managed as non-hospitalised patients.

15.3 Antiviral Therapy

Antivirals are most effective in the early phase of the disease, where there is active viral replication. Whenever indicated, they should ideally be started within 3–5 days of symptom onset and no later than day 10. Remdesivir is the only drug approved for treatment and is used in moderate to severe disease and for high-risk individuals. Nirmatrelvir-ritonavir and molnupiravir are for mild disease in high-risk patients. The antiviral summary is provided in Table 15.1.

Table 15.1 Drugs used for the treatment of COVID-19

Drug	Mechanism of action	Dose and duration	Adverse events	Contraindications	Special remarks
Remdesivir	Inhibits viral RNA-dependent RNA polymerase → halts replication	200 mg IV on Day 1, then 100 mg IV daily for 5–10 days	Elevated liver enzymes, bradycardia, nausea	eGFR <30 mL/min (relative); severe hepatic dysfunction	Most effective *if started within 7 days of symptom onset*; not useful late in the disease with predominant inflammation
Nirmatrelvir-ritonavir (Paxlovid)	Nirmatrelvir: protease inhibitor; Ritonavir: CYP3A4 inhibitor (boosts nirmatrelvir levels)	300/100 mg orally BID × 5 days (adjust in renal impairment)	Diarrhoea, dysgeusia, drug interactions	Severe renal (<30 mL/min) or hepatic impairment; drugs metabolised by CYP3A4	Use within *5 days of symptom onset* in high-risk outpatients; *significant drug–drug interactions*—Requires medication reconciliation
Molnupiravir	Prodrug of NHC; causes lethal mutagenesis in viral RNA	800 mg orally BID × 5 days	Diarrhoea, dizziness, rash	Pregnancy (teratogenicity); <18 years (growth cartilage concerns)	Less effective than Paxlovid; *used when Paxlovid and remdesivir are not options*
Dexamethasone	Glucocorticoid; anti-inflammatory via gene suppression	6 mg IV/PO daily × up to 10 days	Hyperglycaemia, infections, GI bleeding, myopathy	Uncontrolled infections, caution in diabetics, peptic ulcer	*Only indicated in patients requiring oxygen*; harmful if given early in mild cases
Methylprednisolone		0.5–1 mg/kg/day IV/PO (mod); up to 2 mg/kg/day (severe) × 5–10 days			Preferred in *severe COVID-19 pneumonia or ARDS*; higher lung tissue penetration
Prednisolone		Equivalent dose ~40 mg/day × 5–10 days			Used when IV steroids are not feasible: *PO alternative* to dexamethasone

(continued)

Table 15.1 (continued)

Drug	Mechanism of action	Dose and duration	Adverse events	Contraindications	Special remarks
Tocilizumab	IL-6 receptor antagonist; suppresses cytokine storm	8 mg/kg IV (max 800 mg), once; may repeat in 12–24 h	↑Infections, ↑LFTs, GI perforation, neutropenia	Active infections, diverticulitis, latent TB	Given in *severe COVID-19 with high IL-6 markers* and increasing oxygen requirement despite steroids
Sarilumab		400 mg IV once			Alternative to tocilizumab when not available; *similar efficacy*
Baricitinib	JAK1/JAK2 inhibitor; reduces cytokine signalling	4 mg PO daily × up to 14 days	Infections, thrombosis, ↑LFTs, cytopenias	eGFR <15, active TB/ serious infections	Used when *IL-6 inhibitors are unavailable* or contraindicated; avoid combining with IL-6 blockers

15.3.1 Remdesivir

- *Remdesivir* is a nucleotide analogue prodrug that acts by inhibiting the RNA-dependent RNA polymerase of SARS-CoV-2. It is metabolised into an active triphosphate form, which competes with adenosine triphosphate and is incorporated into the viral genome, resulting in the premature termination of viral RNA synthesis. This subsequently halts viral replication, making it effective during the early phase of the disease [6].
- The drug has been shown to decrease time to recovery for hospitalised patients requiring oxygen therapy and decrease the progression to severe disease for high-risk, nonhospitalised patients.
- The drug has to be administered within 7 days of symptom onset. In patients who need oxygen therapy, it is given in conjunction with steroids and/or other immunomodulators. Indications for remdesivir include hospitalised patients with moderate-to-severe COVID-19 infection and high-risk patients with mild disease [1, 2, 5]. Doses and duration are outlined in Box 15.3. Remdesivir is associated with hepatitis and can cause severe hepatic dysfunction, which one should monitor [7].

Box 15.3: Dose and Duration of Remdesivir [2, 5]

Dosing of Remdesivir

- Day 1: 200 mg IV single dose.
- Day 2–5: 100 mg IV Q24H.

For high-risk individuals

- Day 1: 200 mg IV single dose.
- Day 2–3: 100 mg IV q24h.

15.3.2 Nirmatrelvir-Ritonavir (Paxlovid)

- *Nirmatrelvir-ritonavir* is a combination of viral protease inhibitors. Proteases are the enzymes which cleave non-functional polypeptides formed after translation into functional proteins required for viral maturation [8].
- Nirmatrelvir is the primary drug and blocks viral replication by preventing cleavage of viral polyproteins necessary for viral maturation. Ritonavir acts as a booster and acts as a pharmacokinetic enhancer by inhibiting cytochrome P450 3A (CYP3A)-mediated metabolism of nirmatrelvir, thereby increasing and prolonging its plasma concentration [8].
- It has shown to reduce the need for hospitalisation and death in high-risk patients, when given early. Hence, it is used only for patients with mild disease who are at risk of progression to severe disease.

- Dosing of Molnupiravir is mentioned in Box 15.4. This drug comes with a risk of drug interactions, and one has to be cautious while administering it to patients on multiple medications. Common adverse effects include altered taste, diarrhoea and nausea [9].

Box 15.4: Dosing of Nirmatrelvir-Ritonavir

- The drug comes as nirmatrelvir 150 mg tablet and ritonavir 100 mg tablet.
- The drug is given as 300 mg of nirmatrelvir (2 tablets) and 100 mg of ritonavir (1 tablet) together, twice daily for 5 days.

15.3.3 Molnupiravir

- *Molnupiravir* is a nucleoside analogue and acts by inhibiting viral RNA-dependent RNA polymerase. It is metabolised to its active form 'β-D-N4-hydroxycytidine' and is incorporated into viral RNA. This leads to termination of viral replication [10].
- Molnupiravir modestly reduces the risk of hospitalisation and death in high-risk patients when given early. Dosing of Molnupiravir is mentioned in Box 15.5.
- The common adverse events include diarrhoea, nausea and dizziness. There is a concern about genotoxicity and potential effects on bone and cartilage development.
- Molnupiravir is to be avoided in patients aged <18 years, during pregnancy and in breastfeeding women. Indications for use are the same as those of nirmatrelvir-ritonavir and should be used when nirmatrelvir-ritonavir and/or remdesivir is unavailable or contraindicated [11].

Box 15.5: Dosing of Molnupiravir

- The drug comes as a 200 mg capsule.
- It is administered as 800 mg (4 capsules) twice daily for 5 days.

15.4 Anti-inflammatory or Immunomodulatory Treatment

- As the phase of viral replication subsides, most of the patients recover. However, some patients can progress to severe disease. During this phase, immune dysregulation favours pro-inflammatory cytokine production, leading to a hyperinflammatory state and a cytokine storm. Hence, anti-inflammatory agents and immunomodulators are used.
- The use of anti-inflammatory agents and immunomodulators should be restricted to all patients showing features of severe disease, like hypoxia requiring supplemental oxygen, acute respiratory distress syndrome (ARDS), elevated inflammatory markers and hypotension.

- Systemic corticosteroids in combination with/without interleukin-6 (IL-6) inhibitors or with Janus Kinase (JAK) inhibitors are used. These are usually given for 14 days or until hospital discharge, whichever comes first. It is not recommended to use these agents in the early stage or in patients with mild disease. The use of immunomodulators in COVID-19 is summarised in Table 15.1.

15.4.1 Corticosteroids

- Corticosteroids are one of the key drugs used in the treatment of COVID-19, as demonstrated by the landmark RECOVERY Trial [12]. They are used for their anti-inflammatory and immunomodulatory actions. These drugs are used to suppress the excessive immune response during the hyperinflammatory state of COVID-19 illness. It is used in patients with moderate to severe disease who require supplemental oxygen or those with ADRS.
- Corticosteroids should be avoided in patients with mild or asymptomatic disease, as they tend to worsen the outcomes. It has been shown to have decreased mortality for patients requiring oxygen therapy, and is associated with more adverse effects in the patients not requiring oxygen therapy [12]. Box 15.6 mentions the indications and dosing of corticosteroids in COVID-19.
- Post-prandial hyperglycaemia is common and should be promptly managed with insulin. A significant concern with steroid use in COVID-19 is the risk of secondary bacterial infections and fungal infections, including pulmonary aspergillosis and mucormycosis [13, 14].

Box 15.6: Indications and Dosing for the Use of Corticosteroids in COVID-19

Indications for the use of corticosteroids

- Peripheral oxygen saturation (SpO_2) <94% on room air.
- Need for supplemental oxygen.
- Mechanical ventilation.
- ARDS.

Dosing of corticosteroids

- Dexamethasone 6 mg/day.
- Methylprednisolone 32 mg/day.
- Prednisolone 40 mg/day.

15.5 Interleukin-6 Inhibitors

- Interleukin-6 is a proinflammatory cytokine produced by macrophages, T cells and fibroblasts. It aids in regulating the immune response and inflammation. In the early phase, it is raised transiently and helps to mount an antiviral response. In later stages, high IL-6 levels drive the cytokine storm and inflammation, which can progress to ARDS, coagulopathy, DIC, shock, and multi-organ failure, as observed in severe COVID-19 illness. This makes IL-6 a key driver of cytokine storm [15].
- The use of IL-6 inhibitors, as demonstrated by RECOVERY and REM-CAP trials, has been shown to result in shorter recovery time and reduced all-cause mortality [16, 17].
- Current guidelines recommend the use of IL-6 inhibitors in addition to dexamethasone [2, 4]. Two of the IL-6 inhibitors, tocilizumab and sarilumab, are currently in use. They block the downstream IL-6 cytokine signalling pathway. Dosing of IL-6 inhibitors in COVID-19 is mentioned in Box 15.7. Patients on IL-6 inhibitors are at risk of hepatitis and secondary bacterial infections. It is also associated with reactivation of TB and HBV [18].

Box 15.7: Dosing of IL-6 Inhibitors in COVID-19

1. Tocilizumab
    - 8 mg/kg iv over 1 h
    - Usually a single dose.
    - Second dose is given after 8 h if clinical improvement is not seen.
2. Sarilumab
    - 400 mg IV single dose.

15.6 Janus Kinase Inhibitors

- Janus kinase (JAK) is an intracellular tyrosine kinase involved in cytokine signalling and immune regulation via the JAK-STAT pathway. JAKs are activated when cytokines, like IL-6, bind to their receptor. This results in phosphorylation of STAT proteins, which then enter the nucleus and regulate gene expression [19]. In the cytokine storm phase of COVID-19, JAK inhibitors downregulate this cytokine signalling pathway, thereby reducing inflammation. They are used in addition to corticosteroids in hospitalised adults requiring supplemental oxygen, noninvasive or invasive mechanical ventilation, or extracorporeal membrane oxygenation (ECMO).
- Baricitinib is the drug currently used, given as 4 mg OD for up to 14 days. It requires renal dose adjustment. Use of Baricitinib is associated with severe bacterial infections, reactivation of TB, invasive fungal infections, hepatitis, cytopenia, and thrombosis [2, 4, 20].

- Tofacitinib can be used as an alternative to baricitinib. It is given as a 10 mg tablet twice daily. It also requires renal dose modification and has adverse effects similar to baricitinib [21].

15.7 Anticoagulation and Antithrombotic Therapy

- COVID-19 is a prothrombotic state because of underlying thromboinflammation and is associated with raised D-dimer [22]. All patients admitted for COVID-19 should be screened and monitored for coagulation abnormalities, which include PT, aPTT, D-dimer, and fibrinogen [23].
- When clinically indicated, especially if there is suspicion of deep vein thrombosis, one should get a venous doppler scan of both the lower limbs and a Pulmonary Angiogram for Pulmonary Venous Thromboembolism.
- Unless contraindicated, all patients requiring hospitalisation because of COVID-19 disease should receive thromboprophylaxis. For patients who do not require hospitalisation or are hospitalised for other indications, thromboprophylaxis is given only if there is an alternative indication. Unfractionated heparin (UFH) or low molecular weight heparin (LMWH) can be used. However, LMWH is preferred over UFH [24].
- Therapeutic anticoagulation is used if the patient is already taking anticoagulation therapy for other medical conditions or if the patient develops venous thromboembolism (VTE) or deep vein thrombosis (DVT). If clinically or haemodynamically unstable, UFH is used. Whereas LMWH or direct oral anticoagulants (DOAC) can be used if the patient is stable and without any organ dysfunction. Fibrinolytics are reserved for specific conditions (Box 15.8).

Box 15.8: Indications for Fibrinolytics (Reserved for the Following)
- Limb-threatening DVT.
- Massive pulmonary embolism.
- Acute stroke.
- Acute MI.

15.8 Oxygen Support and Respiratory Therapy

- All patients with SpO_2 of <93% will require oxygen therapy. The target SpO_2 is 94–96%. Over oxygen therapy should be avoided. The flow and type of therapy will depend on the severity of the illness, tolerance to the treatment and sensorium [25].
- Oxygenation can be provided through low- or high-flow systems [26]. Although many improve with increased respiratory support to room air, some can deteriorate and may require mechanical ventilation. The titration of oxygen delivery should be based on clinical requirements, guided by arterial blood gas analysis (Table 15.2).

Table 15.2 Oxygen therapy in COVID-19

Indications	Device	Flow	FiO_2 delivered	Remarks
Mild oxygen requirement	Nasal cannula	1–5 L/min	24–35%	Comfortable Limited flow Unreliable FiO_2 Can easily get dislodged
Moderate oxygen requirements	Simple face mask	5–10 L/min	35–60%	Discomforting Can cause CO_2 retention Size may not fit
	Venturi mask	5–15 L/min	24–50%	Precise oxygen delivery High flow Discomforting
High oxygen requirements	Nonrebreather mask (NRBM)	10–15 L/min	60–90%	Has high FiO_2 Used in emergency (when HFNC is not available or during preoxygenation) Requires close monitoring
	High-flow nasal cannula (HFNC)	15–60 L/min	30–100%	Provides high FiO_2 Provides modest PEEP (helps improve functional residual capacity) Used in type 1 respiratory failure Can cause dry mouth Costly and requires experts to set up and monitor
Ventilation	Non-invasive ventilation		21–100%	Used as transition from or to invasive ventilation Preferred over HFNC in patients with CO_2 retention and with pulmonary oedema Uncomfortable and associated with pneumothorax
	Mechanical ventilation		21–100%	Used in severe ARDS Can give controlled ventilation The patient is sedated Can cause pneumothorax Substantial risk of VAP

- Respiratory therapy, in addition to oxygenation, is supported by nebulisations and prone positioning. Prone positioning refers to the patient being in a prone position while undergoing oxygen therapy. Proning helps in the recruitment of the lungs by reducing the difference between dorsal and ventral perfusion pressures, thereby improving lung perfusion. It can be done in all modalities of respiratory therapy [27].
- ECMO (extracorporeal membrane oxygenation) can be used as a rescue therapy in severe COVID-19 patients with refractory hypoxaemia or cardiac failure despite optimal conventional treatment, including mechanical ventilation and

prone positioning. It provides temporary cardiopulmonary support by oxygenating blood outside the body, allowing the heart and lungs time to recover [28].

15.9 Supportive and Adjuvant Care

- In addition to COVID-19-specific therapy, supportive care is also essential. One should provide adequate nutrition and hydration, as well as prophylaxis for gastrointestinal ulcers and pressure ulcers. The patient should be encouraged to mobilise early. Patients are also at risk for developing ICU psychosis and will need mental health support and management [29].

15.10 Management of COVID-19 Based on Disease Severity

The management of COVID-19 is based on the severity of the illness and its associated complications. The summary of COVID-19 management based on clinical severity is presented in Table 15.3 [1, 2, 5].

Table 15.3 Management of COVID-19

Disease severity		Management	Remarks
Mild disease	No high risk for severe disease	Home isolation Social distancing Symptomatic management Self-monitoring of temperature and SpO_2 Patient should seek immediate medical attention if they experience persistent symptoms or when they develop shortness of breath	Avoid antibiotics No anticoagulation, antivirals or immunomodulators
	High risk for severe disease	Patient can be admitted for observation Symptomatic treatment Patient can be initiated on Oral nirmatrelvir-ritonavir 300/100 mg orally BID × 5 days or Inj. remdesivir 200 mg iv on day 1 and 100 mg iv on day 2 and 3 or Tab molnupiravir 800 mg orally BID × 5 days (if nirmatrelvir-ritonavir and remdesivir is unavailable or contraindicated)	Prophylactic heparin can be used, unless contraindicated
	Hospitalized for reasons other than COVID-19	Observe for the progress of the disease Symptomatic management Prophylactic heparin can be given, unless contraindicated	Avoid antibiotics No antivirals, anti-inflammatory or immunomodulators

(continued)

Table 15.3 (continued)

Disease severity		Management	Remarks
Hospitalisation and requiring conventional oxygen	Most patients	Inj. dexamethasone 6 mg iv OD for 10 days or until discharge, whichever comes first, PLUS Inj. remdesivir 200 mg IV once, 100 mg IV once daily for 4 days or until hospital discharge, whichever comes first Prophylactic anticoagulation Awake prone positioning Symptomatic management	If dexamethasone is not available, an equivalent dose of another corticosteroid may be used
	Worsening on corticosteroids (increasing oxygen requirement or inflammation)	In addition to dexamethasone plus remdesivir and prophylactic anticoagulation, add: Tocilizumab 8 mg/kg actual body weight (up to 800 mg) administered as a single IV dose, OR Baricitinib 4 mg PO daily × up to 14 days or until hospital discharge, whichever comes first, OR Sarilumab 400 mg in 100 cc 0.9% NaCl and administer as an IV infusion over 1 h, OR Tofacitinib 10 mg PO twice daily for up to 14 days or until hospital discharge, whichever comes first	Repeat dose of tocilizumab can be given after 8 h if no improvement in the clinical condition Sarilumab, baricitinib and tofacitinib need renal dose adjustment Use sarilumab or tofacitinib only if tocilizumab or baricitinib is not available Continue prone ventilation
Hospitalisation and requiring HFNC, NIV, MV or ECMO	All patients	Inj. dexamethasone 6 mg iv OD for 10 days or until discharge, whichever comes first, PLUS If not already started, inj. remdesivir 200 mg IV once, 100 mg IV once daily for 4 days or until hospital discharge, whichever comes first, PLUS Tocilizumab 8 mg/kg actual body weight (up to 800 mg) administered as a single IV dose, OR Baricitinib 4 mg PO daily × up to 14 days or until hospital discharge, whichever comes first, OR Sarilumab 400 mg in 100 cc 0.9% NaCl and administer as an IV infusion over 1 h, OR Tofacitinib 10 mg PO twice daily for up to 14 days or until hospital discharge, whichever comes first	

15.11 Treatments to be Avoided in COVID-19

- One should avoid using lopinavir-ritonavir, hydroxychloroquine, Ivermectin, neutralising monoclonal antibody, convalescent plasma, and favipiravir.
- Empirical antibiotics are discouraged unless there is clear evidence of bacterial co-infection, helping to prevent antimicrobial resistance [1].

15.12 Conclusions

The management of COVID-19 continues to rely on a layered approach that combines vaccination, personal protective equipment (PPE), antiviral therapy, and supportive care. Vaccination remains the cornerstone of prevention, with updated boosters recommended for older adults, individuals with weakened immune systems, and frontline workers to protect against emerging variants. PPE, especially masks, gloves, gowns, and eye protection, remains essential in healthcare settings and during outbreaks, helping to reduce the transmission of infectious diseases. For high-risk patients, early antiviral treatment with agents like nirmatrelvir/ritonavir (Paxlovid) or remdesivir can significantly lower the risk of hospitalisation and severe disease. Supportive care, including oxygen therapy, corticosteroids, and anticoagulation, is tailored to the severity of the disease. Meanwhile, public health measures such as ventilation, hand hygiene, and isolation continue to serve as community-level protections. Collectively, these strategies form a dynamic and responsive framework for minimising COVID-19's impact across diverse populations.

References

1. IDSA guidelines on the treatment and management of patients with COVID-19 [Internet]. [cited 2025 Jul 19]. Available from: https://www.idsociety.org/practice-guideline/covid-19-guideline-treatment-and-management/.
2. Gulick RM, Pau AK, Daar E, Evans L, Gandhi RT, Tebas P, et al. National Institutes of Health COVID-19 treatment guidelines panel: perspectives and lessons learned. Ann Intern Med. 2024;177(11):1547–57.
3. Martono, Fatmawati F, Mulyanti S. Risk factors associated with the severity of COVID-19. Malays J Med Sci. 2023;30(3):84–92.
4. CDC. COVID-19. 2025 [cited 2025 Jul 19]. People with certain medical conditions and COVID-19 risk factors. Available from: https://www.cdc.gov/covid/risk-factors/index.html.
5. ClinicalGuidanceforManagementofAdultCOVID19Patientsupdatedason05thjan2023.pdf [Internet]. [cited 2025 Jul 19]. Available from: https://covid19dashboard.mohfw.gov.in/pdf/ClinicalGuidanceforManagementofAdultCOVID19Patientsupdatedason05thjan2023.pdf.

6. Gordon CJ, Tchesnokov EP, Woolner E, Perry JK, Feng JY, Porter DP, et al. Remdesivir is a direct-acting antiviral that inhibits RNA-dependent RNA polymerase from severe acute respiratory syndrome coronavirus 2 with high potency. J Biol Chem. 2020;295(20):6785–97.
7. Pan H, Peto R, Henao Restrepo AM, Preziosi MP, Sathiyamoorthy V, Karim QA, et al. Remdesivir and three other drugs for hospitalised patients with COVID-19: final results of the WHO Solidarity randomised trial and updated meta-analyses. Lancet. 2022;399(10339):1941–53.
8. Owen DR, Allerton CMN, Anderson AS, Aschenbrenner L, Avery M, Berritt S, et al. An oral SARS-CoV-2 Mpro inhibitor clinical candidate for the treatment of COVID-19. Science. 2021;374(6575):1586–93.
9. Hammond J, Leister-Tebbe H, Gardner A, Abreu P, Bao W, Wisemandle W, et al. Oral nirmatrelvir for high-risk, nonhospitalized adults with Covid-19. N Engl J Med. 2022;386(15):1397–408.
10. Kabinger F, Stiller C, Schmitzová J, Dienemann C, Kokic G, Hillen HS, et al. Mechanism of molnupiravir-induced SARS-CoV-2 mutagenesis. Nat Struct Mol Biol. 2021;28(9):740–6.
11. Singh AK, Singh A, Singh R, Misra A. Molnupiravir in COVID-19: a systematic review of literature. Diabetes Metab Syndr. 2021;15(6):102329.
12. The RECOVERY Collaborative Group. Dexamethasone in hospitalized patients with Covid-19. N Engl J Med. 2021;384(8):693–704.
13. Bahsoun A, Fakih Y, Zareef R, Bitar F, Arabi M. Corticosteroids in COVID-19: pros and cons. Front Med. 2023;10:1202504.
14. Søvik S, Barratt-Due A, Kåsine T, Olasveengen T, Strand MW, Tveita AA, et al. Corticosteroids and superinfections in COVID-19 patients on invasive mechanical ventilation. J Infect. 2022;85(1):57–63.
15. Wang X, Tang G, Liu Y, Zhang L, Chen B, Han Y, et al. The role of IL-6 in coronavirus, especially in COVID-19. Front Pharmacol [Internet]. 2022 [cited 2025 Jul 19];13. Available from: https://www.frontiersin.org/articles/10.3389/fphar.2022.1033674/full.
16. Abani O, Abbas A, Abbas F, Abbas M, Abbasi S, Abbass H, et al. Tocilizumab in patients admitted to hospital with COVID-19 (RECOVERY): a randomised, controlled, open-label, platform trial. Lancet. 2021;397(10285):1637–45.
17. The REMAP-CAP Investigators. Interleukin-6 receptor antagonists in critically ill patients with Covid-19. N Engl J Med. 2021;384(16):1491–502.
18. Hu J, Sun Y, Zuo X, Zou Y. Assessment of adverse events related to anti-interleukin-6 receptor monoclonal antibodies using the FDA adverse event reporting system: a real-world pharmacovigilance study. Expert Opin Drug Saf. 2024;23(10):1327–39.
19. Shawky AM, Almalki FA, Abdalla AN, Abdelazeem AH, Gouda AM. A comprehensive overview of globally approved JAK inhibitors. Pharmaceutics. 2022;14(5):1001.
20. Marconi VC, Ramanan AV, De Bono S, Kartman CE, Krishnan V, Liao R, et al. Efficacy and safety of baricitinib for the treatment of hospitalised adults with COVID-19 (COV-BARRIER): a randomised, double-blind, parallel-group, placebo-controlled phase 3 trial. Lancet Respir Med. 2021;9(12):1407–18.
21. Guimarães PO, Quirk D, Furtado RH, Maia LN, Saraiva JF, Antunes MO, et al. Tofacitinib in patients hospitalized with Covid-19 pneumonia. N Engl J Med. 2021;385(5):406–15.
22. Spyropoulos AC, Bonaca MP. Studying the coagulopathy of COVID-19. Lancet. 2022;399(10320):118–9.
23. Ichikawa J, Okazaki R, Fukuda T, Ono T, Ishikawa M, Komori M. Evaluation of coagulation status using clot waveform analysis in general ward patients with COVID-19. J Thromb Thrombolysis. 2022;53(1):118–22.
24. Barco S, Voci D, Held U, Sebastian T, Bingisser R, Colucci G, et al. Enoxaparin for primary thromboprophylaxis in symptomatic outpatients with COVID-19 (OVID): a randomised, open-label, parallel-group, multicentre, phase 3 trial. Lancet Haematol. 2022;9(8):e585–93.
25. Gottlieb J, Volk T, Fühner T. Oxygen treatment in Covid-19. Dtsch Arztebl Int. 2021;118(22):375–6.

26. Rengasamy S, Nassef B, Bilotta F, Pugliese F, Nozari A, Ortega R. Administration of supplemental oxygen. Ingelfinger JR, editor. N Engl J Med [Internet]. 2021 [cited 2025 Jul 19];385(3). Available from: http://www.nejm.org/doi/10.1056/NEJMvcm2035240.
27. Gattinoni L, Camporota L, Marini JJ. Prone position and COVID-19: mechanisms and effects. Crit Care Med. 2022;50(5):873–5.
28. Tisminetzky M, Ferreyro BL, Fan E. Extracorporeal membrane oxygenation in COVID-19. Crit Care Clin. 2022;38(3):535–52.
29. Sweeney DA, Malhotra A. Supportive care in patients with critical coronavirus disease 2019. Infect Dis Clin N Am. 2022;36(4):777–89.

COVID-19 and Pregnancy

16

M. A. Ashwini and Vijayalakshmi Reddy

16.1 Introduction

Pregnancy is a complex physiological state marked by significant changes in various systems, including the immune, cardiovascular, respiratory, gastrointestinal, and urinary systems. These adaptive changes, while essential for supporting foetal development, also make pregnant individuals more susceptible to infections and associated complications. The emergence of the severe acute respiratory syndrome coronavirus 2 (SARS-CoV-2), causative agent of COVID-19, posed unique challenges in obstetric care and management. Pregnant women represent a vulnerable group with a distinct clinical profile, and special management considerations are necessary for a favourable outcome with respect to maternal and foetal health. This chapter explores the relationship between COVID-19 and pregnancy, encompassing maternal and foetal outcomes, vaccination safety, and implications for obstetric care.

16.2 Epidemiology of COVID-19 in Pregnancy

Since the early stages of the COVID-19 pandemic, the infection has affected pregnant individuals across all geographic regions and socio-economic strata. Several studies have documented infection rates among pregnant women comparable to the general population [1, 2]. However, variations in testing protocols, access to care, and surveillance mechanisms have also contributed to underreporting in many countries [3].

M. A. Ashwini (✉) · V. Reddy
Department of Neurovirology, National Institute of Mental Health and Neurosciences, Bengaluru, Karnataka, India

S. R. Prabhu et al. (eds.), *COVID-19 in Dental Practice*,
https://doi.org/10.1007/978-3-032-26000-0_16

Pregnancy itself does not increase the risk of acquiring SARS-CoV-2 infection, but once infected, pregnant women are at a higher risk of developing severe disease, particularly in the second and third trimesters. SARS-CoV-2 infection in pregnant women can lead to adverse maternal and foetal outcomes [4, 5]. Hospitalisation rates and intensive care unit (ICU) admissions have been higher among pregnant women compared to non-pregnant women of reproductive age [6]. The differences in disease progression and outcome in this group underscore the need for heightened vigilance and prioritisation of preventive and management strategies.

16.3 Immunopathogenesis

SARS-CoV-2 infection during pregnancy is characterised by complex immune dysregulation involving maternal, placental, and neonatal compartments. Pregnancy-associated immune adaptations predispose infected women to altered antiviral responses, with reductions in $CD4^+$ and $CD8^+$ T-cell numbers and functionality, features of T-cell exhaustion, and diminished regulatory T-cell responses, particularly in severe disease, thereby compromising maternal–foetal immune tolerance and increasing the risk of adverse outcomes such as preeclampsia, preterm birth, foetal growth restriction, and stillbirth [7]. While certain T-cell subsets, such as $\gamma\delta$T and Th17 cells, may show enhanced activity in mild disease, severe COVID-19 is marked by exaggerated NF-κB–driven inflammation and a distinct IFN-λ- driven antiviral signalling profile [8, 9]. At the maternal–foetal interface, SARS-CoV-2 induces a pro-inflammatory placental milieu with elevated cytokine and chemokine levels, including IL-1β, IL-6, IL-8, CXCL9, and CXCL10, contributing to endothelial dysfunction and placental pathology, despite the rarity of direct placental infection or vertical transmission [10]. Systemically, infected pregnant women exhibit elevated levels of inflammatory cytokines such as IL-8, IL-10, and IL-15, while neonates exposed in utero demonstrate mild but measurable inflammatory responses, including increased IL-8 and the induction of T-cell–associated cytokines [7]. Collectively, these findings highlight that COVID-19 in pregnancy primarily drives immune-mediated pathology rather than direct viral effects, with lasting implications for maternal and neonatal health, emphasising the importance of continued monitoring of mother–infant dyads following in utero SARS-CoV-2 exposure.

16.4 Clinical Features, Laboratory, and Imaging Findings

The clinical presentation of COVID-19 in pregnant women is similar to that seen in the general population, including non-pregnant adults. Most commonly reported symptoms include fever, nasal congestion, and cough, followed by myalgia and chills. Other symptoms reported include headache, fatigue, anosmia, ageusia, dyspnoea, diarrhoea, nausea, vomiting, and haemoptysis [11, 12]. A large proportion of pregnant women remain asymptomatic or have mild disease but may be associated with long-term complications [13].

However, a subset can progress to moderate or severe illness, requiring supplemental oxygen or ventilatory support. This is also attributed to the presence of overlapping symptoms between COVID-19 and pregnancy, which leads to delayed diagnosis and treatment. Physiological dyspnoea and abnormally low blood oxygen saturation levels in COVID-19 patients, labelled often as ‘silent hypoxia’, can occur in the absence of dyspnoea, which can lead to the delayed diagnosis and treatment [14]. Moreover, conditions like preeclampsia, hyperemesis gravidarum, or physiological oedema can complicate timely diagnosis and intervention. This necessitates a careful and multidisciplinary assessment of symptomatic pregnant patients, especially in high-risk or late gestation periods.

16.5 Post-acute Sequelae of COVID-19 (PASC) in Pregnancy

Post-acute sequelae of COVID-19 (PASC), also known as long COVID, refers to a range of symptoms that persist for weeks or months after recovery from the acute infection. In pregnant women, the prevalence of PASC ranges from 9.3% to 93%. Common persistent symptoms include fatigue, gastrointestinal complaints, cognitive difficulties (such as poor concentration and memory), respiratory symptoms, and psychological issues like anxiety and depression. Risk factors for developing PASC during pregnancy include severe acute COVID-19 illness, obesity, pre-existing mental health conditions, and lack of COVID-19 vaccination. Pregnant women with PASC are at a higher risk of adverse maternal and neonatal outcomes, including preterm birth, low birth weight, and an increased need for intensive care for both the mother and the newborn. The severity of the initial COVID-19 infection is considered the most important predictor of long COVID, with severe cases associated with prolonged complications such as liver dysfunction and thromboembolic events [2, 15].

16.6 Maternal Outcomes

Existing evidence suggests that pregnant women with symptomatic COVID-19 are more likely to experience complications such as caesarean delivery, intrauterine growth restriction (IUGR), low birth weight, and preterm birth [11, 16].

Poor maternal outcomes in pregnant women are most commonly associated with risk factors including advanced maternal age, obesity, hypertension, diabetes, and late presentation to healthcare facilities. These women have higher risk of maternal morbidity including placental disruption, preeclampsia, and eclampsia [11].

Additionally, moderate or severe SARS-CoV-2 infection during the second and third semesters are associated with a higher risk of maternal and foetal complications [4].

Postpartum complications including fever, hypoxia, the need for invasive ventilation, and hospital readmission are observed more frequently in patients with COVID-19 compared to those without the infection [17].

16.7 Foetal and Neonatal Outcomes

The majority of the infections in neonates occur post-partum, with the horizontal mode of transmission from infected mothers in the early post-natal period being common. Though infrequent, vertical transmission of SARS-CoV-2 has been documented. Further transmission through breastfeeding does not seem to be associated with transmission of the virus [18].

The most common symptoms reported in infected neonates include respiratory distress, fever, and feeding difficulties. Neonatal ARDS is very rare. Gastrointestinal manifestations include diarrhoea, vomiting, while neurological features like hypertonia and irritability have also been reported. Other include tachycardia, hypotension, conjunctivitis, and cutaneous rash. Neonatal intensive care unit (NICU) admissions were most common when they were symptomatic or tested positive for viral RNA [19]. However, all the neonates in NICU may not have needed critical care, and this was implemented in the early stages of the pandemic, as NICU represents only area where isolation of neonates is possible [18].

Studies have observed notable rise in congenital abnormalities, especially those linked to early gestational infections and specific cardiac conditions. However, there is no definitive evidence directly connecting maternal SARS-CoV-2 infection to congenital malformations [20]. In general, the vast majority of neonates do well clinically, and there is no conclusive evidence of congenital malformations linked to maternal SARS-CoV-2 infection.

16.8 Maternal and Perinatal Outcomes Associated with SARS-CoV-2 Variants in Pregnancy

Evidence consistently demonstrates that pregnancy outcomes vary by SARS-CoV-2 variant, with the Delta variant associated with the most adverse maternal and perinatal outcomes [21]. Compared with Alpha, wild-type, and Omicron infections, Delta infection in pregnancy has been linked to higher rates of severe maternal morbidity, ICU admission, preterm birth, stillbirth, and NICU admission. Maternal deaths related to COVID-19 remain rare across all variants, but inflammatory and coagulation markers, including CRP, IL-6, D-dimer, and transaminases, are notably elevated in Delta infections, reflecting greater disease severity. Delta has also been associated with poorer neonatal outcomes, including small-for-gestational-age infants and lower Apgar scores, as well as increased placental SARS-CoV-2 detection [22]. In contrast, Omicron infections appear to be associated with milder maternal disease and fewer severe pregnancy complications [22]. Collectively, these findings highlight the variant-specific impact of COVID-19 in pregnancy and underscore the need for ongoing surveillance and research as new variants continue to emerge.

16.9 Diagnostic Considerations in Pregnancy

Diagnosis of COVID-19 in pregnancy follows the same principles as in the general population, with real-time reverse transcription PCR (RT-PCR) and computed tomography (CT) scans used most commonly for confirmation of the infection, and these, when used together, provide an accurate diagnosis [23]. Detection of SARS-CoV-2 RNA by RT-PCR in respiratory samples is considered the gold standard. However, chest radiography and CT scans should not be contraindicated in pregnant women if required. Chest radiography findings in pregnant women are similar to those of non-pregnant individuals, with airspace opacities, multi-lobar infiltrates, and ground-glass opacities [24].

IgM antibody assays in conjunction with RT-PCR have been found to be a very sensitive method for diagnosis and can be considered as a non-radiation-based alternative to imaging [25]. Additionally, rapid antigen tests can be considered for screening of suspected pregnant women [26].

Blood markers, including C-reactive protein (CRP), D-dimer, ferritin, and lymphocyte counts, are routinely used to evaluate disease severity [27]. However, physiological changes in pregnancy can influence these parameters, necessitating pregnancy-specific interpretation.

16.10 Management and Treatment

The management of COVID-19 in pregnancy is generally similar to that in non-pregnant patients, with key considerations such as maintaining peripheral oxygen saturation (SpO_2) $\geq 94\%$ to ensure adequate placental oxygen transfer [28, 29]. Optimal care requires a multidisciplinary team including obstetricians, respiratory physicians, anaesthetists, virologists, midwives, and intensivists [29]. Pharmacological treatment is shown in Table 16.1.

Table 16.1 Pharmacological management of COVID-19 in pregnancy

Types	Drugs	Period	Indication	Remarks
Corticosteroids	Prednisolone 40 mg OD, hydrocortisone 80 mg BD, or methylprednisolone 1 mg/kg BD for 5–7 days followed by OD for 5–7 days	10 days or until discharge from hospital	SpO_2—<94% or oxygen requirement	Dexamethasone—Associated with neurocognitive and sensory disorders in childhood
IL-6 receptor antagonists	Tocilizumab 8 mg/kg Sarilumab 400 mg	Once by IV infusion	Hypoxia (SpO_2—<94% or oxygen requirement) or CRP ≥75 mg/L or admitted to ICU	May have adverse consequences with live vaccines
Neutralising monoclonal antibodies	Sotrovimab 500 mg	Single IV infusion—30 min	Non-hospitalised patients with mild/moderate disease and one risk factor for progression	Ongoing symptoms within 5 days of a SARS-CoV-2 positive test, treated pre-emptively
	Tixagevimab 300 mg IM Cilgavimab 300 mg IM	Separate consecutive IM injections	Not routinely given; only when expected benefits outweigh the potential risks	Safety data within pregnancy are lacking, have potential to cross the placenta
Antiviral	Remdesivir	3 day IV: Day 1—200 mg; Days 2 and 3—100 mg	Not routinely used Only in worsening stage after standard management	Useful in non-omicron genotype
VTE prophylaxis	LMWH	Inpatient admission and 10 days post discharge	Outpatient management should undergo VTE risk assessment	Last dose should be withheld for 12 h (prophylaxis) and 24 h (treatment) before spinal/epidural procedures

SpO_2 Oxygen saturation, *VTE* Venous thromboembolism, *BCG* bacille Calmette-Guerin, *LMWH* Low molecular weight heparin, *MDT* Multidisciplinary team, *OD* Once in a day, *BD* Twice in a day, *IM* Intramuscular, *IV* Intravenous, *IL* Interleukin, *ICU* Intensive care unit, *CRP* C reactive protein

16.11 Delivery and Postnatal Care

The timing of delivery in pregnant women with COVID-19 should be individualised, taking into account the severity of infection, maternal condition, comorbidities, gestational age, and overall risks and benefits to both mother and foetus [17]. This decision must be made through shared decision-making involving the patient, family, and the multidisciplinary care team. COVID-19 infection itself is not an absolute indication for delivery [28–30]. Indications for timely delivery include respiratory distress, refractory hypoxaemia ($SpO_2 < 94\%$), arterial partial pressure of oxygen (PaO_2)/fraction of inspired oxygen (FiO_2) ≤ 300 mmHg or worsening critical illness [17, 30]. The mode of delivery, whether induction of vaginal delivery or caesarean section, should be guided by the severity of the disease and institutional capabilities [30].

Postpartum women should be managed in isolation with close monitoring of vital signs. Breastfeeding is encouraged for its well-established benefits for both the mother and the neonate. In cases where mother and baby are separated, expressed breast milk may be offered as an alternative [28, 30].

16.12 Antenatal Surveillance Post-infection

Antenatal surveillance after a COVID-19 infection requires closer monitoring due to an increased risk of complications such as preeclampsia, preterm birth, IUGR, and oligohydramnios [31]. The specific surveillance plan should be individualised and determined by a multidisciplinary healthcare team. The key monitoring areas are as follows:

- *Foetal Growth and Amniotic Fluid*: Regular monitoring of foetal growth via ultrasound is recommended, often after the resolution of acute COVID-19 illness, to rule out placental abnormalities and oligohydramnios.
- *Maternal Complications*: Healthcare providers should be vigilant for the development or worsening of pregnancy-related conditions, including:

  1. *Preeclampsia and Hypertension*: COVID-19 can exacerbate or mimic symptoms of preeclampsia, so blood pressure monitoring is vital.
  2. *Thromboembolism*: COVID-19 further increases the risk of a prothrombotic state in pregnancy. Prophylactic low molecular weight heparin (LMWH) may be considered on a case-by-case basis during hospitalisation or for at least 10 days postpartum.
  3. *Respiratory Distress*: Even after initial recovery, there is a risk of developing respiratory morbidity. Ongoing monitoring of oxygen saturation and respiratory symptoms is important.
  4. *Post-COVID Sequelae (Long COVID)*: Pregnant women should be monitored for persistent symptoms like fatigue, shortness of breath, and brain fog, which

can overlap with normal pregnancy symptoms but may indicate a post-COVID syndrome.

5. *Mental Health*: Both the pandemic and the infection can increase anxiety and depression. Mental health support and screening should be a routine part of all antenatal contacts.
6. *Timing and Mode of Delivery*: COVID-19 infection alone is not an indication for an immediate or specific mode of delivery. Decisions should be based on standard obstetric indications and the overall maternal and foetal condition, following a multidisciplinary assessment.
7. *Neonatal Care*: While vertical transmission to the baby is considered rare, newborns of mothers who had COVID-19 may have a higher chance of needing neonatal unit admission due to complications like preterm birth or feeding issues [31, 32].

16.13 Vaccination in Pregnancy

COVID-19 vaccination significantly reduces the risk of infection and, importantly, the severity of disease if a breakthrough infection occurs. All available evidence supports the safety and efficacy of administering currently approved SARS-CoV-2 vaccines during pregnancy [17, 33]. Studies have shown no increased risk of miscarriage, congenital anomalies, or other adverse maternal or foetal outcomes following vaccination [34–36].

Both mRNA vaccines (Pfizer-BioNTech and Moderna) and non-replicating viral vector vaccines (Covishield) have been used safely in pregnant populations [37, 38]. Vaccination during pregnancy may also confer passive immunity to the newborn, as maternal antibodies generated post-vaccination can cross the placenta and provide protection in the early neonatal period [39, 40]. Similarly, antibodies are present in breast milk, offering additional immune benefits to the infant [41].

16.14 Conclusion/Summary

- Pregnant individuals are at increased risk of severe COVID-19 and poor maternal outcomes.
- Vertical transmission of SARS-CoV-2 is rare.
- Infection increases the likelihood of pregnancy-related complications such as pre-eclampsia, preterm birth, and stillbirth.
- Clinical management should not be altered solely due to pregnancy; early treatment is crucial.
- Pregnant women with moderate to severe COVID-19 are at the highest risk of developing post-acute sequelae of COVID-19 (PASC), especially with pre-existing comorbidities, which is associated with increased adverse maternal and neonatal outcomes.

- Mental health support should be provided to all pregnant women affected by COVID-19 to reduce psychological impacts such as anxiety and depression.
- COVID-19 vaccination during pregnancy is safe, effective, and provides passive immunity to the newborn.
- Addressing vaccine hesitancy through informed counselling is critical to improving vaccine uptake among pregnant individuals.

References

1. Overton EE, Goffman D, Friedman AM. The epidemiology of COVID-19 in pregnancy. Clin Obstet Gynecol. 2022,65(1):110–22.
2. Metz TD, Clifton RG, Hughes BL, Sandoval G, Saade GR, Grobman WA, et al. Disease severity and perinatal outcomes of pregnant patients with coronavirus disease 2019 (COVID-19). Obstet Gynecol. 2021;137(4):571–80.
3. Prevalence of COVID-19 among pregnant women and its impact on childbirth in March 2021: data from the French National Perinatal Survey - ScienceDirect [Internet]. [cited 2025 July 4]. Available from: https://www.sciencedirect.com/science/article/abs/pii/S2468784724000357.
4. Eh K, Mamv C, Av C, Aancr R, Amb C, Ns S, et al. Impact of clinical severity on maternal and perinatal outcome across trimesters in COVID 19 pregnancies: a prospective cohort study. J Adv Med Med Res. 2024;36(2):63–76.
5. Ellington S, Strid P, Tong VT, Woodworth K, Galang RR, Zambrano LD, et al. Characteristics of women of reproductive age with laboratory-confirmed SARS-CoV-2 infection by pregnancy status — United States, January 22–June 7, 2020. Morb Mortal Wkly Rep. 2020;69(25):769–75.
6. Lipińska-Gediga M, Goździk W, Śmiechowicz J, Adamik B. Pregnancy and COVID-19: comparing ICU outcomes for pregnant and nonpregnant women. Viruses. 2025;17(1):51.
7. Garcia-Flores V, Romero R, Xu Y, Theis KR, Arenas-Hernandez M, Miller D, et al. Maternal-fetal immune responses in pregnant women infected with SARS-CoV-2. Nat Commun. 2022;13(1):320.
8. Tartaglia E, Bordoni V, Oliva A, Vergori A, Girardi E, Antinori A, et al. T helper profile in pregnant women recovered from COVID-19. J Reprod Immunol. 2022;153:103661.
9. Foo SS, Cambou MC, Mok T, Fajardo VM, Jung KL, Fuller T, et al. The systemic inflammatory landscape of COVID-19 in pregnancy: extensive serum proteomic profiling of mother-infant dyads with in utero SARS-CoV-2. Cell Rep Med. 2021;2(11):100453.
10. Lu-Culligan A, Chavan AR, Vijayakumar P, Irshaid L, Courchaine EM, Milano KM, et al. Maternal respiratory SARS-CoV-2 infection in pregnancy is associated with a robust inflammatory response at the maternal-fetal interface. Med. 2021;2(5):591–610.e10.
11. Jafari M, Pormohammad A, Sheikh Neshin SA, Ghorbani S, Bose D, Alimohammadi S, et al. Clinical characteristics and outcomes of pregnant women with COVID-19 and comparison with control patients: a systematic review and meta-analysis. Rev Med Virol. 2021;31(5):e2208.
12. Dawood FS, Varner M, Tita A, Newes-Adeyi G, Gyamfi-Bannerman C, Battarbee A, et al. Incidence and clinical characteristics of and risk factors for severe acute respiratory syndrome coronavirus 2 (SARS-CoV-2) infection among pregnant individuals in the United States. Clin Infect Dis. 2022;74(12):2218–26.
13. Abuova G, Ayazbekov A, Nurkhasimova R, Shaimardenova G, Kulbaeva S, Nurmagambet S. Asymptomatic forms of COVID-19 in pregnant women: long-term consequences. Int J Infect Dis. 2022;116:S46.

14. Machluf Y, Rosenfeld S, Ben Shlomo I, Chaiter Y, Dekel Y. The misattributed and silent causes of poor COVID-19 outcomes among pregnant women. Front Med. 2021;8:745797.
15. Georgakopoulou VE, Taskou C, Spandidos DA, Sarantaki A. Long COVID-19 and pregnancy: a systematic review. Biomed Rep. 2025;22(1):15.
16. Schwartz DA, Graham AL. Potential maternal and infant outcomes from (Wuhan) coronavirus 2019-nCoV infecting pregnant women: lessons from SARS, MERS, and other human coronavirus infections. Viruses. 2020;12(2):194.
17. Rasmussen SA, Jamieson DJ. COVID-19 and pregnancy. Infect Dis Clin N Am. 2022;36(2):423–33.
18. Raschetti R, Vivanti AJ, Vauloup-Fellous C, Loi B, Benachi A, De Luca D. Synthesis and systematic review of reported neonatal SARS-CoV-2 infections. Nat Commun. 2020;11:5164.
19. Jeganathan K, Paul AB. Vertical transmission of SARS-CoV-2: a systematic review. Obstet Med. 2022;15(2):91–8.
20. Ren H, Zhang X, Zhang S, Pan J, Wang W. The association of increased incidence of congenital heart disease in newborns with maternal COVID-19 infection during pregnancy. Sci Rep. 2024;14(1):24866.
21. Incognito GG, Distefano REC, Campo G, Gulino FA, Gulisano C, Gullotta C, et al. Comparison of maternal and neonatal outcomes between SARS-CoV-2 variants: a retrospective, monocentric study. J Clin Med [Internet]. 2023 Oct 1 [cited 2026 Jan 2];12(19). Available from: https://www.mdpi.com/2077-0383/12/19/6329.
22. Feng Q, Cui Q, Xiao Z, Liu Z, Fan S. Maternal and perinatal outcomes of SARS-CoV-2 and variants in pregnancy. Matern Fetal Med. 2023;5(2):104–14.
23. Uygun-Can B, Acar-Bolat B. Clinical properties and diagnostic methods of COVID-19 infection in pregnancies: meta-analysis. Biomed Res Int. 2020;2020:1708267.
24. Nana M, Hodson K, Lucas N, Camporota L, Knight M, Nelson-Piercy C. Diagnosis and management of covid-19 in pregnancy 2022 [cited 2025 July 9]; Available from: https://www.bmj.com/content/377/bmj-2021-069739.
25. Profiling Early Humoral Response to Diagnose Novel Coronavirus Disease (COVID-19) - PubMed [Internet]. [cited 2025 July 9]. Available from: https://pubmed.ncbi.nlm.nih.gov/32198501/.
26. Rottenstreich A, Zarbiv G, Kabiri D, Porat S, Sompolinsky Y, Reubinoff B, et al. Rapid antigen detection testing for universal screening for severe acute respiratory syndrome coronavirus 2 in women admitted for delivery. Am J Obstet Gynecol. 2021;224(5):539–40.
27. Maged El-Goly AM, Metwally AA. Diagnosis of COVID-19 infection in pregnancy. In: Covid-19 infect pregnancy; 2021. p. 39–62.
28. El-Goly AMM. Management of COVID-19 infection during pregnancy, labor, and puerperium. In: Covid-19 infect pregnancy; 2021. p. 63–89.
29. Teelucksingh S, Nana M, Nelson-Piercy C. Managing COVID-19 in pregnant women. Breathe (Sheff). 2022;18(2):220019.
30. Wu D, Fang D, Wang R, Deng D, Liao S. Management of pregnancy during the COVID-19 pandemic. Glob Chall. 2021;5(2):2000052.
31. Kurmanova G, Ayazbekov A, Kurmanova A, Rakhimbayeva M, Trimova G, Kulembayeva A. PostCOVID-19 impact on perinatal outcomes. Diagnostics (Basel). 2024;15(1):57.
32. Vousden N, Ramakrishnan R, Bunch K, Morris E, Simpson N, Gale C, et al. Management and implications of severe COVID-19 in pregnancy in the UK: data from the UK obstetric surveillance system national cohort. Acta Obstet Gynecol Scand. 2022;101(4):461–70.
33. Shimabukuro TT, Kim SY, Myers TR, Moro PL, Oduyebo T, Panagiotakopoulos L, et al. Preliminary findings of mRNA Covid-19 vaccine safety in pregnant persons. N Engl J Med. 2021;384(24):2273–82.
34. Magnus MC, Gjessing HK, Eide HN, Wilcox AJ, Fell DB, Håberg SE. Covid-19 vaccination during pregnancy and first-trimester miscarriage. N Engl J Med. 2021;385(21):2008–10.
35. Theiler RN, Wick M, Mehta R, Weaver AL, Virk A, Swift M. Pregnancy and birth outcomes after SARS-CoV-2 vaccination in pregnancy. Am J Obstet Gynecol MFM. 2021;3(6):100467.

36. Blakeway H, Prasad S, Kalafat E, Heath PT, Ladhani SN, Le Doare K, et al. COVID-19 vaccination during pregnancy: coverage and safety. Am J Obstet Gynecol. 2022;226(2):236.e1–236.e14.
37. Collier ARY, McMahan K, Yu J, Tostanoski LH, Aguayo R, Ansel J, et al. Immunogenicity of COVID-19 mRNA vaccines in pregnant and lactating women. JAMA. 2021;325(23):2370–80.
38. Kalafat E, Heath P, Prasad S, O Brien P, Khalil A. COVID-19 vaccination in pregnancy. Am J Obstet Gynecol. 2022;227(2):136–47.
39. Flannery DD, Gouma S, Dhudasia MB, Mukhopadhyay S, Pfeifer MR, Woodford EC, et al. Assessment of maternal and neonatal cord blood SARS-CoV-2 antibodies and placental transfer ratios. JAMA Pediatr. 2021;175(6):594–600.
40. Beharier O, Plitman Mayo R, Raz T, Nahum Sacks K, Schreiber L, Suissa-Cohen Y, et al. Efficient maternal to neonatal transfer of antibodies against SARS-CoV-2 and BNT162b2 mRNA COVID-19 vaccine. J Clin Invest. 2021;131(13):e150319.
41. Perl SH, Uzan-Yulzari A, Klainer H, Asiskovich L, Youngster M, Rinott E, et al. SARS-CoV-2-specific antibodies in breast milk after COVID-19 vaccination of breastfeeding women. JAMA. 2021;325(19):2013–4.

Long-Term Effects of COVID-19

17

Amrita Pattanaik

17.1 Introduction

Coronavirus disease 2019 (COVID-19), caused by the severe acute respiratory syndrome coronavirus 2 (SARS-CoV-2), was initially viewed as an acute respiratory infection. However, as the pandemic evolved, it became evident that a significant proportion of individuals do not fully recover even weeks or months after the acute illness. Also, it was seen that multiple organ systems were involved, leading to severe and protracted impairment of function. This phenomenon, now widely referred to as "long COVID" or post-acute sequelae of SARS-CoV-2 infection (PASC), has become a significant public health concern. The other terminologies used to indicate the long-term sequelae of COVID are "post-acute (sequelae of) COVID-19" and "chronic COVID-19". Many clinicians are uncertain about evaluating and managing patients with this condition due to conflicting definitions, the presence of multiple proposed pathophysiological mechanisms, lack of universally accepted biomarkers to indicate the condition for diagnosis and prognosis [1–4].

The term "long COVID" has been used by the public health bodies in the United States as the persistence of signs and symptoms beyond 4 weeks from the onset of acute illness [5]. WHO uses the term "post-COVID condition" and defines it as symptoms persisting for at least 2 months, without an alternative explanation, in individuals with a history of confirmed or probable SARS-CoV-2 infection [6]. The UK health organisations use the term "post-COVID-19 syndrome" and define it as symptoms that persist for more than 12 weeks following acute SARS-CoV-2 infection and cannot be attributed to another diagnosis [7]. The range of symptoms is broad and involves multiple organ systems, reflecting the systemic impact of SARS-CoV-2 infection. Patients may experience fatigue, cognitive impairment, dyspnoea, chest pain, palpitations, and psychological dysfunction, among others. In severe cases, there can be considerable damage to the heart, lungs, kidneys, skin, and brain.

A. Pattanaik (✉)
National Institute of Mental Health and Neuro Sciences (NIMHANS), Bengaluru, India

S. R. Prabhu et al. (eds.), *COVID-19 in Dental Practice*,
https://doi.org/10.1007/978-3-032-26000-0_17

The burden extends beyond clinical symptoms, affecting social functioning and quality of life [8].

This chapter aims to impart a comprehensive overview of the long-term effects of COVID-19. By examining epidemiology, pathophysiology, clinical features, management strategies, and public health implications, it seeks to educate students and healthcare professionals with the essential knowledge to address the evolving challenge of post-COVID sequelae.

17.2 Epidemiology of Long COVID

Long COVID affects a notable proportion of individuals who are diagnosed with SARS-CoV-2 infection. The incidence of the condition varies significantly across studies: 50–85% among unvaccinated hospitalised patients, 10–35% among unvaccinated individuals who were not hospitalised, and 8–12% among vaccinated individuals. The risk appears higher in those who experienced severe acute disease requiring hospitalisation, but even mild or asymptomatic cases have reported persistent symptoms [2].

Various risk factors influence the presentation of long COVID in patients. Specific symptoms such as muscle aches, headaches, fatigue, and shortness of breath in the first week of infection are predictive of long COVID. Other risk factors include older age (higher risk in age >50 years) and comorbidities like obesity, asthma, diabetes, and cardiovascular disease. Women are more likely to develop long COVID. It is also seen that the condition is more prevalent in low socioeconomic and disadvantaged ethnic groups. Vaccination has been shown to reduce, though not eliminate, the risk of long-term sequelae. Re-infection is another significant risk factor for developing long COVID. Emerging data also suggest that certain viral variants may influence the prevalence and presentation of long COVID [2, 9, 10].

From a health systems perspective, the global burden is substantial. Millions worldwide may require ongoing care, placing a strain on healthcare resources, rehabilitation services, and workforce productivity. Recognition of this burden has prompted the development of specialised post-COVID clinics in many countries [11].

17.3 Pathophysiology of Long COVID

The mechanisms underlying long COVID are complex and multifactorial. The pathophysiological pathways are multiple, including the following:

- *Viral Persistence and Reactivation of Latent Viruses*: Fragments of viral RNA and proteins like spike and nucleocapsid protein have been identified in the gut, respiratory tract, and even the central nervous system months after acute infection. Persistent antigenic stimulation may drive chronic immune activation [2, 4, 12, 13].

- *Chronic Inflammation and Immune Dysregulation*: Abnormal immune responses are a key feature. Autoantibody production against self-antigens has been detected, raising concerns about autoimmunity. Persistent elevation of pro-inflammatory cytokines, reduced T-cell function, and impaired viral clearance suggest an immune imbalance [4, 14, 15].
- *Coagulopathy from Endothelial Dysfunction and Microvascular Injury*: SARS-CoV-2 directly infects endothelial cells via ACE2 receptors, disrupting vascular integrity. This leads to a pro-thrombotic state, microvascular inflammation, and impaired oxygenation. Such mechanisms likely explain lingering chest pain, dyspnoea, and symptoms of the Central Nervous System (CNS) [4, 16, 17].
- *Neuroinflammation and Autonomic Dysfunction*: Neuroimaging and biomarker data support that long COVID involves chronic neuroinflammation, particularly in brainstem regions like the dorsolateral inferior medulla, potentially disrupting autonomic centres. Autonomic dysfunction may manifest as postural orthostatic tachycardia syndrome (POTS), orthostatic hypotension, reduced heart rate variability, and other features [4, 18].
- *Gut Dysbiosis*: Gut dysbiosis is characterised by reduced microbial diversity or loss of beneficial bacteria and overgrowth of opportunistic pathogens. This can compromise gut barrier integrity. This disruption may lead to systemic inflammation through microbial translocation, immune dysregulation, and sustained activation of pro-inflammatory pathways, contributing to persistent symptoms of long COVID [4, 19].
- *Mitochondrial and Metabolic Dysfunction*: Long COVID patients frequently report post-exertional malaise and fatigue resembling chronic fatigue syndrome. Impaired mitochondrial function may underlie these symptoms [4, 20].
- *Psychosocial Interplay*: While primarily biological, long COVID is worsened by long-term effects of medical trauma related to isolation, stress, and uncertainty (e.g., post-ICU syndrome, post-traumatic stress disorder (PTSD)). These psychosocial factors can amplify symptom perception and recovery challenges [4, 21].

17.4 Clinical Features and Diagnosis

Long COVID manifests across multiple organ systems, with varied severity and duration.

- *Respiratory*: Long COVID respiratory system manifestations are primarily cough and dyspnoea, with hypoxaemia. Some individuals continue to desaturate on exertion months after acute infection. Pulmonary function tests reveal diffusion impairments in some patients. Imaging may show fibrosis, bronchial wall thickening, or residual ground-glass opacities [4, 22].

- *Neurological and Cognitive*: Cognitive dysfunction or "brain fog" is among the most disabling neurological features seen in long COVID. Patients report memory lapses, poor attention, slowed processing, and impaired execution. Neurocognitive tests support these subjective complaints. Ongoing neuroinflammation is a major driver hypothesised to be the cause of the fatigue/neuropsychiatric symptoms. Other neurological features include anosmia, dysgeusia, neuropathic pain, dizziness, headaches, and sleep disturbances [23–25].
- *Cardiovascular*: The common cardiovascular symptoms in long COVID include palpitation, tachycardia, chest pain, myocarditis, pericarditis, and arrhythmias. Postural orthostatic tachycardia syndrome (POTS) and inappropriate sinus tachycardia are increasingly being recognised. Cardiac MRI has demonstrated lingering myocardial inflammation in a subset of patients, raising concerns about long-term cardiac outcomes. Thromboembolic events, although rare, remain a concern in patients with long COVID [4, 26, 27].
- *Psychological*: Rates of depression, anxiety, and PTSD are significantly higher among Long COVID patients. Insomnia, irritability, and social withdrawal are common. Stigma and disbelief from peers or healthcare providers often exacerbate these mental health issues [4, 21].
- *Musculoskeletal and Systemic*: Fatigue, post-exertional malaise, myalgia, and arthralgia persist for months in many. Patients describe profound weakness, limiting activities of daily living. Some experience joint swelling and stiffness, raising the possibility of autoimmune activation [28, 29].
- *Other Systems*: Gastrointestinal manifestations (abdominal pain, bloating, and diarrhoea), endocrine abnormalities (thyroiditis, menstrual irregularities, and glycaemic fluctuations), renal impairment, dermatological features (alopecia, urticaria, and rashes), and ocular involvement (conjunctivitis and blurred vision) have been documented [30–34].
- *Diagnosis*: Long COVID remains a diagnosis of exclusion. Evaluation requires a detailed clinical history, physical examination, and targeted investigations. Recommended assessments include pulmonary function tests, echocardiography, autonomic function testing, neuropsychological evaluations, MRI for neurological or cardiac symptoms, and relevant blood work (inflammatory, coagulation, and autoimmune profiles) [35, 36].

17.5 Management of Long COVID

Management of long COVID is challenging and requires a holistic, individualised approach.

Multidisciplinary Care Long COVID clinics are emerging worldwide, integrating pulmonologists, cardiologists, neurologists, rheumatologists, psychiatrists, and rehabilitation specialists. This model ensures coordinated evaluation and therapy, thereby reducing care fragmentation [35, 36].

Symptom-Targeted Interventions

- *Respiratory*: Pulmonary rehabilitation programmes focus on breathing techniques, gradual reconditioning, and supplemental oxygen when indicated. Antifibrotic therapies are under trial for post COVID pulmonary fibrosis [2, 4, 38].
- *Neurological*: Cognitive rehabilitation includes memory training, occupational therapy, and structured return-to-work or academic plans. Sleep disorders may require pharmacological management or behavioural interventions. Neuropathic pain can be treated with agents like gabapentin or duloxetine [2, 37].
- *Cardiovascular*: Patients with POTS benefit from increased salt/fluid intake, compression stockings, and graded exercise. Medications like beta-blockers, ivabradine, or midodrine may be used. Regular cardiac monitoring is essential in patients with myocarditis [2, 37].
- *Fatigue and Musculoskeletal Symptoms*: Careful pacing strategies are key, as overexertion can worsen post-exertional malaise. Anti-inflammatory or analgesic medications may provide symptomatic relief [2, 37].
- *Psychological*: Access to counselling, cognitive behavioural therapy (CBT), and psychiatric care is essential. Selective serotonin reuptake inhibitors (SSRIs) and anxiolytics may help in moderate to severe cases. Peer support groups have shown positive outcomes in patient engagement and mental health [2, 37].
- *Other Systems*: In long COVID, gastrointestinal symptoms (abdominal pain, bloating, altered bowel habits) are managed with dietary changes, probiotics, or acid-suppressive therapy. Endocrine disturbances such as thyroiditis, menstrual irregularities, or glycaemic instability are treated via standard protocols with close monitoring. Dermatological issues, including alopecia, urticaria, or rashes, are generally self-limiting but may require topical steroids, antihistamines, or specialist referral. Overall, care remains symptom-targeted and supportive, escalating to speciality input when persistent or severe [2].

Emerging and Experimental Therapies Several pharmacological strategies are under investigation, including antivirals targeting residual viral reservoirs, immunomodulators to correct immune dysregulation, and agents targeting microclots or endothelial dysfunction. Clinical trials are ongoing and hold promise for future standardised therapies [39].

Rehabilitation and Lifestyle Strategies Physical therapy, yoga, mindfulness, and graded return-to-activity programmes have demonstrated benefit. Telemedicine platforms are vital for follow-up, especially in rural or resource-limited areas [2, 40].

17.6 Societal and Public Health Impact

The burden of long COVID extends far beyond individual health, affecting families, communities, and economies. As Greenhalgh et al. note, persistent symptoms such as fatigue, cognitive dysfunction, and post-exertional malaise often impair people's ability to return to work, leading to high rates of absenteeism, reduced productivity, and in severe cases, prolonged disability leave [2]. These effects are not confined to older adults or those with pre-existing conditions—adolescents and young adults are also affected, facing significant academic disruption due to difficulty concentrating, memory lapses, and reduced stamina. The loss of educational and employment opportunities in younger cohorts underscores the long-term socio-economic consequences of the condition.

Healthcare systems, already strained by acute COVID-19 surges, must now absorb the increased demand for multidisciplinary diagnostics, speciality consultations, and prolonged rehabilitation services [2]. This surge includes complex needs such as cardiopulmonary evaluation, neurocognitive assessment, and mental health support. Emerging rehabilitation trials, such as the CICERO study, are testing telehealth-delivered cognitive rehabilitation interventions to address disabling "brain fog" and improve daily functioning [40]. These innovations demonstrate the importance of integrating digital health solutions to expand access, especially in rural or resource-limited settings.

From a policy perspective, long COVID highlights the urgent need for systemic adjustments:

- Workplace accommodations (e.g., flexible hours, remote work options, graded return-to-work programmes) to support employees struggling with fluctuating symptoms.
- Disability recognition frameworks to ensure financial and social protections for those unable to resume employment.
- Guaranteed access to rehabilitation services, including physical therapy, cognitive rehabilitation, and psychological care, to reduce the risk of long-term dependence and marginalisation.

Together, these measures state that long COVID is not merely a clinical challenge but a societal issue demanding coordinated responses across healthcare, education, labour, and social policy domains [2, 40].

17.7 Research and Future Directions

Research priorities in long COVID have been shaped through collaborative efforts involving patients, caregivers, clinicians, and researchers. A recent multi-stakeholder priority-setting partnership identified several critical areas of focus, including defining reliable biomarkers for diagnosis, unravelling the underlying pathophysiological mechanisms, and accelerating the development of targeted therapies. These priorities reflect the lived realities of patients who continue to experience debilitating symptoms years after acute infection and underscore the urgent need for translational research that links mechanistic understanding to effective interventions [41].

Ongoing and planned clinical trials are investigating a wide spectrum of potential therapies. These include antivirals to clear residual viral reservoirs, anti-inflammatory or immunomodulatory agents to address immune dysregulation, and antithrombotic strategies targeting microclots and endothelial dysfunction. Parallel studies are exploring rehabilitation programmes, ranging from structured physical therapy to cognitive and psychological support to optimise functional recovery and improve quality of life [39, 41].

Beyond the laboratory and clinic, long COVID highlights broader implications for pandemic preparedness. The pandemic has revealed critical gaps in health system resilience, particularly in addressing the chronic sequelae of infectious diseases. Health systems must, therefore, be designed not only to manage acute surges but also to support survivors facing long-term morbidity. This includes scaling multidisciplinary care pathways, investing in rehabilitation infrastructure, and embedding patient-centred approaches into routine practice [42].

17.8 Conclusion

Long COVID represents one of the most complex outcomes of the SARS-CoV-2 pandemic. Since it affects multiple organ systems and impairs quality of life, it poses major challenges for patients, clinicians, and health systems alike. While most patients eventually recover, a subset experiences prolonged disability. Early recognition, multidisciplinary care, and tailored rehabilitation are key to improving outcomes. Ongoing research is critical for elucidating pathophysiological mechanisms, identifying effective treatments, and developing preventive strategies.

Summary Table

Long COVID—significant symptoms, diagnosis, and management

Organ system	Common symptoms	Diagnostic tools	Management strategies	References
Respiratory	Dyspnoea, cough, chest tightness, exercise intolerance	Pulmonary function tests, chest CT/X-ray, oximetry	Pulmonary rehab, oxygen therapy, anti-fibrotics (trial)	[2, 4, 37]
Neurological/Cognitive	Brain fog, memory loss, headaches, anosmia, sleep disturbance	Neurocognitive testing, MRI, autonomic testing	Cognitive rehab, sleep hygiene, neuropathic pain medications	[2, 36]
Cardiovascular	Palpitations, chest pain, tachycardia, POTS, myocarditis	ECG, echocardiography, cardiac MRI, Holter monitoring	Beta-blockers, ivabradine, fluids/salt, cardiac monitoring	[2, 36]
Psychological	Depression, anxiety, PTSD, insomnia	Psychiatric evaluation, screening questionnaires	CBT, counselling, SSRIs/anxiolytics, peer support	[2, 36]
Musculoskeletal	Fatigue, myalgia, arthralgia, post-exertional malaise	Functional assessments, inflammatory markers	Pacing, graded activity (individualized), analgesics	[2, 36]

References

1. Kostka K, Roel E, Trinh NTH, Mercadé-Besora N, Delmestri A, Mateu L, et al. The burden of post-acute COVID-19 symptoms in a multinational network cohort analysis. Nat Commun. 2023;14(1):7449. https://doi.org/10.1038/s41467-023-42726-0.
2. Greenhalgh T, Sivan M, Perlowski A, Nikolich JŽ. Long COVID: a clinical update. Lancet. 2024;404(10453):707–24. https://doi.org/10.1016/S0140-6736(24)01136-X.
3. Pattanaik A, Bhandarkar BS, Lodha L, Marate S. SARS-CoV-2 and the nervous system: current perspectives. Arch Virol. 2023;168(6):171. https://doi.org/10.1007/s00705-023-05801-x.
4. Vlaming-van Eijk LE, Tang G, Bourgonje AR, den Dunnen WFA, Hillebrands JL, van Goor H. Post-COVID-19 condition: clinical phenotypes, pathophysiological mechanisms, pathology, and management strategies. J Pathol. 2025;266(4–5):369–89. https://doi.org/10.1002/path.6443.
5. Centers for Disease Control And Prevention. Long COVID [Internet]. Atlanta: CDC; 2025 [cited 2025 Sep 21]. Available from: https://www.cdc.gov/long-covid/about/index.html.
6. Soriano JB, Murthy S, Marshall JC, Relan P, Diaz JV. WHO clinical case definition working group on post-COVID-19 condition. A clinical case definition of post-COVID-19 condition by a Delphi consensus. Lancet Infect Dis. 2022;22(4):e102–7. https://doi.org/10.1016/S1473-3099(21)00703-9.
7. NHS England. Post COVID syndrome (long COVID) [Internet]. London: NHS England; 2025 [cited 2025 Sep 21]. Available from: https://www.england.nhs.uk/coronavirus/post-covid-syndrome-long-covid/.
8. O'Keefe LC. Post-acute COVID-19 syndrome, "long COVID". Workplace Health Saf. 2023;71(5):263. https://doi.org/10.1177/21650799231164605.
9. Turner S, Khan MA, Putrino D, Woodcock A, Kell DB, Pretorius E. Long COVID: pathophysiological factors and abnormalities of coagulation. Trends Endocrinol Metab. 2023;34(6):321–44. https://doi.org/10.1016/j.tem.2023.03.002.
10. Xie Y, Choi T, Al-Aly Z. Postacute sequelae of SARS-CoV-2 infection in the pre-Delta, Delta, and Omicron eras. N Engl J Med. 2024;391(6):515–25. https://doi.org/10.1056/NEJMoa2403211.
11. Al-Aly Z, Davis H, McCorkell L, Soares L, Wulf-Hanson S, Iwasaki A, et al. Long COVID science, research and policy. Nat Med. 2024;30(8):2148–64. https://doi.org/10.1038/s41591-024-03173-6.
12. Craddock V, Mahajan A, Spikes L, Krishnamachary B, Ram AK, Kumar A, et al. Persistent circulation of soluble and extracellular vesicle-linked spike protein in individuals with postacute sequelae of COVID-19. J Med Virol. 2023;95(2):e28568. https://doi.org/10.1002/jmv.28568.
13. Peluso MJ, Ryder D, Flavell RR, Wang Y, Levi J, LaFranchi BH, et al. Tissue-based T cell activation and viral RNA persist for up to 2 years after SARS-CoV-2 infection. Sci Transl Med. 2024;16(754):eadk3295. https://doi.org/10.1126/scitranslmed.adk3295.
14. Garmendia JV, García AH, De Sanctis CV, Hajdúch M, De Sanctis JB. Autoimmunity and immunodeficiency in severe SARS-CoV-2 infection and prolonged COVID-19. Curr Issues Mol Biol. 2022;45(1):33–50. https://doi.org/10.3390/cimb45010003.
15. Saito S, Shahbaz S, Osman M, Redmond D, Bozorgmehr N, Rosychuk RJ, et al. Diverse immunological dysregulation, chronic inflammation, and impaired erythropoiesis in long COVID patients with chronic fatigue syndrome. J Autoimmun. 2024;147:103267. https://doi.org/10.1016/j.jaut.2024.103267.
16. Montezano AC, Camargo LL, Mary S, Neves KB, Rios FJ, Stein R, et al. SARS-CoV-2 spike protein induces endothelial inflammation via ACE2 independently of viral replication. Sci Rep. 2023;13(1):14086. https://doi.org/10.1038/s41598-023-41115-3.
17. Bernard I, Limonta D, Mahal LK, Hobman TC. Endothelium infection and dysregulation by SARS-CoV-2: evidence and caveats in COVID-19. Viruses. 2020;13(1):29. https://doi.org/10.3390/v13010029.

18. Blitshteyn S. Neuroinflammation at the dorsolateral inferior medulla: a possible central nervous system localization for POTS and long COVID. Biomedicine. 2025;13(1):166. https://doi.org/10.3390/biomedicines13010166.
19. Vidal A, Barrows B, Bao G, Goudzwaard A, Papoutsis A, Hazan S. COVID-19 long COVID and gut dysbiosis. Am J Gastroenterol. 2024;119(Suppl 1):S170. https://doi.org/10.14309/01.ajg.0001029304.22881.fe.
20. Macnaughtan J, Chau KY, Brennan E, Toffoli M, Spinazzola A, Hillman T, et al. Mitochondrial function is impaired in long COVID patients. Ann Med. 2025;57(1):2528167. https://doi.org/10.1080/07853890.2025.2528167.
21. Sankar K, Gould MK, Prescott HC. Psychological morbidity after COVID-19 critical illness. Chest. 2023;163(1):139–47. https://doi.org/10.1016/j.chest.2022.09.035.
22. Patton MJ, Benson D, Robison SW, Raval D, Locy ML, Patel K, et al. Characteristics and determinants of pulmonary long COVID. JCI Insight. 2024;9(10):e177518. https://doi.org/10.1172/jci.insight.177518.
23. Braga J, Lepra M, Kish SJ, et al. Neuroinflammation after COVID-19 with persistent depressive and cognitive symptoms. JAMA Psychiatry. 2023;80:787–95.
24. Elboraay T, Ebada MA, Elsayed M, et al. Long-term neurological and cognitive impact of COVID-19: a systematic review and meta-analysis in over 4 million patients. BMC Neurol. 2025;25:250. https://doi.org/10.1186/s12883-025-04174-9.
25. Jennings G, Monaghan A, Xue F, Duggan E, Romero-Ortuño R. Comprehensive clinical characterisation of brain fog in adults reporting long COVID symptoms. J Clin Med. 2022;11(12):3440. https://doi.org/10.3390/jcm11123440.
26. Lingering cardiac involvement in previously well people after mild COVID-19. Nat Med. 2022;28(10):2011–2. https://doi.org/10.1038/s41591-022-02002-y.
27. Ormiston CK, Świątkiewicz I, Taub PR. Postural orthostatic tachycardia syndrome as a sequela of COVID-19. Heart Rhythm. 2022;19(11):1880–9. https://doi.org/10.1016/j.hrthm.2022.07.014.
28. Twomey R, DeMars J, Franklin K, Culos-Reed SN, Weatherald J, Wrightson JG. Chronic fatigue and post-exertional malaise in people living with long COVID. Phys Ther. 2022;102(4):pzac005. https://doi.org/10.1093/ptj/pzac005.
29. Karaarslan F, Güneri FD, Kardeş S. Long COVID: rheumatologic and musculoskeletal symptoms in hospitalized COVID-19 survivors at 3 and 6 months. Clin Rheumatol. 2022;41(1):289–96. https://doi.org/10.1007/s10067-021-05942-x.
30. Choudhury A, Tariq R, Jena A, Vesely EK, Singh S, Khanna S, et al. Gastrointestinal manifestations of long COVID: a systematic review and meta-analysis. Ther Adv Gastroenterol. 2022;15:17562848221118403. https://doi.org/10.1177/17562848221118403.
31. Mourelatos P, Vrettou CS, Diamantopoulos A, Vassiliou AG, Jahaj E, Angelousi A, et al. A prospective study on endocrine function in patients with long COVID symptoms. Hormones (Athens). 2024;23(1):59–67. https://doi.org/10.1007/s42000-023-00511-0.
32. Frediani MM, Ribeiro HS, Busatto GF, Carvalho CRR, Burdmann EA. Renal long COVID: a scoping review. Kidney Med. 2025;7(8):101039. https://doi.org/10.1016/j.xkme.2025.101039.
33. Martora F, Villani A, Fabbrocini G, Battista T. COVID-19 and cutaneous manifestations: a review of the published literature. J Cosmet Dermatol. 2023;22(1):4–10. https://doi.org/10.1111/jocd.15477.
34. Huang D, Xuan W, Li Z. Impact of COVID-19 on ocular surface health: infection mechanisms, immune modulation, and inflammatory responses. Viruses. 2025;17(1):68. https://doi.org/10.3390/v17010068.
35. Bailey J, Lavelle B, Miller J, Jimenez M, Lim PH, Orban ZS, et al. Multidisciplinary center care for long COVID syndrome: a retrospective cohort study. Am J Med. 2025;138(1):108–20. https://doi.org/10.1016/j.amjmed.2023.05.002.
36. Yelin D, Moschopoulos CD, Margalit I, Gkrania-Klotsas E, Landi F, Stahl JP, et al. ESCMID rapid guidelines for assessment and management of long COVID. Clin Microbiol Infect. 2022;28(7):955–72. https://doi.org/10.1016/j.cmi.2022.02.018.

37. Seo JW, Kim SE, Kim Y, Kim EJ, Kim T, Lee SH, et al. Updated clinical practice guidelines for the diagnosis and management of long COVID. Infect Chemother. 2024;56(1):122–57. https://doi.org/10.3947/ic.2024.0024.
38. Shu Y, He L, Liu C. Impact of antifibrotic medications on post-COVID-19 pulmonary fibrosis: a systematic review and meta-analysis. Int J Infect Dis. 2024;147:107193. https://doi.org/10.1016/j.ijid.2024.107193.
39. Bonilla H, Peluso MJ, Rodgers K, Aberg JA, Patterson TF, Tamburro R, et al. Therapeutic trials for long COVID-19: a call to action from the RECOVER initiative. Front Immunol. 2023;14:1129459. https://doi.org/10.3389/fimmu.2023.1129459.
40. Vanova M, Patel AMR, Scott I, et al. Telehealth-delivered cognitive rehabilitation for post-COVID syndrome: CICERO study protocol. Trials. 2024;25:704. https://doi.org/10.1186/s13063-024-08554-3.
41. Grant A, Stage E, Blane D, Goss H, Ormerod J, McIver S, et al. Four years in: research priorities for long COVID. Health Expect. 2024;27(5):e70072. https://doi.org/10.1111/hex.70072.
42. Sundararaman T, Muraleedharan VR, Ranjan A. Pandemic resilience and health systems preparedness: lessons from COVID-19. J Soc Econ Dev. 2021;23(Suppl 2):290–300. https://doi.org/10.1007/s40847-020-00133-x.

COVID-19 in Children

18

Amrita Pattanaik

18.1 Introduction

Coronavirus disease 2019 (COVID-19) is caused by the severe acute respiratory syndrome coronavirus 2 (SARS-CoV-2), a novel beta-coronavirus identified in December 2019 in Wuhan, China. The World Health Organisation declared it a pandemic on March 11, 2020 [1]. While COVID-19 predominantly affects adults, children have been less frequently diagnosed, accounting for approximately 1–5% of confirmed cases [2]. The clinical presentation in children is often milder, with many being asymptomatic or exhibiting mild symptoms such as fever, cough, pharyngeal erythema, and gastrointestinal disorders [2]. However, rare but severe manifestations, such as Multisystem Inflammatory Syndrome in Children (MIS-C), have been observed, characterised by high fever, rash, conjunctivitis, and gastrointestinal symptoms with potential for multiorgan failure [3]. Understanding these unique aspects is crucial for healthcare providers to ensure timely diagnosis and appropriate management.

This chapter aims to equip students with a comprehensive understanding of COVID-19 in children, emphasising the differences in clinical presentation compared to adults. By focusing on the pathophysiology, diagnostic approaches, management strategies, and preventive measures, students will be better prepared to address the challenges posed by the disease in paediatric populations.

A. Pattanaik (✉)
National Institute of Mental Health and Neuro Sciences (NIMHANS), Bengaluru, India

S. R. Prabhu et al. (eds.), *COVID-19 in Dental Practice*,
https://doi.org/10.1007/978-3-032-26000-0_18

18.2 Epidemiology and Transmission of COVID-19 in Children

18.2.1 Global Epidemiology

Globally, children represent a smaller proportion of confirmed COVID-19 cases, typically ranging from 1–13% depending on the region. In high-income countries, paediatric cases surged during variant waves (e.g., Delta and Omicron), while low- and middle-income countries often reported lower testing rates, potentially underestimating the actual paediatric burden [4].

18.2.2 Age Distribution

COVID-19 affects all paediatric age groups, but disease severity and presentation vary. Infants (<1 year) are more vulnerable to hospitalisation, while children aged 5–11 generally experience mild or asymptomatic illness [2]. Adolescents show higher infection rates compared to younger children, likely due to increased mobility and social interaction [5, 6]. Milder disease in young children is hypothesised to stem from lower ACE2 receptor expression, which SARS-CoV-2 uses for cell entry, and more robust innate immune responses. Additionally, pre-existing cross-reactive immunity from frequent exposures to common cold coronaviruses may play a protective role [7].

18.2.3 Transmission Dynamics

Children, particularly when asymptomatic or mildly symptomatic, contribute significantly to SARS-CoV-2 household transmission [8]. While early in the pandemic, they were considered less likely to drive community spread, later studies revealed comparable viral loads to adults. School outbreaks demonstrated efficient in-group transmission, although mitigation strategies (e.g., masking, ventilation) reduced spread. Preschool-aged children typically transmit the virus to caregivers rather than peers, whereas older children and adolescents more frequently initiate household clusters. The role of asymptomatic carriers, especially among the younger age groups, underscores the importance of widespread testing and contact tracing [9, 10].

18.2.4 Risk Factors

While most children experience mild COVID-19, certain pre-existing conditions increase the risk of severe outcomes. Asthma and obesity are the most frequently identified comorbidities associated with hospitalisation. Immunocompromised children, including those undergoing chemotherapy or with primary immunodeficiencies, face increased risk of prolonged illness and complications. Neurological conditions and chronic cardiac disease also correlate with higher ICU admission rates. Despite this, mortality remains low in paediatric populations. Ethnic and socioeconomic disparities further influence outcomes, with marginalised groups experiencing higher disease burden and limited access to care [11–13].

18.3 Pathophysiology of COVID-19 in Children

18.3.1 Viral Entry and Immune Response

SARS-CoV-2 infects host cells via the angiotensin-converting enzyme 2 (ACE2) receptor, with cellular entry facilitated by the serine protease TMPRSS2. Paediatric populations exhibit lower ACE2 expression in nasal and pulmonary epithelium, which may reduce viral entry efficiency. Additionally, children show a more robust innate immune response, including heightened expression of pattern-recognition receptors and interferon pathways, which contribute to early viral control. Frequent viral exposures in early life may prime the immune system, promoting rapid clearance of SARS-CoV-2. These immunological factors collectively contribute to the generally milder clinical course observed in children [11, 14].

18.3.2 Differential Pathogenesis

Compared to adults, children with COVID-19 typically experience a milder disease course, likely due to differences in immune response and vascular function. Adults are more prone to dysregulated immune activation, including the cytokine storm, which contributes to severe lung injury and multi-organ dysfunction. In contrast, children demonstrate a more regulated immune activation with limited pro-inflammatory cytokine release. Endothelial integrity, which diminishes with age, also plays a protective role in younger populations. Moreover, the lower prevalence of comorbidities such as cardiovascular disease and diabetes in children further reduces the risk of severe outcomes [15, 16].

18.3.3 Multisystem Inflammatory Syndrome in Children (MIS-C)

MIS-C is a rare but serious complication that typically arises 2–6 weeks after SARS-CoV-2 infection. It is characterised by systemic hyperinflammation affecting multiple organs, including the heart, gastrointestinal tract, and nervous system. The pathogenesis is hypothesised to involve a post-viral autoimmune or autoinflammatory response, distinct from acute COVID-19. Diagnostic criteria, as defined by the CDC, include fever, laboratory markers of inflammation, multisystem involvement, and recent SARS-CoV-2 infection or exposure [17]. Management involves supportive care and immunomodulatory therapy such as intravenous immunoglobulin (IVIG), corticosteroids, and, in severe cases, biologics like anakinra [18].

18.3.4 Long COVID in Children

Emerging evidence indicates that a subset of children experiences persistent symptoms—termed "long COVID"—after resolution of acute infection. Symptoms include fatigue, cognitive difficulties, mood disturbances, and exercise intolerance, lasting weeks to months. While the prevalence appears lower than in adults, long COVID can significantly impact quality of life and school attendance. Pathophysiological mechanisms may include immune dysregulation, autonomic dysfunction, and viral persistence. Ongoing cohort studies are refining case definitions and identifying risk factors, such as older age, female sex, and initial symptom burden [19]. Multidisciplinary care is recommended for affected children, with individualised rehabilitation plans [20].

18.4 Clinical Features and Diagnosis

18.4.1 Common Symptoms in Children

Children with COVID-19 commonly present with mild to moderate symptoms. Respiratory symptoms such as fever, cough, nasal congestion, and shortness of breath are most frequently reported. Gastrointestinal manifestations, including diarrhoea, vomiting, and abdominal pain, are more prevalent in children than adults and may occur even in the absence of respiratory symptoms. Atypical presentations—such as conjunctivitis, rash, or neurological symptoms like anosmia, headaches, and fatigue—have also been documented. Infants may display non-specific signs such as poor feeding or irritability. These varied presentations can delay diagnosis and complicate clinical decision-making in paediatric settings [21, 22].

18.4.2 Severe Disease Manifestations

Although most paediatric cases are mild, a minority develop severe disease. Acute respiratory distress syndrome (ARDS), viral pneumonia, and sepsis-like syndromes are observed in severe cases, particularly among children with comorbidities. Chest imaging may show bilateral ground-glass opacities, consolidation, or pleural effusions in severe disease. In critically ill children, complications can include myocarditis, coagulopathy, and multiorgan failure. Admission to paediatric intensive care units (PICUs) is generally low, but those requiring ventilation or inotropic support have higher morbidity. Risk factors for severe outcomes include obesity, chronic lung disease, and immunosuppression [11, 23].

18.4.3 MIS-C: Clinical Presentation and Timing

Multisystem Inflammatory Syndrome in Children (MIS-C) is a post-infectious complication typically occurring 2–6 weeks after SARS-CoV-2 exposure. Clinical features include persistent high fever, abdominal pain, vomiting, rash, conjunctivitis, and mucocutaneous inflammation. Cardiac involvement—such as myocarditis, pericardial effusion, or coronary artery dilation—is common, and echocardiography is critical for evaluation. Laboratory findings include elevated inflammatory markers (CRP, ESR, ferritin), lymphopenia, and elevated troponin or BNP. Differentiation from Kawasaki disease and septic shock is essential, and a history of recent COVID-19 infection or positive serology supports diagnosis [18].

18.4.4 Diagnostic Approach

The primary diagnostic method for acute COVID-19 is real-time reverse transcription PCR (RT-PCR), typically performed on nasopharyngeal swabs. Antigen testing offers rapid results but has lower sensitivity, especially in asymptomatic individuals. Serologic testing may aid in identifying past infection or MIS-C. Imaging plays a key role: chest X-rays can detect pneumonia, while CT scans are reserved for complex cases due to radiation risks. Echocardiography is recommended for patients with suspected MIS-C to assess myocardial function and coronary arteries. Laboratory panels assessing inflammation, coagulation, and organ function help guide management in moderate-to-severe disease [18, 23–25].

18.4.5 Differential Diagnosis

Differential diagnoses include respiratory syncytial virus (RSV), influenza, adenovirus, and other viral illnesses. RSV and influenza may present similarly with fever, cough, and respiratory distress but tend to show distinct seasonality and clinical courses. PCR-based multiplex panels can aid differentiation, and MIS-C must be distinguished from bacterial sepsis or Kawasaki disease [26–28].

18.5 Management of COVID-19 in Paediatric Patients

18.5.1 Mild-to-Moderate Cases

Most paediatric COVID-19 cases are mild and can be managed at home with supportive care. This includes ensuring adequate hydration, administering antipyretics for fever, and monitoring symptoms. Parents should be counselled on warning signs such as respiratory distress, persistent fever, and decreased oral intake. Outpatient follow-up is advised for children with underlying health conditions or persistent symptoms. High-risk groups, such as infants under 3 months and immunocompromised children, may require more frequent reassessment. Isolation measures and household precautions should be emphasised to prevent transmission [29].

18.5.2 Severe Cases and Hospitalisation

Children with Hypoxia, Respiratory Distress, or Multisystem Involvement Require Hospitalisation [24]. Oxygen supplementation is the first-line intervention for hypoxic patients. Remdesivir is authorised for use in select hospitalised paediatric patients with confirmed SARS-CoV-2 infection and evidence of lower respiratory tract disease. Corticosteroids, such as dexamethasone, are indicated for children requiring respiratory support. Additional therapies, including anticoagulation, tocilizumab, or baricitinib, may be considered on a case-by-case basis under guidance from infectious disease or critical care specialists [30, 31]. Care should be individualised, considering age, comorbidities, and disease severity, and multidisciplinary collaboration is essential in managing complex cases [29, 31].

18.5.3 MIS-C Management

Management of MIS-C requires a multidisciplinary team, including cardiology, infectious disease, rheumatology, and intensive care. First-line immunomodulatory therapy includes intravenous immunoglobulin (IVIG) and corticosteroids. In refractory cases, biologics such as anakinra or infliximab may be employed. Cardiovascular monitoring is critical, with serial echocardiography to detect coronary artery abnormalities or myocardial dysfunction. Laboratory markers should be monitored regularly to guide treatment response and tapering of immunosuppression. Supportive care, including fluid management and inotropic support when needed, is essential. Most children respond well to treatment, but long-term cardiac follow-up is recommended due to potential sequelae [18].

18.5.4 Post-acute Care and Rehabilitation

Children recovering from COVID-19, particularly those with long COVID, may experience fatigue, cognitive disturbances, and exercise intolerance. Rehabilitation includes physical therapy, psychological support, and academic reintegration plans. Follow-up should be individualised based on symptom persistence and functional limitations, ideally within a multidisciplinary paediatric long COVID clinic [20, 32].

18.6 Preventive Measures and Infection Control in Paediatric Settings

18.6.1 Transmission Prevention in Paediatric Care Settings

In paediatric care environments, rigorous infection control practices are critical to preventing nosocomial transmission of SARS-CoV-2. Personal protective equipment (PPE)—including N95 respirators or surgical masks, gloves, gowns, and eye protection—is essential for healthcare workers managing suspected or confirmed cases. Paediatric patients with COVID-19 should be isolated in negative-pressure rooms when available or in dedicated COVID-19 units [33, 34]. Hand hygiene, environmental disinfection, and physical distancing in waiting areas reduce the risk of transmission. Staff cohorting and routine screening protocols help identify asymptomatic carriers, who play a significant role in paediatric settings. Training and adherence to guidelines remain key to minimising spread [35].

18.6.2 Impact of School Closures and Remote Learning

School closures, implemented early in the pandemic, played a role in limiting transmission but had significant consequences for children's mental health, social development, and academic achievement. Children from low-income families were disproportionately affected due to limited access to digital learning tools [36, 37]. Evidence now supports school reopening with mitigation strategies, including masking, ventilation, cohorting, and vaccination of eligible populations [38]. Public health policy must balance the risk of transmission with the adverse effects of prolonged closures, prioritising in-person learning where safe. Targeted closures should be based on community transmission levels and school-specific outbreaks [39, 40].

18.6.3 Vaccination Strategies

Vaccination remains a cornerstone of COVID-19 prevention. Several vaccines have been authorised for paediatric use. mRNA vaccines (like Pfizer-BioNTech vaccine) are approved for children aged 6 months and older in age-appropriate doses, administered in a two- or three-dose series depending on age and risk status. Clinical trials have shown favourable safety profiles and strong immunogenicity in children, with rare adverse events such as myocarditis occurring predominantly in adolescent males [41–43]. Protein subunit vaccines are known to elicit strong neutralising-antibody responses and provide reasonable protection against symptomatic infection, with favourable tolerability. Inactivated vaccines have demonstrated high real-world effectiveness in preventing severe disease and hospitalisation in children, even during waves of immune-evasive variants. Viral-vector vaccines elicit robust cellular immunity and provide sustained protection against severe outcomes, though their effectiveness against mild infections declines more rapidly [44–46].

Vaccination has been shown to reduce SARS-CoV-2 transmission within households and communities, indirectly protecting vulnerable groups such as immunocompromised children and those under 6 months of age who are not yet vaccine-eligible [47]. Additionally, vaccinated children are less likely to develop severe disease or MIS-C [48]. School-based vaccination programmes and community outreach are effective at increasing vaccination uptake, particularly among underserved populations. Vaccine equity and parental education are essential to improving coverage and reducing disparities. Booster doses are recommended for children at high risk or during surges of immune-evasive variants. Integrating COVID-19 vaccination into routine immunisation schedules may enhance long-term control of the virus in paediatric populations [49, 50].

18.7 Ongoing Research and Future Directions

18.7.1 Emerging Variants

The emergence of SARS-CoV-2 variants such as Delta and Omicron has altered the epidemiological landscape, with implications for paediatric disease severity and transmission. The Omicron variant, while generally associated with milder disease, led to a significant surge in paediatric hospitalisations due to increased transmissibility [51]. Emerging subvariants with immune escape potential, such as XBB.1.5 and BA.2.86, pose challenges for current vaccine and treatment strategies. Ongoing surveillance is essential to detect variant-specific impacts on paediatric outcomes and guide the development of targeted interventions, especially as younger children remain more vulnerable due to lower vaccination rates and immature immune responses [51, 52].

18.7.2 Current Research

Clinical trials are actively evaluating updated vaccine formulations for broader variant coverage in children, including bivalent and next-generation mRNA vaccines [53]. Research is also focused on refining paediatric treatment protocols, including optimal use of antivirals and immunomodulators for MIS-C. Longitudinal studies are tracking the effects of COVID-19 on paediatric physical and neurodevelopmental health, with early evidence suggesting a subset of children experience persistent symptoms months after recovery. Integrating findings into public health strategies will improve preparedness and care for paediatric patients in future waves or pandemics [54].

18.7.3 Lessons for Future Pandemics

The COVID-19 pandemic underscored the importance of rapid paediatric inclusion in clinical trials, robust public health infrastructure, and real-time data sharing [55]. It highlighted disparities in healthcare access and digital learning tools, which must be addressed in preparedness plans. Future pandemic responses should prioritise school continuity, mental health services, and equity in vaccine distribution [56]. Multidisciplinary collaboration, including paediatrics, infectious disease, and public health, is critical in creating adaptable, child-specific guidelines [57]. Strengthening international research networks and pandemic simulation exercises will help anticipate and mitigate the next global health crisis affecting children [55].

18.8 Conclusion

The COVID-19 pandemic has reshaped paradigms in paediatric infectious diseases, revealing important insights into the epidemiology, clinical spectrum, and outcomes of SARS-CoV-2 infection in children. Although illness in paediatric populations has generally been milder than in adults, the disease burden remains significant, particularly with the emergence of highly transmissible variants and the occurrence of serious complications such as multisystem inflammatory syndrome in children (MIS-C) and long COVID, with children having comorbidities at increased risk of severe outcomes. Diagnostic approaches have evolved rapidly, with molecular testing and imaging playing key roles in identifying typical and atypical presentations while distinguishing COVID-19 from other viral respiratory infections. Management strategies now range from supportive outpatient care for mild illness to hospitalisation and immunomodulatory therapies for severe disease and MIS-C, with growing recognition of the need for rehabilitation and long-term follow-up in children with post-acute sequelae. Preventive measures, including infection control practices in healthcare and educational settings and paediatric vaccination programmes, have been central to reducing transmission and protecting vulnerable groups. At the same time, ongoing research remains critical to address emerging variants and optimise paediatric care. Collectively, these lessons underscore the importance of early paediatric inclusion in research, equitable access to healthcare, and resilient health and education systems to strengthen preparedness for future pandemics.

References

1. World Health Organization. Coronavirus disease (COVID-19) pandemic. 2020. Accessed 20 Apr 2025. https://www.who.int/emergencies/diseases/novel-coronavirus-2019.
2. Ludvigsson JF. Systematic review of COVID-19 in children shows milder cases and a better prognosis than adults. Acta Paediatr. 2020;109(6):1088–95. https://doi.org/10.1111/apa.15270. Epub 2020 Apr 14. PMID: 32202343; PMCID: PMC7228328.
3. La Torre F, Elicio MP, Monno VA, Chironna M, Moramarco F, Campanozzi A, Civino A, Cecinati V, Vairo U, Giordano M, Milella L, Loconsole D, Cardinale F. Incidence and

prevalence of multisystem inflammatory syndrome in children (MIS-C) in Southern Italy. Children (Basel). 2023;10(5):766. https://doi.org/10.3390/children10050766. PMID: 37238314; PMCID: PMC10217079.

4. Eastin C, Eastin T. Epidemiological characteristics of 2143 pediatric patients with 2019 coronavirus disease in China. J Emerg Med. 2020;58(4):712–3.
5. Leidman E, Duca LM, Omura JD, Proia K, Stephens JW, Sauber-Schatz EK. COVID-19 trends among persons aged 0–24 years — United States, March 1–December 12, 2020. MMWR Morb Mortal Wkly Rep. 2021;70:88–94. https://doi.org/10.15585/mmwr.mm7003e1.
6. Schneiderman M, Rumain B, Kaganovskiy L, Geliebter A. Incidence and relative risk of COVID-19 in adolescents and youth compared with older adults in 19 US States, Fall 2020. JAMA Netw Open. 2022;5(7):e2222126. https://doi.org/10.1001/jamanetworkopen.2022.22126.
7. Dioguardi M, Cazzolla AP, Arena C, Sovereto D, Caloro GA, Dioguardi A, Crincoli V, Laino L, Troiano G, Lo Muzio L. Innate immunity in children and the role of ACE2 expression in SARS-CoV-2 infection. Pediatr Rep. 2021;13(3):363–82. https://doi.org/10.3390/pediatric13030045. PMID: 34287338; PMCID: PMC8293341.
8. Funk A, Florin TA, Kuppermann N, Finkelstein Y, Kazakoff A, Baldovsky M, Tancredi DJ, Breslin K, Bergmann KR, Gardiner M, Pruitt CM, Liu DR, Neuman MI, Wilkinson M, Ambroggio L, Pang X-L, Cauchemez S, Malley R, Klassen TP, Lee BE, Payne DC, Mahmud SM, Freedman SB, on behalf of the Pediatric Emergency Research Network (PERN). Household transmission dynamics of asymptomatic SARS-CoV-2–infected children: a multinational, controlled case-ascertained prospective study. Clin Infect Dis. 2024;78(6):1522–30. https://doi.org/10.1093/cid/ciae069.
9. Bayhan Gİ, Özkubat Korkmaz I, Şahiner ES, Tekeli N, Akdağ AG, Uyan Erten AZ, Taşbaşı AB, Göre B, Doğru M, Kırca F, Dinç B. Are SARS-CoV-2 viral loads in children lower than in adults? J Infect. 2023;86(1):e13–4. https://doi.org/10.1016/j.jinf.2022.08.025. Epub 2022 Aug 24. PMID: 36029921; PMCID: PMC9398939.
10. Paul LA, Daneman N, Schwartz KL, et al. Association of age and pediatric household transmission of SARS-CoV-2 infection. JAMA Pediatr. 2021;175(11):1151–8. https://doi.org/10.1001/jamapediatrics.2021.2770.
11. Choi JH, Choi SH, Yun KW. Risk factors for severe COVID-19 in children: a systematic review and meta-analysis. J Korean Med Sci. 2022;37(5):e35. https://doi.org/10.3346/jkms.2022.37.e35. PMID: 35132841; PMCID: PMC8822112.
12. Ungar SP, Solomon S, Stachel A, Shust GF, Clouser KN, Bhavsar SM, Lighter J. Hospital and ICU admission risk associated with comorbidities among children with COVID-19 ancestral strains. Clin Pediatr (Phila). 2023;62(9):1048–58. https://doi.org/10.1177/00099228221150605. Epub 2023 Jan 20. PMID: 36661087; PMCID: PMC9895283.
13. Dennis-Heyward EA, Shah SN. Pediatric COVID-19 disparities and prioritizing equity—children are not spared. JAMA Pediatr. 2021;175(9):898–900. https://doi.org/10.1001/jamapediatrics.2021.1682.
14. Bunyavanich S, Do A, Vicencio A. Nasal gene expression of angiotensin-converting enzyme 2 in children and adults. JAMA. 2020;323(23):2427–9. https://doi.org/10.1001/jama.2020.8707.
15. Shang Z, Huang L, Qin S. The underlying mechanism behind the different outcomes of COVID-19 in children and adults. Front Immunol. 2025;16:1440169. https://doi.org/10.3389/fimmu.2025.1440169. PMID: 40370452; PMCID: PMC12075420.
16. Molloy EJ, Bearer CF. COVID-19 in children and altered inflammatory responses. Pediatr Res. 2020;88:340–1. https://doi.org/10.1038/s41390-020-0881-y.
17. Centers for Disease Control and Prevention. Clinical overview of multisystem inflammatory syndrome in children (MIS-C). 2025. Accessed October 20, 2025. https://www.cdc.gov/mis/hcp/clinical-overview/index.html.
18. Feleszko W, Okarska-Napierała M, Buddingh EP, Bloomfield M, Sediva A, Bautista-Rodriguez C, Brough HA, Eigenmann PA, Eiwegger T, Eljaszewicz A, Eyerich S, Gomez-Casado C, Fraisse A, Janda J, Jiménez-Saiz R, Kallinich T, Krohn IK, Mortz CG, Riggioni C, Sastre J,

Sokolowska M, Strzelczyk Z, Untersmayr E, Tramper-Stranders G, Immunology Section and Working Group Infections of the EAACI. Pathogenesis, immunology, and immune-targeted management of the multisystem inflammatory syndrome in children (MIS-C) or pediatric inflammatory multisystem syndrome (PIMS): EAACI Position Paper. Pediatr Allergy Immunol. 2023;34(1):e13900. https://doi.org/10.1111/pai.13900. PMID: 36705045.

19. Lopez-Leon S, Wegman-Ostrosky T, Ayuzo Del Valle NC, Perelman C, Sepulveda R, Rebolledo PA, Cuapio A, Villapol S. Long-COVID in children and adolescents: a systematic review and meta-analyses. Sci Rep. 2022;12(1):9950. https://doi.org/10.1038/s41598-022-13495-5. PMID: 35739136; PMCID: PMC9226045.
20. Noij L, Terheggen-Lagro S, Muselaers E, Whittaker E, Gosling J, Brackel C, Oostrom K, Alsem M. A multidisciplinary approach: management and rehabilitation of children with pediatric post-COVID-19 condition. Pediatr Infect Dis J. 2024;43(9):880–4. https://doi.org/10.1097/INF.0000000000004408. Epub 2024 May 29. PMID: 38808972; PMCID: PMC11319073.
21. Melo MM, Neta MMR, Neto ARS, Carvalho ARB, Magalhães RLB, Valle ARMC, Ferreira JHL, Aliaga KMJ, Moura MEB, Freitas DRJ. Symptoms of COVID-19 in children. Braz J Med Biol Res. 2022;55:e12038. https://doi.org/10.1590/1414-431X2022e12038. PMID: 35703681; PMCID: PMC9200047.
22. Christophers B, Gallo Marin B, Oliva R, et al. Trends in clinical presentation of children with COVID-19: a systematic review of individual participant data. Pediatr Res. 2022;91:494–501. https://doi.org/10.1038/s41390-020-01161-3.
23. Kurian J, Blumfield E, Levin TL, Liszewski MC. Imaging findings in acute pediatric coronavirus disease 2019 (COVID-19) pneumonia and multisystem inflammatory syndrome in children (MIS-C). Pediatr Radiol. 2022;52(10):1985–97. https://doi.org/10.1007/s00247-022-05393-9. Epub 2022 May 26. PMID: 35616701; PMCID: PMC9132751.
24. Kortz TB, Connolly E, Cohen CL, Cook RE, Jonas JA, Lipnick MS, Kissoon N. Diagnosis and acute management of COVID-19 and multisystem inflammatory syndrome in children. Pediatr Emerg Care. 2021;37(10):519–25. https://doi.org/10.1097/PEC.0000000000002538. PMID: 34591810; PMCID: PMC8855974.
25. World Health Organization. Multisystem inflammatory syndrome in children and adolescents temporally related to COVID-19 [Scientific brief]. 2020. https://www.who.int/news-room/commentaries/detail/multisystem-inflammatory-syndrome-in-children-and-adolescents-with-covid-19.
26. Brigadoi G, Demarin GC, Boracchini R, Pierantoni L, Rossin S, Barbieri E, Tirelli F, Cantarutti A, Tempo G, Giaquinto C, Lanari M, Da Dalt L, Donà D. Comparison between the viral illness caused by SARS-CoV-2, influenza virus, respiratory syncytial virus and other respiratory viruses in pediatrics. Viruses. 2024;16(2):199. https://doi.org/10.3390/v16020199. PMID: 38399975; PMCID: PMC10891516.
27. Hernández García M, Roldan Berengue E, Guitart C, Girona-Alarcón M, Argüello G, Pino R, de Sevilla MF, García-García JJ, Jordan I. Multisystem inflammatory syndrome in children (MIS-C) and sepsis differentiation by a clinical and analytical score: MISSEP score. Eur J Pediatr. 2023;182(11):5109–18. https://doi.org/10.1007/s00431-023-05168-w. Epub 2023 Sep 7. PMID: 37676491; PMCID: PMC10640430.
28. Noval Rivas M, Arditi M. Kawasaki disease and multisystem inflammatory syndrome in children: common inflammatory pathways of two distinct diseases. Rheum Dis Clin North Am. 2023;49(3):647–59. https://doi.org/10.1016/j.rdc.2023.03.002. Epub 2023 Mar 17. PMID: 37331738; PMCID: PMC10020039.
29. American Academy of Pediatrics. Outpatient COVID-19 management strategies in children and adolescents [Clinical guidance]. 2022. Available from: https://aap oc.org/wp-content/uploads/2022/10/Outpatient-COVID-19-Management-Strategies-in-Children-and-Adolescents.pdf.
30. Klučka J, Klabusayová E, Kratochvíl M, Musilová T, Vafek V, Skříšovská T, Kosinová M, Havránková P, Štourač P. Critically Ill pediatric patient and SARS-CoV-2 infection. Children. 2022;9(4):538. https://doi.org/10.3390/children9040538.

31. COVID-19 Treatment Guidelines Panel. Coronavirus Disease 2019 (COVID-19) Treatment Guidelines [Internet]. Washington (DC): National Institutes of Health; 2022 [cited 2025 Dec 26]. Available from: https://www.atrainceu.com/sites/default/files/media/2022-12/Covid%2019%20Treatment%20Guidelines%20Oct%2019%2C%202022%20Update.pdf.
32. Goicoechea-Calvo A, Coll-Fernández R, Navarro Expósito N, Colomer Giralt M, González-Aumatell A, Méndez-Hernández M, Carreras-Abad C, Pallarès Fontanet N, Tebe Cordomi C, Durà Mata MJ, et al. Effects of paediatric post-COVID-19 condition on physical function and daily functioning: a cross-sectional study. Children. 2025;12(9):1216. https://doi.org/10.3390/children12091216.
33. Reich P, Elward A. Infection prevention during the coronavirus disease 2019 pandemic. Infect Dis Clin North Am. 2022;36(1):15–37. https://doi.org/10.1016/j.idc.2021.12.002. PMID: 35168708; PMCID: PMC8837397.
34. Kim SC, Kong SY, Park GJ, Lee JH, Lee JK, Lee MS, Han HS. Effectiveness of negative pressure isolation stretcher and rooms for SARS-CoV-2 nosocomial infection control and maintenance of South Korean emergency department capacity. Am J Emerg Med. 2021;45:483–9. https://doi.org/10.1016/j.ajem.2020.09.081. Epub 2020 Oct 1. PMID: 33039226; PMCID: PMC7528735.
35. Pham TM, Tahir H, van de Wijgert JHHM, Van der Roest BR, Ellerbroek P, Bonten MJM, Bootsma MCJ, Kretzschmar ME. Interventions to control nosocomial transmission of SARS-CoV-2: a modelling study. BMC Med. 2021;19(1):211. https://doi.org/10.1186/s12916-021-02060-y. PMID: 34446011; PMCID: PMC8390112.
36. El Jaouhari M, Edjoc R, Waddell L, Houston P, Atchessi N, Striha M, Bonti-Ankomah S. Impact of school closures and re-openings on COVID-19 transmission. Can Commun Dis Rep. 2021;47(12):515–23. https://doi.org/10.14745/ccdr.v47i12a02. PMID: 35018139; PMCID: PMC8699400.
37. Cortés-Albornoz MC, Ramírez-Guerrero S, García-Guáqueta DP, Vélez-Van-Meerbeke A, Talero-Gutiérrez C. Effects of remote learning during COVID-19 lockdown on children's learning abilities and school performance: a systematic review. Int J Educ Dev. 2023;101:102835. https://doi.org/10.1016/j.ijedudev.2023.102835. Epub 2023 Jun 14. PMID: 37361921; PMCID: PMC10266495.
38. Dewan M, Sharma N, Panda PS, Banerjee P. School reopening: back to classroom. A systematic review of strategies and their implementation during COVID-19 pandemic. J Family Med Prim Care. 2022;11(8):4273–9. https://doi.org/10.4103/jfmpc.jfmpc_23_22. Epub 2022 Aug 30. PMID: 36352990; PMCID: PMC9638583.
39. McGee RS, Homburger JR, Williams HE, Bergstrom CT, Zhou AY. Model-driven mitigation measures for reopening schools during the COVID-19 pandemic. Proc Natl Acad Sci U S A. 2021;118(39):e2108909118. https://doi.org/10.1073/pnas.2108909118. PMID: 34518375; PMCID: PMC8488607.
40. Walsh S, Chowdhury A, Braithwaite V, Russell S, Birch JM, Ward JL, Waddington C, Brayne C, Bonell C, Viner RM, Mytton OT. Do school closures and school reopenings affect community transmission of COVID-19? A systematic review of observational studies. BMJ Open. 2021;11(8):e053371. https://doi.org/10.1136/bmjopen-2021-053371. PMID: 34404718; PMCID: PMC8375447.
41. Sabu JM, Zahid I, Jacob N, Alele FO, Malau-Aduli BS. Effectiveness of the BNT162b2 (Pfizer-BioNTech) vaccine in children and adolescents: a systematic review and meta-analysis. Vaccines (Basel). 2022;10(11):1880. https://doi.org/10.3390/vaccines10111880. PMID: 36366387; PMCID: PMC9698079.
42. Muñoz FM, Sher LD, Sabharwal C, Gurtman A, Xu X, Kitchin N, Lockhart S, Riesenberg R, Sexter JM, Czajka H, Paulsen GC, Maldonado Y, Walter EB, Talaat KR, Englund JA, Sarwar UN, Hansen C, Iwamoto M, Webber C, Cunliffe L, Ukkonen B, Martínez SN, Pahud BA, Munjal I, Domachowske JB, Swanson KA, Ma H, Koury K, Mather S, Lu C, Zou J, Xie X, Shi PY, Cooper D, Türeci Ö, Şahin U, Jansen KU, Gruber WC, C4591007 Clinical Trial Group. Evaluation of BNT162b2 Covid-19 vaccine in children younger than 5 years of age. N Engl

J Med. 2023;388(7):621–34. https://doi.org/10.1056/NEJMoa2211031. PMID: 36791162; PMCID: PMC9947923.
43. Jeremiah SS, Das P, Venkatesan M, Albinzayed R, Ahmed A, Stevenson NJ, Corbally M, Alqahtani M, Al-Wedaie F, Farid E, et al. Humoral and innate immunological profile of paediatric recipients of Pfizer-BioNTech BNT162b2 mRNA vaccine. Microorganisms. 2024;12(7):1389. https://doi.org/10.3390/microorganisms12071389.
44. Jara A, Undurraga EA, Zubizarreta JR, González C, Acevedo J, Pizarro A, Vergara V, Soto-Marchant M, Gilabert R, Flores JC, Suárez P, Leighton P, Eguiguren P, Ríos JC, Fernandez J, García-Escorza H, Araos R. Effectiveness of CoronaVac in children 3–5 years of age during the SARS-CoV-2 Omicron outbreak in Chile. Nat Med. 2022;28(7):1377–80. https://doi.org/10.1038/s41591-022-01874-4. Epub 2022 May 23. PMID: 35605637; PMCID: PMC9307483.
45. Áñez G, Dunkle LM, Gay CL, Kotloff KL, Adelglass JM, Essink B, Campbell JD, Cloney-Clark S, Zhu M, Plested JS, Roychoudhury P, Greninger AL, Patel N, McGarry A, Woo W, Cho I, Glenn GM, Dubovsky F, 2019nCoV-301–Pediatric Expansion Study Group. Safety, immunogenicity, and efficacy of the NVX-CoV2373 COVID-19 vaccine in adolescents: a randomized clinical trial. JAMA Netw Open. 2023;6(4):e239135. https://doi.org/10.1001/jamanetworkopen.2023.9135. PMID: 37099299; PMCID: PMC10536880.
46. Folegatti PM, Ewer KJ, Aley PK, Angus B, Becker S, Belij-Rammerstorfer S, Bellamy D, Bibi S, Bittaye M, Clutterbuck EA, Dold C, Faust SN, Finn A, Flaxman AL, Hallis B, Heath P, Jenkin D, Lazarus R, Makinson R, Minassian AM, Pollock KM, Ramasamy M, Robinson H, Snape M, Tarrant R, Voysey M, Green C, Douglas AD, AVS H, Lambe T, Gilbert SC, Pollard AJ, Oxford COVID Vaccine Trial Group. Safety and immunogenicity of the ChAdOx1 nCoV-19 vaccine against SARS-CoV-2: a preliminary report of a phase 1/2, single-blind, randomised controlled trial. Lancet. 2020;396(10249):467–78. https://doi.org/10.1016/S0140-6736(20)31604-4. Epub 2020 Jul 20. Erratum in: Lancet. 2020 Aug 15;396(10249):466. 10.1016/S0140-6736(20)31687-1. Erratum in: Lancet. 2020 Dec 12;396(10266):1884. 10.1016/S0140-6736(20)32597-6. PMID: 32702298; PMCID: PMC7445431.
47. Godoy P, Martínez-Baz I, Parron I, García-Cenoz M, Ferras J, Carol M, Bes N, Guillaumes M, Godoy S, Toledo D, et al. Vaccinated COVID-19 index cases are less likely to transmit SARS-CoV-2 to their household contacts: a cohort study. Vaccines. 2024;12(3):240. https://doi.org/10.3390/vaccines12030240.
48. Hamad Saied M, van der Griend L, van Straalen JW, Wulffraat NM, Vastert S, Jansen MHA. The protective effect of COVID-19 vaccines on developing multisystem inflammatory syndrome in children (MIS-C): a systematic literature review and meta-analysis. Pediatr Rheumatol Online J. 2023;21(1):80. https://doi.org/10.1186/s12969-023-00848-1. PMID: 37550719; PMCID: PMC10405572.
49. Nguyen KH, McChesney C, Rodriguez C, Vasudevan L, Bednarczyk RA, Corlin L. Child and adolescent COVID-19 vaccination coverage by educational setting, United States. Public Health. 2024;229:126–34. https://doi.org/10.1016/j.puhe.2024.01.029. Epub 2024 Mar 1. PMID: 38430658; PMCID: PMC10961195.
50. Fayad D, Frenck RW Jr. COVID-19 vaccines in children. J Clin Med. 2024;13(1):87. https://doi.org/10.3390/jcm13010087.
51. Pokorska-Śpiewak M, Pawłowska M, Ciechanowski P, Peregrym M, Dobrzeniecka A, Sobolewska-Pilarczyk M, Franczak J, Majda-Stanisławska E, Szczepańska B, Zaleska I, Flisiak R. Differences in clinical presentation of COVID-19 in children hospitalized during domination of early (BA.1, BA.2) and late (BA.5, BA.2.75, BQ.1 and XBB.1.5) SARS-CoV-2 Omicron Subvariants. Pediatr Infect Dis J. 2024;43(2):149–54. https://doi.org/10.1097/INF.0000000000004167. Epub 2023 Nov 3. PMID: 37922516; PMCID: PMC11500694.
52. Lewnard JA, Mahale P, Malden D, et al. Immune escape and attenuated severity associated with the SARS-CoV-2 BA.2.86/JN.1 lineage. Nat Commun. 2024;15:8550. https://doi.org/10.1038/s41467-024-52668-w.
53. Centers for Disease Control and Prevention. Effectiveness of bivalent mRNA vaccines in preventing COVID-19–associated emergency department and urgent care encounters and

hospitalizations among adults — United States, September–November 2023. MMWR Morb Mortal Wkly Rep. 2025;74(40):607–14. Available from: https://www.cdc.gov/mmwr/volumes/74/wr/mm7440a1.htm.
54. Wang LJ, Tsai CS, Chou WJ, Li CJ, Lee SY, Chen YC, Lin IC. Medical outcomes of children with neurodevelopmental disorders after SARS-CoV-2 vaccination: a six-month follow-up study. Vaccine. 2023;41(29):4267–73. https://doi.org/10.1016/j.vaccine.2023.05.067. Epub 2023 May 29. PMID: 37271705; PMCID: PMC10225977.
55. Fleming PF, Gale C, Molloy EJ, et al. Paediatric research in the times of COVID-19. Pediatr Res. 2021;90:267–71. https://doi.org/10.1038/s41390-021-01479-6.
56. von Rhein M, Dratva J, Seiler M. Editorial: COVID-19 - lessons learned in pediatrics. Front Pediatr. 2025;13:1737801. https://doi.org/10.3389/fped.2025.1737801. PMID: 41357805; PMCID: PMC12678310.
57. Cheng TL, Devaskar SU, Pediatric Policy Council. Pediatric research today and tomorrow post-COVID-19. Pediatr Res. 2021;90(1):13–5. https://doi.org/10.1038/s41390-021-01520-8. Epub 2021 Apr 13. PMID: 33850294; PMCID: PMC8042618.

COVID-19 and Flu: Similarities and Differences

19

Lonika Lodha

19.1 Introduction and Epidemiology

The influenza virus has caused multiple deadly pandemics over the past century but has recently been overshadowed by the COVID-19 pandemic. Currently, in the post-pandemic era, both viruses co-circulate and often cause similar clinical syndromes, but they differ markedly in their pathogenesis, epidemiology, and clinical management. However, it is essential to identify and differentiate between these two infections for individual patient care and public health decision-making, especially vaccination policies. A comparative discussion of these two infections is crucial for clinicians, public health professionals, and policymakers, as it provides valuable insights into disease diagnosis, prevention, and control strategies.

Influenza A, B, and C viruses cause a spectrum of respiratory illnesses ranging from asymptomatic or mild upper respiratory infection to severe and lethal pneumonia, occasionally complicated by non-respiratory manifestations. Influenza D virus has so far only been isolated from animals [1]. COVID-19 is the name given to the pandemic that began in late 2019 and was caused by a novel beta-coronavirus, SARS-CoV-2. The virus is thought to have originated from bats and is now known to cause acute as well as chronic manifestations, mainly affecting the respiratory system but ultimately impacting all major organs and organ systems [2].

Both SARS-CoV-2 and influenza viruses are enveloped. The genome of influenza viruses is single-stranded, positive-sense, segmented RNA, and is shorter (13.5 kb) than SARS-CoV-2 [2]. A wide variety of species, including domestic mammals, poultry, and wild birds, act as reservoirs of influenza A viruses. Influenza A virus is responsible for the recurring pandemics resulting from genomic reassortment, while B and C subtypes do not possess this attribute [1].

L. Lodha (✉)
Department of Neurovirology, National Institute of Mental Health and Neurosciences (NIMHANS), Bengaluru, Karnataka, India

S. R. Prabhu et al. (eds.), *COVID-19 in Dental Practice*,
https://doi.org/10.1007/978-3-032-26000-0_19

The World Health Organisation (WHO) estimates that approximately 1 billion seasonal influenza cases occur globally each year, with 3–5 million severe cases and up to 650,000 deaths [3, 4]. On the other hand, the COVID-19 pandemic has resulted in more than 7 million deaths as of May 2025 [5].

Much like COVID-19, influenza infection is also more likely to cause severe illness or complications in individuals at extremes of age, those with chronic medical conditions, immunosuppressed persons, and pregnant women [3, 6]. Other common risk factors of increased likelihood of hospitalisation and ICU admission are non-white race, low socioeconomic status, and comorbidities, including asthma, interstitial lung disease, chronic obstructive pulmonary disease (COPD), cardiac disease, and chronic kidney disease [7]. Some differential risk factors for COVID-19 and influenza have also been identified; for example, obesity and diabetes are more critical for COVID-19 than for flu [7, 8].

Influenza A viruses are classified into subtypes based on HA and NA glycoproteins, with 16 HA and 9 NA types, and are categorised as human or avian flu strains. Only H1, H2, and H3 subtypes have been confirmed to spread in humans, leading to major pandemics. The 1918 H1N1 "Spanish influenza" was highly lethal, infecting 500 million people globally. Subsequent pandemics caused by variants of the 1918 virus included the 1957 H2N2 "Asian influenza", the 1968 H3N2 "Hong Kong flu", and the 2009 H1N1 "swine flu", with decreasing mortality over time. The 2009 H1N1 strain emerged from reassortment among swine, human, and avian influenza viruses and continues to circulate alongside H3N2, reflecting the ongoing evolution and impact of influenza A on public health [2].

The genetic evolution of SARS-CoV-2 is much more complex than that of influenza A. The WHO categorised variants into variants of interest (VOIs) and variants of concern (VOCs) based on their impact on transmissibility and immune evasion. Early variants such as Alpha, Beta, Gamma, and Delta contributed to global waves of infection, with Delta proving highly contagious. In November 2021, Omicron was identified in South Africa and rapidly spread worldwide due to its increased infectivity and partial vaccine resistance. Omicron led to more reinfections and breakthrough cases, prompting recommendations for booster vaccinations [2].

19.2 Clinical Features and Outcomes

The incubation period of influenza A virus is 1–7 days, while that of SARS-CoV-2 is 2–14 days [2]. In general, COVID-19 leads to more severe illness than influenza across groups of patients, including adults, children, and even immunocompromised patients. Patients with COVID-19 are more likely to require hospitalisation, ICU admission, and mechanical ventilation than patients with influenza. Patients with COVID-19 are also more likely to require extended hospitalisation and/or longer ICU stays, which may be up to twice as long as those of patients with influenza. COVID-19 is also shown to be more likely to result in the development of acute respiratory distress syndrome and is associated with higher mortality rates compared to the flu [7–19].

However, it is essential to note that the severity of COVID-19 was affected by the variant in circulation at that time (some of which were found to be less or equally severe than the influenza strains circulating simultaneously), along with the vaccination status of the study populations, and also appeared to decrease as the pandemic declined [13–15, 20–23].

Studies indicate that the Omicron variant is associated with milder symptoms and a decreased likelihood of hospitalisation, ICU admission, and mortality following vaccination, despite exhibiting greater transmissibility than the Delta variant. Compared with Omicron, the Delta variant resulted in more severe clinical presentations. Earlier variants, including Alpha and Delta, were linked to increased severity, as evidenced by higher rates of hospitalisation and mortality. An extensive study across two respiratory viral seasons has shown that, during the 2022 to 2023 season, COVID-19 carried a moderately higher mortality risk than influenza, while similar risks were observed in the 2023–2024 season. Hospitalisation rates for COVID-19 and influenza were nearly equivalent during the latter season. Across both seasons, the cumulative incidence of COVID-19 mortality remained higher than that of influenza during follow-up. The elevated risk of long-term mortality relative to influenza persisted at both 90-day and 180-day intervals. Notably, among individuals vaccinated against either infection during the 2022–2023 season, no significant difference in 30-day hospitalisation risk was observed between COVID-19 and influenza [24–26].

Children diagnosed with COVID-19 tend to experience fewer symptoms, such as cough, fever, and dyspnoea, than those with influenza. Their haemoglobin levels are also notably higher than those of paediatric influenza patients. However, both groups show similar rates of sore throat, platelet, neutrophil and lymphocyte counts, (depending on the variant of SARS CoV 2), and similar outcomes, including mortality, ICU admission, mechanical ventilation, and duration of hospital stay. Research on influenza in community and hospital settings found that 67.7% of children under five who tested positive for influenza had symptoms, with 16.2% developing acute lower respiratory illness (ALRI). Among these, 17.4% had chest wall indrawing, and 14.2% needed hospitalisation. Conversely, up to half of children with COVID-19 may not show symptoms, and overall, the disease tends to be milder in children than in adults. Hospitalisation rates for children with COVID-19 range from 0.1% to 2%, with deaths being sporadic, though they can reach up to 1% among hospitalised cases. Approximately 30% of young patients admitted to critical care for COVID-19 exhibit signs of acute respiratory distress syndrome. However, viral bronchiolitis or asthma flare-ups are uncommon with COVID-19; their presence should prompt consideration of co-infection with other viruses. Certain complications occur specifically in children, depending on the infection: benign acute childhood myositis (BACM) is linked to influenza A, while multisystem inflammatory syndrome in children (MIS-C) is associated with COVID-19 [17, 27–29].

Although laboratory investigations are not helpful in differentiating between influenza and COVID-19, a few probable differential haematological and biochemical markers have been identified for the two infections. Total leucocyte counts are significantly lower in COVID-19 compared to influenza; in fact, leukopenia has been recognised as one of the hallmarks of COVID-19 [30–32]. However, this finding may not always be seen in paediatric patients [17]. Elevated aspartate transaminase, lactate dehydrogenase, creatine kinase MB, and C-reactive protein levels have been reported in both influenza and COVID-19, with no consensus regarding their use as differential markers [17, 31].

Viral clearance, as evidenced by a negative result on nucleic acid detection test, is likely to occur earlier in influenza than in COVID-19 [31, 33]. However, in the long term (12 weeks post-infections), the likelihood of ongoing symptoms or functional impairment is the same for influenza and COVID-19 [34].

Both influenza and COVID-19 are associated with extra-respiratory complications, including cardiac, gastrointestinal, musculoskeletal, renal, and neurological syndromes, along with the immunological phenomenon known as "cytokine storm" [35–37]. Of note, several peculiar characteristics have been associated with COVID-19, such as anosmia, ageusia, psychiatric manifestations, and long-term persistence of the disease in the form of "long-COVID" [36].

19.3 Management

The most crucial difference between the management of COVID-19 and influenza is the availability of specific antivirals for influenza. COVID-19 treatment includes empirical and symptomatic approaches. Various drugs, including oseltamivir, ganciclovir, chloroquine, hydroxychloroquine, lopinavir/ritonavir, remdesivir, and arbidol, have been investigated for efficacy, with mixed results. While corticosteroids such as dexamethasone reduced 28-day mortality in severe cases, WHO guidelines advise against their use in mild cases. Passive antibody infusion with convalescent plasma may provide short-term immunity, and traditional therapies such as oxygen support and ECMO remain options for severe cases. Despite global efforts to develop effective treatments, no definitive antiviral drug has been universally approved for COVID-19 [38].

In contrast, antiviral therapy is the mainstay of influenza treatment, with neuraminidase inhibitors (NAIs) such as oseltamivir, zanamivir, laninamivir, and peramivir being widely used, whereas M2 inhibitors, such as amantadine, have been withdrawn due to resistance. Other treatments include HA inhibitors like arbidol and virus RNA polymerase inhibitors such as ribavirin. Resistance to oseltamivir and zanamivir is rare. NAIs are part of international guidelines for influenza management, though corticosteroid therapy has not been shown to improve survival rates and may even increase mortality. New therapies now focus on targeting inflammation, such as using the mTOR inhibitor rapamycin to reduce inflammatory activity. Plasma immunotherapy and other supportive treatments are administered based on patient needs [38].

19.4 Interactions Between COVID-19 and Flu

Coinfection with SARS-CoV-2 and influenza presents significant epidemiological challenges, as both viruses share transmission routes and tend to coincide during seasonal peaks. While SARS-CoV-2 does not always align exactly with influenza A's peak, it frequently overlaps with flu season, increasing healthcare burdens and misdiagnosis rates. Coinfected individuals generally (but not always) experience worse health outcomes, including increased risks of hospitalisation, respiratory failure, cardiac injury, and other complications. Coinfected patients also experience severe lymphopenia, weaker antibody responses, and increased inflammation. Furthermore, influenza A virus has been found to enhance SARS-CoV-2 infectivity by increasing ACE2 expression in respiratory cells, further exacerbating disease severity. Ultimately, understanding the mechanisms behind dual infections can improve disease management, support integrated surveillance systems, and inform preventive measures, such as expanded vaccination campaigns and targeted interventions for vulnerable populations [9, 30, 39–41].

Interestingly, cross-protection has been demonstrated between COVID-19 and influenza vaccinations. Antibodies against the delta variant of SARS-CoV-2 cross-react with the influenza A virus, while prior influenza vaccination reduces susceptibility to COVID-19 and the likelihood of adverse COVID-19 outcomes [42–46].

19.5 Conclusion

Conclusive diagnostic testing for identification of the aetiology is required in view of common transmission routes and overlapping clinical syndromes caused by the influenza virus and SARS-CoV-2, with a specific antiviral being available for only one of these, i.e., oseltamivir for the influenza virus. Combination vaccines against circulating variants of both viruses should be considered, as both are likely to continue co-circulating, and cross-protection has been demonstrated.

References

1. Krammer F, Smith GJD, Fouchier RAM, Peiris M, Kedzierska K, Doherty PC, et al. Influenza. Nat Rev Dis Primers. 2018;4:3. https://doi.org/10.1038/S41572-018-0002-Y
2. Wang X, Li J, Liu H, Hu X, Lin Z, Xiong N. SARS-CoV-2 versus influenza a virus: characteristics and co-treatments. Microorganisms. 2023;11:580. https://doi.org/10.3390/MICROORGANISMS11030580.
3. Influenza (seasonal) n.d.. https://www.who.int/news-room/fact-sheets/detail/influenza-(seasonal). Accessed 15 May 2025.

4. Iuliano AD, Roguski KM, Chang HH, Muscatello DJ, Palekar R, Tempia S, et al. Estimates of global seasonal influenza-associated respiratory mortality: a modelling study. Lancet. 2017;391:1285. https://doi.org/10.1016/S0140-6736(17)33293-2.
5. COVID-19 deaths | WHO COVID-19 dashboard n.d.. https://data.who.int/dashboards/covid19/deaths?n=o. Accessed 24 May 2025
6. Hanage WP, Schaffner W. Burden of acute respiratory infections caused by influenza virus, respiratory syncytial virus, and SARS-CoV-2 with consideration of older adults: a narrative review. Infect Dis Ther. 2024;14:5. https://doi.org/10.1007/S40121-024-01080-4.
7. Branche A, Ramesh M, Francis B. A narrative review of key risk factors for severe illness following SARS-CoV-2, influenza virus, and respiratory syncytial virus infection. Infect Dis Ther. 2024;14:39. https://doi.org/10.1007/S40121-024-01081-3.
8. Els F, Kleynhans J, Wolter N, du Plessis M, Moosa F, Tempia S, et al. Comparing adults with severe SARS-CoV-2 or influenza infection: South Africa, 2016–2021. S Afr J Infect Dis. 2024:39. https://doi.org/10.4102/SAJID.V39I1.574.
9. Vieceli T, Croda J, Bastos LSL, Bozza FA, Ranzani OT. The burden, clinical features and outcomes of SARS-CoV-2, influenza and co-infections during concurrently out-of-season outbreaks in Brazil. Public Health. 2025;238:101–7. https://doi.org/10.1016/j.puhe.2024.10.016.
10. Atamna A, Berkov E, Drozdinsky G, Shochat T, Ben Zvi H, Eliakim-Raz N, et al. Clinical outcomes of hospitalized patients with SARS-CoV-2 omicron variant vs. influenza A during influenza season 2021 to 2022: a retrospective observational study. Isr Med Assoc J. 2023;25:585–9.
11. Hedberg P, Valik JK, Abdel-Halim L, Alfvén T, Nauclér P. Outcomes of SARS-CoV-2 omicron variant infections compared with seasonal influenza and respiratory syncytial virus infections in adults attending the emergency department: a multicenter cohort study. Clin Infect Dis. 2024;78:900–7. https://doi.org/10.1093/CID/CIAD660.
12. Spindel J, Furmanek S, Chandler T, Ramirez JA, Cavallazzi R. In patients hospitalized for community-acquired pneumonia, SARS-CoV-2 is associated with worse clinical Outcomes when compared to influenza. Pathogens. 2023;12:571. https://doi.org/10.3390/PATHOGENS12040571/S1.
13. Dickow J, Gunawardene MA, Willems S, Feldhege J, Wohlmuth P, Bachmann M, et al. Higher in-hospital mortality in SARS-CoV-2 omicron variant infection compared to influenza infection—insights from the CORONA Germany study. PLoS One. 2023:18. https://doi.org/10.1371/JOURNAL.PONE.0292017.
14. Portmann L, De Kraker MEA, Fröhlich G, Thiabaud A, Roelens M, Schreiber PW, et al. Hospital outcomes of community-acquired SARS-CoV-2 omicron variant infection compared with influenza infection in Switzerland. JAMA Netw Open. 2023;6:E2255599. https://doi.org/10.1001/JAMANETWORKOPEN.2022.55599.
15. Boon H, Meinders AJ, van Hannen EJ, Tersmette M, Schaftenaar E. Comparative analysis of mortality in patients admitted with an infection with influenza A/B virus, respiratory syncytial virus, rhinovirus, metapneumovirus or SARS-CoV-2. Influenza Other Respir Viruses. 2024;18:13237. https://doi.org/10.1111/IRV.13237.
16. Mendoza MA, Motoa G, Raja MA, Frattaroli P, Fernandez A, Anjan S, et al. Difference between SARS-CoV-2, seasonal coronavirus, influenza, and respiratory syncytial virus infection in solid organ transplant recipients. Transpl Infect Dis. 2022;25:e13998. https://doi.org/10.1111/TID.13998.
17. Lin F, Chen MT, Zhang L, Wu M, Xie H, Guan ZX, et al. Resurgence of influenza A after SARS-CoV-2 omicron wave and comparative analysis of hospitalized children with COVID-19 and influenza A virus infection. Front Med (Lausanne). 2023;10:1289487. https://doi.org/10.3389/FMED.2023.1289487.
18. Zhong Z, Wang X, Guo J, Li X, Han Y. Comparison of clinical characteristics and outcomes in intensive care units between patients with coronavirus disease 2019 (COVID-19) and patients with influenza: a systematic review and meta-analysis. J Intensive Care Med. 2024;39:840–52. https://doi.org/10.1177/08850666241232888.
19. Pormohammad A, Ghorbani S, Khatami A, Razizadeh MH, Alborzi E, Zarei M, et al. Comparison of influenza type a and B with COVID-19: a global systematic review and

meta-analysis on clinical, laboratory and radiographic findings. Rev Med Virol. 2021;31 https://doi.org/10.1002/RMV.2179.
20. Bechmann L, Esser T, Färber J, Kaasch A, Geginat G. Outcomes of influenza and COVID-19 inpatients in different phases of the SARS-CoV-2 pandemic: a single-centre retrospective case–control study. J Hosp Infect. 2023;138:1. https://doi.org/10.1016/J.JHIN.2023.04.014.
21. Liu C, He F. Systematic review and meta-analysis of randomized controlled trials comparing the clinical outcomes of SARS-CoV-2 and influenza in pediatric patients. Adv. Clin Exp Med. 2025;34:1267–76. https://doi.org/10.17219/ACEM/192224.
22. Athina P, Stavroula L, Despoina Zoe MT, Stavroula K, Maria KG. The clinical burden of SARS-CoV-2 compared to influenza a in the same cohort of paediatric outpatients; increased influenza severity and potential insights. J Paediatr Child Health. 2025;61 https://doi.org/10.1111/JPC.70014.
23. Brigadoi G, Demarin GC, Boracchini R, Pierantoni L, Rossin S, Barbieri E, et al. Comparison between the viral illness caused by SARS-CoV-2, influenza virus, respiratory syncytial virus and other respiratory viruses in pediatrics. Viruses. 2024;16:199. https://doi.org/10.3390/V16020199/S1.
24. Seyedalinaghi S, Afsahi AM, Mirzapour P, Afzalian A, Shahidi R, Dashti M, et al. Comparison of omicron and delta variants of SARS-CoV-2: a systematic review of current evidence. Infect Disord Drug Targets. 2024;24:21–57. https://doi.org/10.2174/0118715265279242240216114548.
25. Livieratos A, Gogos C, Akinosoglou K. SARS-CoV-2 variants and clinical outcomes of special populations: a scoping review of the literature. Viruses. 2024;16:1222. https://doi.org/10.3390/V16081222.
26. Bajema KL, Bui DP, Yan L, Li Y, Rajeevan N, Vergun R, et al. Severity and long-term mortality of COVID-19, influenza, and respiratory syncytial virus. JAMA Intern Med. 2025;185:324–34. https://doi.org/10.1001/JAMAINTERNMED.2024.7452.
27. Yu B, Chen HH, Hu XF, Mai RZ, He HY. Comparison of laboratory parameters, clinical symptoms and clinical outcomes of COVID-19 and influenza in pediatric patients: a systematic review and meta-analysis. World J Clin Cases. 2022;10:10516. https://doi.org/10.12998/WJCC.V10.I29.10516.
28. He L, Weng J, Zhu F, Zhang Y, Chen J, Chen S, et al. The morbidity spectrum of influenza, respiratory syncytial virus, human metapneumovirus and human parainfluenza virus in young children by age and country income level: a systematic review and meta-analysis. Int J Infect Dis. 2025:157. https://doi.org/10.1016/j.ijid.2025.107938.
29. Zachariah P. COVID-19 in children. Infect Dis Clin N Am. 2022;36:1–14. https://doi.org/10.1016/j.idc.2021.11.002.
30. Asseri AA, Al-Qahtani SM, Alzaydani IA, Al-Jarie A, Alyazidi NS, Alrmelawi AA, et al. Clinical and epidemiological characteristics of respiratory syncytial virus, SARS-CoV-2 and influenza paediatric viral respiratory infections in Southwest Saudi Arabia. Ann Med. 2024;57:2445791. https://doi.org/10.1080/07853890.2024.2445791.
31. Zhong W, Wu Y, Yue W, Fang J, Xie B, Xu N, et al. Distinguishing COVID-19 from seasonal influenza in patients under age 65 years—a retrospective observational cohort study comparing the 2009 influenza A (H1N1) and 2022 SARS-CoV-2 pandemics. Front Cell Infect Microbiol. 2023;13:1179552. https://doi.org/10.3389/FCIMB.2023.1179552.
32. Dabaja-Younis H, Fuchs E, Shorbaji N, Appel T, Carmon N, Shachor-Meyouhas Y, et al. SARS-CoV-2 and seasonal influenza: similarities and disparities. Arch Virol. 2022;167:2761. https://doi.org/10.1007/S00705-022-05615-3.
33. Stone EC, Okasako-Schmucker DL, Taliano J, Schaefer M, Kuhar DT. Risk period for transmission of SARS-CoV-2 and seasonal influenza: a rapid review. Infect Control Hosp Epidemiol. 2025;46:227. https://doi.org/10.1017/ICE.2025.11.
34. Brown M, Gerrard J, McKinlay L, Marquess J, Sparrow T, Andrews R. Ongoing symptoms and functional impairment 12 weeks after testing positive for SARS-CoV-2 or influenza in Australia: an observational cohort study. BMJ Public Health. 2023;1:e000060. https://doi.org/10.1136/BMJPH-2023-000060.

35. Uyeki TM, Hui DS, Zambon M, Wentworth DE, Monto AS. Influenza Lancet. 2022;400:693. https://doi.org/10.1016/S0140-6736(22)00982-5.
36. El-Kassas M, Alboraie M, Elbadry M, El Sheemy R, Abdellah M, Afify S, et al. Non-pulmonary involvement in COVID-19: a systemic disease rather than a pure respiratory infection. World J Clin Cases. 2023;11:493. https://doi.org/10.12998/WJCC.V11.I3.493.
37. Gu Y, Zuo X, Zhang S, Ouyang Z, Jiang S, Wang F, et al. The mechanism behind influenza virus cytokine storm. Viruses. 2021;13:1362. https://doi.org/10.3390/V13071362.
38. Bai Y, Tao X. Comparison of COVID-19 and influenza characteristics. J Zhejiang Univ Sci B. 2021;22:87. https://doi.org/10.1631/JZUS.B2000479.
39. Huang Y, Li S, Ye W, Wang H, Su J, Gao L, et al. Viral infections in elderly individuals: a comprehensive overview of SARS-CoV-2 and influenza susceptibility, pathogenesis, and clinical treatment strategies. Vaccines (Basel). 2025;13:431. https://doi.org/10.3390/VACCINES13040431.
40. Qi CH, Lim R, Pung R. Excess respiratory hospitalisations associated with influenza, respiratory syncytial virus and SARS-CoV-2 in Singapore from 2015 to 2023. Influenza Other Respir Viruses. 2025;19:e70098. https://doi.org/10.1111/IRV.70098.
41. Yan X, Li K, Lei Z, Luo J, Wang Q, Wei S. Prevalence and associated outcomes of coinfection between SARS-CoV-2 and influenza: a systematic review and meta-analysis. Int J Infect Dis. 2023;136:29–36. https://doi.org/10.1016/j.ijid.2023.08.021.
42. Alam MM, Salauddin A, Moni S, Limon MBH, Musarrat R, Bosu S, et al. Cross-neutralization of influenza a by SARS-CoV-2 specific neutralizing antibodies and polyclonal plasma: is pre-exposure to SARS-CoV-2 protective against influenza A? Heliyon. 2024;10:e40638. https://doi.org/10.1016/J.HELIYON.2024.E40638.
43. Teluguakula N, Chow VTK, Pandareesh MD, Dasegowda V, Kurrapotula V, Gopegowda SM, et al. SARS-CoV-2 and influenza co-infection: fair competition or sinister combination? Viruses. 2024;16:793. https://doi.org/10.3390/V16050793.
44. Jiang B, Huang Q, Jia M, Xue X, Wang Q, Yang W, et al. Association between influenza vaccination and SARS-CoV-2 infection and its outcomes: systematic review and meta-analysis. Chin Med J. 2022;135:2282. https://doi.org/10.1097/CM9.0000000000002427.
45. Tayar E, Abdeen S, Abed Alah M, Chemaitelly H, Bougmiza I, Ayoub HH, et al. Effectiveness of influenza vaccination against SARS-CoV-2 infection among healthcare workers in Qatar. J Infect Public Health. 2022;16:250. https://doi.org/10.1016/J.JIPH.2022.12.016.
46. Mosaed R, Fasihi H, Norouzi A, Anjomanian V, Ardalan MA, Noodeh FA, et al. Influenza vaccine and COVID-19 pandemic: could this vaccine help limit the potential adverse consequences of SARS-CoV-2? Iran J Pharma Res. 2022:21. https://doi.org/10.5812/IJPR-127032.

COVID-19 Vaccination

20

Lonika Lodha

20.1 Introduction

The outbreak of COVID-19 spurred remarkable progress in vaccine technology, driving a rapid expansion of global vaccine manufacturing across diverse platforms. Beginning in December 2020, just months after the identification of SARS-CoV-2, COVID-19 vaccines moved swiftly through clinical trials and became widely accessible. Massive vaccination programmes were rolled out across nations, playing a crucial role in curbing the pandemic and ultimately leading to the official conclusion of the Public Health Emergency of International Concern (PHEIC) in May 2023.

20.2 Correlates of Protection

Correlates of Protection (CoP) are biomarkers above a defined threshold that can replace clinical outcomes as primary endpoints, predicting vaccine effectiveness to support the approval of new vaccines or follow-up studies [1].

Neutralising antibodies (NAbs) and spike-binding IgG have been identified as strong predictors of clinical protection against SARS-CoV-2 infection. Through integrative analyses, their roles as species- and vaccine-independent CoP have been demonstrated. Binding and neutralising antibodies have been recognised as reliable markers for clinical protection, with high NAb titres best predicting clinical outcomes, while elevated spike-binding IgG titres have been shown to correlate with lower viral loads in both throat and lung samples. Furthermore, all four IgG subclasses and spike-binding IgM have emerged as predictors of protection, with children's heightened IgM responses suggested to contribute to their milder COVID-19 presentations [2, 3].

L. Lodha (✉)
Department of Neurovirology, National Institute of Mental Health and Neurosciences (NIMHANS), Bengaluru, Karnataka, India

S. R. Prabhu et al. (eds.), *COVID-19 in Dental Practice*,
https://doi.org/10.1007/978-3-032-26000-0_20

Although it remains difficult to pinpoint a protective mechanism for T cells that does not also involve their role in helping antibody production in individuals with antibody responses, there is evidence that T cells contribute to protection against SARS-CoV-2, as some people experience asymptomatic COVID-19 without developing detectable antibodies, and individuals with immunoglobulin deficiencies have also been observed to be protected, both situations showing T cell activity [3].

20.3 Types of Vaccines and Their Efficacy

Multiple platforms have been utilised to produce COVID-19 vaccines, and the approved formulations are given either parenterally or through the intranasal (mucosal) route (Table 20.1). Parenteral vaccines offer strong systemic immunity but require healthcare professionals to administer them, are costly, and elicit weaker

Table 20.1 Approved COVID-19 vaccines

Type of vaccine (route of administration)	Name (Manufacturer)
Modified mRNA encoding S protein (parenteral)	BNT162b2 (ancestral); bivalent version with Omicron (BioNTech SE, Pfizer Inc.)
	mRNA-1273 (Moderna)
Modified adenovirus vector encoding S protein (parenteral)	ChAdOx1-nCoV-19 (AstraZeneca, University of Oxford)
	ChAdOx1 nCoV-19 (Serum Institute of India)
	Ad26CoV2.S (Johnson & Johnson)
	Ad5-nCoV (CanSino Biologics Inc.)
	Sputnik V (Gamaleya Research Institute of Epidemiology and Microbiology)
Inactivated SARS-CoV-2 (parenteral)	BBIBP-CorV (Sinopharm)
	CoviVac (Russian Academy of Sciences)
	CoronaVac (Sinovac Biotech Ltd.)
	BBV152 (Bharat Biotech)
	VLA2001 (Valneva)
Adjuvanted protein subunit (parenteral)	ZF2001 (Chinese Academy of Sciences)
	PHH-1 V (HIPRA)
Peptide subunit (parenteral)	EpiVacCorona (Vektor State Research Centre, Russia)
Recombinant S protein nanoparticle (parenteral)	NVX-CoV2373/Nuvaxovid: Ancestral; Nuvaxovid: Omicron XBB1.5 (Novavax)
	NVX-CoV2373/Covovax (Serum Institute of India)
Recombinant S protein subunit (parenteral and intranasal)	RAZI-COV PARS (RAZI Vaccine and Serum Research Institute)
Viral vector (replicating) (intranasal)	dNS1-RBD (Beijing Wantai)
	BBV154 (Bharat Biotech International Limited)
Viral vector (non-replicating) (intranasal)	Ad5-nCoV-IH (CanSinoBio)
	Sputnik V/Gam-COVIDVac (The Gamaleya Research Institute of Epidemiology and Microbiology)

mucosal responses. Mucosal vaccines are non-invasive, cost-effective, easy to administer, and stimulate both mucosal and systemic immunity yet face challenges such as short nasal residence times and the need for adequate delivery devices. Both types can be affected by pre-existing immunity against viral vectors. It has been suggested that the "prime-boost" strategy, i.e., a primer of parenteral vaccination followed by a mucosal booster vaccination, might enhance vaccination effectiveness against COVID-19 [4, 5].

Notwithstanding the impact of demography and geography on vaccine effectiveness, overall, mRNA vaccines have shown higher efficacy, ranging from 52% to 80% after the first dose and rising to approximately 95% after the second dose. Inactivated vaccines showed relatively lower efficacy of 50–60% after one dose and 51–84% after two doses [6].

The three vaccines with the largest body of data behind them are the BNT162b2, mRNA-1273, and AZD1222. All three demonstrated a comparable average vaccine efficacy (VE) of more than 77% against symptomatic infections, albeit with wide variation, ranging from 44% to 100%, depending on the variants of concern (VOC) studied, the age of the study participants, and prior infections. Notably, the VE against serious outcomes of COVID-19 (hospitalisation and death) was very high at more than 90%, irrespective of the circulating VOC, and was also maintained in the elderly population [7].

Across the various COVID-19 vaccine platforms, notable differences were observed in the immune responses generated. The mRNA-based vaccines induced a stronger anti-spike IgG response, while subunit vaccines produced comparatively higher neutralising antibody titres. Each vaccine type demonstrated distinct profiles for both anti-spike IgG and neutralising antibodies, with seroconversion rates exceeding 98% among vaccinated individuals. Both inactivated and subunit vaccines led to a robust production of neutralising antibodies and were associated with fewer commonly reported adverse reactions than other platforms [8].

People who had previously contracted SARS-CoV-2 consistently exhibited higher median levels of IgG antibodies than those without prior infections—a trend supported by numerous studies. Although antibody concentrations gradually declined over time in both groups, the initial difference remained evident. Importantly, for those with a history of infection, receiving a single dose of an mRNA vaccine provided substantial additional protection against infection, symptomatic disease, and hospitalisation, as well as hospitalisation or death, supplementing the immunity gained from natural infection. This enhanced protection was observed both before and during the Omicron variant's predominance [2, 9].

Nevertheless, no vaccine guarantees absolute protection against symptomatic COVID-19. In research studies, between 0.1% and 3.8% of vaccinated participants contracted COVID-19 during follow-up periods ranging from 144 to 302 days, with similar outcomes reported in observational studies [2].

20.4 Impact of Viral Variants on Vaccine Efficacy

The first vaccine (BNT162b2) was developed against the B.1 strain. Still, the Alpha variant began spreading just as vaccines were being rolled out, and neutralisation studies showed they retained their effectiveness. On the contrary, vaccine effectiveness against the Delta variant was lower than that against the Alpha variant [10].

Many variants were shown, by serologic testing, to escape neutralising antibodies, including Alpha, Beta, Delta, and Omicron variants along with their subvariants BA.1, BA.1.1, BA.2, BA.2.12.1, BA.4, BA.5, and more recently, XBB.1.5, EG.5.1, HV.1, and JN.1. Consequently, there has been considerable diminution of VE against symptomatic illness. Notably, hospitalisation and mortality rates remain stable among vaccinated individuals, suggesting that existing COVID-19 vaccines still offer strong protection against severe illness, even when neutralising antibody levels are low [11].

The duration of vaccine effectiveness (VE) against symptomatic infection was found to have a half-life of 87 days for the Omicron variant, compared with 316 days for the Delta variant. Comparable rates of decline in VE were observed across various age groups [12]. The emergence of the Omicron variant prompted the first significant revision to COVID-19 vaccines. Towards the end of 2022, bivalent vaccines were rolled out, designed to target both the original virus and Omicron BA.1. Subsequently, a new bivalent booster was approved, aimed at the Omicron BA.4 and BA.5 subvariants as well as the initial strain. In September 2023, the FDA granted authorisation for a new monovalent mRNA vaccine targeting XBB.1.5. As new coronaviruses with the potential to cause illness in humans are expected to continue emerging, it is increasingly vital to develop a universal vaccine that can provide protection against a wide range of coronaviruses. Current research is focused on developing a vaccine that provides comprehensive protection against the coronavirus family, including SARS-CoV-2 and MERS-CoV [10].

20.5 Considerations in Special Populations

Among people living with HIV (PLWH), a combined serological response rate of 87.09% was observed following SARS-CoV-2 vaccination, based on data from 10,343 individuals. Achieving robust immunogenicity in this group is closely linked to receiving a third vaccine dose and maintaining effective HIV treatment [13].

In patients with chronic kidney disease (CKD) undergoing dialysis, COVID-19 vaccines also demonstrated strong immune efficacy and safety, with an 80% seropositivity rate. Those who had previously contracted COVID-19 showed even higher rates of antibody response. The most frequently reported side effects were localised pain at the injection site and fatigue, but the overall safety profile remained high [14].

Allogeneic haematopoietic cell transplant (alloHCT) recipients exhibited a pooled antibody response rate of 74% after three vaccine doses. Notably, among patients who did not respond to the initial two doses, just under half (49%)

developed antibodies after a third dose. Factors such as male sex and a shorter interval between the transplant and the third dose were associated with a reduced likelihood of responding to the third dose [15].

In the case of autoimmune hepatitis (AIH) patients, immune responses to COVID-19 vaccination were diminished, particularly in those on specific immunosuppressive treatments like steroids and mycophenolate mofetil (MMF) [16]. For individuals with autoimmune neurological disorders, COVID-19 vaccines were generally well-tolerated, with few reports of adverse events or worsening of pre-existing conditions [17].

In liver transplant recipients (LTR), the rate of seroconversion after at least two vaccine doses was 53% among those transplanted within the past 7 years, compared with 83% among those transplanted more than 7 years ago. The vaccine response in these patients was influenced by factors such as vaccine type, immunosuppressive therapy, body mass index (BMI), leukopenia, comorbidities, and time since transplant [18].

Meta-analyses in solid organ transplant recipients revealed that the favourable antibody response rates increased with each subsequent mRNA vaccine dose: 10.4% after the first dose, 44.9% after the second, 63.1% after the third, and 85% after the fourth dose, underscoring the importance of repeated boosters for this group [19, 20].

Among pregnant women, when evaluating VE across multiple COVID-19 variants, mRNA vaccines showed a VE of 72%, viral vector vaccines 49%, and inactivated vaccines 61%, irrespective of the vaccination schedule. There was no evidence linking COVID-19 vaccination (even a single dose) during pregnancy to negative pregnancy or infant outcomes, regardless of the trimester or vaccine type. Some evidence, though considered of low certainty, suggests that maternal vaccination may decrease the risk of severe or hospitalised COVID-19 in infants [21].

20.6 Adverse Effects

In general, the approved COVID-19 vaccines are rarely associated with severe adverse effects. The frequently reported adverse events are mild and self-resolving, including pain at the injection site, fatigue, myalgia, fever, chills, headache, etc. [22, 23].

Oral side effects following COVID-19 vaccinations are relatively uncommon, with the most frequently observed symptoms including changes in taste such as dysgeusia and ageusia, hypersensitivity reactions like glossitis, swelling of the lips and mouth, and sensory disturbances such as oral paraesthesia. Lichenoid lesions are the most common adverse events reported in the oral cavity, with other symptoms including oral paraesthesia, lip swelling, ageusia, dysgeusia, hypogeusia, hypaesthesia, xerostomia, and inflammation of the tongue. Notably, dysgeusia and xerostomia are more frequently associated with adenoviral vector vaccines compared to mRNA-based vaccines.

Analysing the occurrence of oral adverse effects by vaccine type, the highest proportion of cases were reported following administration of the mRNA BNT162b2 (Pfizer-BioNTech) vaccine, followed by the ChAdOX1 (AstraZeneca) vaccine, the mRNA-1273/Moderna vaccine, and Ad26.COV2.5 (Johnson & Johnson). Furthermore, oral side effects appear to be more prevalent in females [24–26].

Guillain Barre Syndrome (GBS), a rare profound adverse effect of COVID-19 vaccination, is reported to occur more frequently with adenoviral vectored vaccines compared to mRNA vaccines. It has also been observed that, in contrast to the typical presentation of GBS, the variant occurring after COVID-19 vaccination tends to manifest with more pronounced symptoms and is more likely to result in hemiparesis [27, 28].

Skin-related side effects were most commonly seen as reactions at the injection site, followed by general rashes or unspecified skin eruptions, urticarial rashes, swelling such as angioedema, shingles (herpes zoster), and various types of red rashes, including morbilliform, maculopapular, and erythematous macular eruptions, as well as pityriasis rosea and similar presentations. Less frequent skin reactions were also noted. Additionally, flare-ups of existing skin conditions have been observed. Overall, cutaneous side effects following SARS-CoV-2 vaccination appear to be diverse, relatively rare, and generally not serious [29].

The occurrence of acute myocarditis and/or pericarditis following COVID-19 vaccination is rare, with rates reported between 1 and 10.7 per 100,000, varying according to factors such as age, sex, and the specific vaccine used. Although cases of myocarditis are more frequent after mRNA COVID-19 vaccines than before the pandemic, those affected generally experience favourable outcomes [30, 31].

While reports exist regarding endocrine and reproductive side effects, the literature examined does not conclusively demonstrate a direct causal link between COVID-19 vaccination and endocrine complications. The emergence of endocrine disorders following mass vaccination campaigns might be attributed to causality bias rather than being a consequence of the vaccines themselves [32, 33].

20.7 Post-pandemic Vaccination Recommendations

The CDC recommends the latest COVID-19 vaccine for most adults aged 18 and older. For children aged 6 months to 17 years, the benefits of vaccination should be discussed with a healthcare provider. Particular importance is placed on receiving the 2024–2025 COVID-19 vaccine if individuals are aged 65 and older, are at high risk for severe COVID-19, or have not previously received a COVID-19 vaccine [34].

The World Health Organisation (WHO) recommendations for COVID-19 vaccination prioritise high-risk groups, including older adults, health workers, pregnant people, and individuals with comorbidities or immunocompromising conditions. These groups are advised to receive 1–3 doses of the vaccine at the first dose, followed by revaccination 6–12 months later. Revaccination after the primary regimen is not recommended for healthy adults, adolescents, and children [35].

References

1. O'Reilly S, Byrne J, Feeney ER, Mallon PWG, Gautier V. Navigating the landscape of B cell mediated immunity and antibody monitoring in SARS-CoV-2 vaccine efficacy: tools, strategies and clinical trial insights. Vaccines (Basel). 2024;12:1089. https://doi.org/10.3390/VACCINES12101089.
2. Bylica I, Jachowicz-Matczak E, Brodowicz J, Sułkowska J, Bociąga-Jasik M, Heczko P, et al. SARS-CoV-2 vaccine-induced humoral immunity in immunocompetent European adults: a systematic review. Microorganisms. 2025;13:535. https://doi.org/10.3390/MICROORGANISMS13030535/S1.
3. Brady C, Tipton T, Carnell O, Longet S, Gooch K, Hall Y, et al. A systems biology approach to define SARS-CoV-2 correlates of protection. NPJ Vaccines. 2025;10:1–15. https://doi.org/10.1038/S41541-025-01103-2;SUBJMETA.
4. Tscherne A, Sun W, Liu STH, Krammer F. Mucosal COVID-19 vaccines in clinical development. Vaccine. 2025;63:127602. https://doi.org/10.1016/J.VACCINE.2025.127602.
5. Tobias J, Steinberger P, Wilkinson J, Klais G, Kundi M, Wiedermann U. SARS-CoV-2 vaccines: the advantage of mucosal vaccine delivery and local immunity. Vaccines (Basel). 2024;12:795. https://doi.org/10.3390/VACCINES12070795/S1.
6. Azeem M, Cancemi P, Mukhtar F, Marino S, Peri E, Di Prima G, et al. Efficacy and limitations of SARS-CoV-2 vaccines – a systematic review. Life Sci. 2025;371:123610. https://doi.org/10.1016/J.LFS.2025.123610.
7. Chuenkitmongkol S, Solante R, Burhan E, Chariyalertsak S, Chiu NC, Do-Van D, et al. Expert review on global real-world vaccine effectiveness against SARS-CoV-2. Expert Rev Vaccines. 2022;21:1255–68. https://doi.org/10.1080/14760584.2022.2092472.
8. Mirzakhani M, Bayat M, Dashti M, Tahmasebi S, Rostamtabar M, Esmaeili Gouvarchin Ghaleh H, et al. The assessment of anti–SARS-CoV-2 antibodies in different vaccine platforms: a systematic review and meta-analysis of COVID-19 vaccine clinical trial studies. Rev Med Virol. 2024;34 https://doi.org/10.1002/RMV.2579.
9. Volkman HR, Nguyen JL, Mustapha MM, Yang J, Jodar L, McLaughlin JM. Effectiveness of a single COVID-19 mRNA vaccine dose in individuals with prior SARS-CoV-2 infection: a systematic review. Commun Med. 2025;5:151. https://doi.org/10.1038/S43856-025-00882-Y.
10. Angius F, Puxeddu S, Zaimi S, Canton S, Nematollahzadeh S, Pibiri A, et al. SARS-CoV-2 evolution: implications for diagnosis, treatment, vaccine effectiveness and development. Vaccines (Basel). 2024;13:17. https://doi.org/10.3390/VACCINES13010017.
11. Mahrokhian SH, Tostanoski LH, Vidal SJ, Barouch DH. COVID-19 vaccines: immune correlates and clinical outcomes. Hum Vaccin Immunother. 2024;20:2324549. https://doi.org/10.1080/21645515.2024.2324549.
12. Menegale F, Manica M, Zardini A, Guzzetta G, Marziano V, D'Andrea V, et al. Evaluation of waning of SARS-CoV-2 vaccine–induced immunity: a systematic review and meta-analysis. JAMA Netw Open. 2023;6:e2310650. https://doi.org/10.1001/JAMANETWORKOPEN.2023.10650.
13. Søndergaard MH, Thavarajah JJ, Churchill Henson H, Wejse CM. SARS-CoV-2 vaccine immunogenicity for people living with HIV: a systematic review and meta-analysis. HIV Med. 2024;25:16–37. https://doi.org/10.1111/HIV.13537.
14. Li K, Xia Y, Ye H, Sun X, Shi B, Wu J. Effectiveness and safety of immune response to SARS-CoV-2 vaccine in patients with chronic kidney disease and dialysis: a systematic review and meta-analysis. Biomed Rep. 2024;20:78. https://doi.org/10.3892/BR.2024.1766.
15. Rubin M, Suelzer E, Ulschmid C, Thapa B, Szabo A, Abid MB. Efficacy of SARS-CoV-2 vaccine doses in allogeneic hemopoietic stem cell recipients: a systematic review and meta-analysis. Asian Pac J Cancer Prev. 2024;25:393. https://doi.org/10.31557/APJCP.2024.25.2.393.
16. Tian Z, Chen Y, Yao Y, Chen L, Zhu X, Shen Z, et al. Immunogenicity and risk factors for poor humoral immune response to SARS-CoV-2 vaccine in patients with autoimmune hepatitis: a systematic review and meta-analysis. Rev Esp Enferm Dig. 2024;116:671–9. https://doi.org/10.17235/REED.2024.10053/2023.

17. Ning F, Cao X-Q, Wang Q-Q, Li Z-Y, Ruan Z, Chang T. Safety of SARS-CoV-2 vaccine in patients with autoimmune neurological conditions: a systematic review and meta-analysis. Heliyon. 2023;10:e23944. https://doi.org/10.1016/J.HELIYON.2023.E23944.
18. Luo X, Lessomo FYN, Yu Z, Xie Y. Factors influencing immunogenicity and safety of SARS-CoV-2 vaccine in liver transplantation recipients: a systematic review and meta-analysis. Front Immunol. 2023;14:1145081. https://doi.org/10.3389/FIMMU.2023.1145081/FULL.
19. Manothummetha K, Chuleerarux N, Sanguankeo A, Kates OS, Hirankarn N, Thongkam A, et al. Immunogenicity and risk factors associated with poor humoral immune response of SARS-CoV-2 vaccines in recipients of solid organ transplant: a systematic review and meta-analysis. JAMA Netw Open. 2022;5:e226822. https://doi.org/10.1001/JAMANETWORKOPEN.2022.6822.
20. Mu Y, Wu H, Jiang Z, Liu K, Xue X, Zhang W, et al. Serological responses after a fourth dose of SARS-CoV-2 vaccine in solid organ transplant recipients: a systematic review and meta-analysis. Vaccines (Basel). 2023;11:1130. https://doi.org/10.3390/VACCINES11071130.
21. Ciapponi A, Berrueta M, Argento FJ, Ballivian J, Bardach A, Brizuela ME, et al. Safety and effectiveness of COVID-19 vaccines during pregnancy: a living systematic review and meta-analysis. Drug Saf. 2024;47:991. https://doi.org/10.1007/S40264-024-01458-W.
22. Magalhães BAP, Medeiros Minasi J, Lobato RC, Lemos LC, de Britto LS, Barros RM, et al. Globally approved vaccines for COVID-19: a systematic review. Braz J Microbiol. 2025;56:511–27. https://doi.org/10.1007/S42770-024-01600-X/METRICS.
23. Pimenta PC, de Aquino Lima TC, Geraldine VGS, Tourinho FS, do Nascimento MC, Novaes RD, et al. COVID-19 vaccine adverse events by country income level: a systematic review and meta-analysis of randomized controlled trials. Am J Health Promot. 2025; https://doi.org/10.1177/08901171251365229.
24. Sharma P, Malik S, Wadhwan V, Sharma R. Pathophysiology of oral lesions subsequent to SARS-CoV-2 vaccination: a systematic review. J Oral Maxillofac Pathol. 2024;28:443. https://doi.org/10.4103/JOMFP.JOMFP_511_23.
25. López-Carriches C, Santana-Torres T, Bahram-Taheri R, Leco-Berrocal MI. Systematic review of the oral manifestations produced by the SARS-CoV-2 vaccine. J Clin Exp Dent. 2023;15:e578. https://doi.org/10.4317/JCED.60688.
26. Tsuchiya H, Mizogami M. Characteristics of oral adverse effects following COVID-19 vaccination and similarities with oral symptoms in COVID-19 patients: taste and saliva secretory disorders. Med Princ Pract. 2024;34:101. https://doi.org/10.1159/000543182.
27. Censi S, Bisaccia G, Gallina S, Tomassini V, Uncini A. Guillain–Barré syndrome and COVID-19 vaccination: a systematic review and meta-analysis. J Neurol. 2024;271:1063. https://doi.org/10.1007/S00415-024-12186-7.
28. Sadowski J, Huk J, Otulak S, Zawiło J, Klaudel T, Roszak M, et al. Association between Guillain-Barré syndrome and SARS-CoV-2 virus infection, including the impact of COVID-19 vaccination in the context of the development and general clinical characteristics of the disease. J Neurovirol. 2025;31:333. https://doi.org/10.1007/S13365-025-01267-6.
29. Avallone G, Quaglino P, Cavallo F, Roccuzzo G, Ribero S, Zalaudek I, et al. SARS-CoV-2 vaccine-related cutaneous manifestations: a systematic review. Int J Dermatol. 2022;61:16063. https://doi.org/10.1111/IJD.16063.
30. Sousa JP, Roque D, Guerreiro C, Teixeira R. Anti-SARS-CoV-2 vaccine-induced myocarditis—real but, in general, rare and mild: a consensus statement from the Studies Committee of the Portuguese Society of Cardiology. Rev Port Cardiol. 2023;42:161. https://doi.org/10.1016/J.REPC.2023.01.003.
31. Ishisaka Y, Watanabe A, Aikawa T, Kanaoka K, Takagi H, Wiley J, et al. Overview of SARS-CoV-2 infection and vaccine associated myocarditis compared to non-COVID-19-associated myocarditis: a systematic review and meta-analysis. Int J Cardiol. 2024:395. https://doi.org/10.1016/j.ijcard.2023.131401.
32. Ishay A, Oleinikov K, Chertok Shacham E. SARS-CoV-2-vaccine-related endocrine disorders: an updated narrative review. Vaccines (Basel). 2024;12:750. https://doi.org/10.3390/VACCINES12070750/S1.

33. Zhu S, Luan C, Zhang S, Wang X, Long F, Zhang Q, et al. Effect of SARS-CoV-2 infection and vaccine on ovarian reserve: a systematic review. Eur J Obstetr Gynecol Reprod Biol. 2024;292:63–70. https://doi.org/10.1016/j.ejogrb.2023.10.029.
34. Staying Up to Date with COVID-19 Vaccines | COVID-19 | CDC n.d.. https://www.cdc.gov/covid/vaccines/stay-up-to-date.html. Accessed 5 Oct 2025.
35. COVID-19 Vaccines Advice n.d.. https://www.who.int/emergencies/diseases/novel-coronavirus-2019/covid-19-vaccines/advice. Accessed 5 Oct 2025.

Part IV

Oral Lesions Associated with COVID-19

21 The Oral Cavity as a Potential Reservoir and the Route of Entry of SARS-CoV-2

Pedro Miguel dos Santos Abrantes

21.1 The Oral Cavity as a Route of Entry for SARS-CoV-2

The oral cavity serves as a portal of entry and replication site for various viral infections, including severe acute respiratory syndrome coronavirus 2 (SARS-CoV-2). SARS-CoV-2 typically enters the host by infecting respiratory epithelial cells through contaminated aerosols or droplets [1] and is known to infect various structures of the oral cavity, allowing it to replicate, damage infected tissues, and disseminate locally.

Various oral sites, including mucosal tissues (gingivae, palate, lips, and cheeks), dental pulp, the tongue, minor and major salivary glands, as well as sulcular and periodontal pocket epithelia, express angiotensin-converting enzyme 2 (ACE2) cellular receptors, Furin cellular protein convertase, and transmembrane serine protease 2 (TMPRSS2) [2]. ACE2 functions as a receptor for SARS-CoV-2 spike proteins, while Furin and TMPRSS2 enhance the binding between ACE2 and SARS-CoV-2 by facilitating viral fusion with the cell membrane [3]. In the absence of sufficient TMPRSS2, the virus can enter host cells via endocytosis, supported by the host's cathepsin B (CTSB) and cathepsin L (CTSL) proteases, which are present in salivary glands and gingivae [4, 5]. Besides TMPRSS2, which is highly important for SARS-CoV-2 infection [6], membrane proteases TMPRSS4 and TMPRSS11D (primarily found in the intestinal and respiratory mucosae, respectively) can also facilitate viral entry [7], while TMPRSS3, TMPRSS5, and TMPRSS7 have been found to correlate with ACE2 expression in salivary glands [8].

ACE2 and TMPRSS2 are widely distributed in the oral mucosa, with both being present in the tongue, oral mucosal surfaces, tonsils, salivary glands, and oral blood vessels [7, 9], as well as in dental pulp [10]. ACE2 is also found in oral epithelial

P. M. dos Santos Abrantes (✉)
Department of Medical Biosciences, Faculty of Natural Sciences, University of the Western Cape, Bellville, South Africa
e-mail: pabrantes@uwc.ac.za

S. R. Prabhu et al. (eds.), *COVID-19 in Dental Practice*,
https://doi.org/10.1007/978-3-032-26000-0_21

cells, while TMPRSS2 can be located in the sulcular epithelium. On the other hand, TMPRSS4 and TMPRSS11D have been identified in most oral mucosal surfaces, salivary glands, and tonsils but are not present in the taste buds, labial mucosa, or oral blood vessels [7]. Furin is broadly distributed across the oral mucosa but is mainly concentrated in the epithelial cells of the tongue [9], only being absent from the tonsils [7]. These factors facilitate the attachment, infection, replication, and spread of SARS-CoV-2 within oral tissues. This process is especially prominent in older patients, who exhibit higher levels of ACE2, Furin, and TMPRSS2 [11, 12], which, together with SARS-CoV-2's ability to evade the host's innate immune responses [13] and the declining immunity typically seen in older individuals, increases their susceptibility to severe SARS-CoV-2 infection.

21.2 The Oral Cavity as a Reservoir of SARS-CoV-2

21.2.1 Oral SARS-CoV-2 Niches and the Role of Saliva

Evidence of the oral cavity as a SARS-CoV-2 reservoir includes its detection in salivary glands, saliva, the tongue (including taste buds), oral mucosal surfaces, dental caries lesions, dental calculus, dental plaque, gingivocrevicular fluid, sulcular and periodontal pockets, and periodontal tissues of infected patients [2, 14]. SARS-CoV-2 can infect and replicate in different layers of keratinized (gingiva and palate) and non-keratinized (lip and cheek) oral mucosae, with viral replication occurring in shed epithelial cells that are then dispersed in saliva [4, 15]. In addition to oral mucosal surfaces, the virus also attaches to the openings of salivary gland ducts [16], where it can replicate [17] and cause cellular damage [18]. The resulting inflammatory reactions can, in some cases, lead to sialadenitis [19], potentially causing secretory dysfunction and xerostomia [5, 20].

Since saliva contains various antimicrobial peptides and compounds [21], hyposalivation results in a weakened oral innate immune response and increases susceptibility to infection by different opportunistic microorganisms, including viruses, bacteria, and yeasts of the *Candida* genus [21], which are usually controlled in the mouth by salivary histatins [22]; furthermore, hyposalivation can potentially disrupt the surfaces of the oral and airway mucosa, facilitating greater SARS-CoV-2 colonization and adhesion [23]. Hyposalivation related to SARS-CoV-2 infection may continue even after the patient recovers, possibly due to initial virus-induced damage to salivary gland cells [24]. Additionally, zinc deficiency, which is common in patients infected with SARS-CoV-2, results in impaired saliva secretion [25]. Damage to the salivary gland tissues can lead to fibrosis during repair, causing further hyposalivation and obstruction of the salivary ducts [7].

Viral shedding from infected tissues occurs in saliva, enabling SARS-CoV-2 to spread through respiratory droplets [26]. There also appears to be a delay in the host's response in the mouth, as SARS-CoV-2 viral RNA is detected in saliva earlier than the host's SARS-CoV-2 antigens [27]. This, combined with SARS-CoV-2's ability to disrupt the host's antiviral responses, permits the virus to replicate and spread during the early stages of infection continuously and to induce an abnormal pro-inflammatory state [13]. The presence of SARS-CoV-2 from infected salivary glands has been observed in cell-free saliva [4], further facilitating SARS-CoV-2 dissemination within the oral mucosa, including in oral biofilms [28, 29], which can be difficult to eradicate without proper oral hygiene. SARS-CoV-2-infected ciliated cells (originally from the respiratory tract) can also be present in saliva, potentially serving as a mechanism for cross-infection and viral persistence due to increased viral loads between these two anatomical sites [30] and possibly allowing the virus to enter the lower respiratory and gastrointestinal tracts [16].

21.2.2 SARS-CoV-2 and the Periodontium

Periodontitis is characterized by the destruction of tooth-supporting tissues, triggered by an imbalance of the gingival and periodontal bacterial flora and a proinflammatory host response. The development of periodontitis-associated periodontal pockets enables both host inflammatory responses and periodontopathogens to interact with the rest of the oral mucosa, acting as a gateway to the respiratory and circulatory systems [31].

Periodontal disease is strongly linked to increased susceptibility to SARS-CoV-2 and more severe disease outcomes [32]. The presence of SARS-CoV-2 in gingivo-crevicular fluid—along with the expression of ACE2 receptors and TMPRSS2 in sulcular and periodontal pocket epithelia, areas that are anatomically distinct and typically better protected compared to other oral tissues—facilitates viral entry and replication in these oral niches [5, 33, 34]. Patients with SARS-CoV-2 who also have periodontal disease tend to experience higher mortality rates than those with a healthy periodontium [35, 36], likely due to the production of periodontitis-related proinflammatory cytokines (e.g., IL-1β and TNF-α) that heighten the risk of severe COVID-19 [37]. These proinflammatory cytokines can also promote an increase in bacteria such as *Porphyromonas gingivalis*, *Fusobacterium nucleatum*, and *Prevotella intermedia*, leading to acute periodontitis [38]. Such periodontopathogens are known to secrete enzymes that facilitate viral adhesion [38]. In contrast, *F. nucleatum* has been shown to upregulate ACE2 expression in human alveolar epithelial cells [39] and exacerbate alveolar epithelial inflammation by producing the matrix metalloproteinase 9 enzyme in lung tissues [40]. It has also been proposed that individuals with periodontal disease are more susceptible to viral adhesion and persistent infection due to the expression of Gal-3, a pro-inflammatory protein [41]. Disruption of the oral microbiome and oral epithelial interactions, alongside impaired oral immune responses, are also suspected factors [38]. These elements may contribute to the development of necrotizing periodontal disease, characterized by necrosis of alveolar bone, gingiva, and periodontal tissues, which has been reported in SARS-CoV-2 patients and is associated with immunosuppression and oral pathogens such as *F. nucleatum* and *P. intermedia* [42].

Periodontal disease is a known risk factor for the development of various systemic conditions, which in turn can increase SARS-CoV-2 disease severity [43] due to preexisting systemic inflammation [44]. The overexpression of pro-inflammatory cytokines and metalloproteinases has been associated with chronic periodontitis and severe SARS-CoV-2 disease [42]. Periodontopathogens can be aspirated into the respiratory tract [45, 46], which, together with the migration of proinflammatory cytokines from gingivocrevicular fluid to potentially virus-infected saliva and their subsequent aspiration, can lead to infection and inflammation of the lower respiratory tract [47, 48]. Increased SARS-CoV-2 disease severity in the lungs can ensue due to the expression of pro-inflammatory cytokines and ACE2 in the lower respiratory tract [39], with an increase in periodontopathogen-associated pro-inflammatory cytokines reported in alveolar, bronchial, and pharyngeal epithelial cells [49]. Viral spread to the periodontal capillary blood supply could also enable SARS-CoV-2 to reach the circulatory system and distant organs [1], potentially causing systemic disease.

21.2.3 Oral Microbiome Changes and Host Predisposition to Infection Due to SARS-CoV-2

Infection by SARS-CoV-2 is associated with a reduction in the variety of oral bacteria, a significant decrease in the numbers of immunomodulatory organisms (associated with a healthy oral microbiome), and a shift to a dysbiotic environment characterized by a higher presence of opportunistic bacteria and fungi [50], which can cause or exacerbate lower respiratory and gastrointestinal tract infections.

Poor oral health is known to be linked with respiratory diseases [51], with SARS-CoV-2 adhesion to the respiratory epithelium being possibly mediated by a dysbiotic pathogen-induced cytokine response [52]. Oral inflammation is also understood to lead to gut inflammation [53], with oral SARS-CoV-2 infection being associated with gut microbiome dysbiosis [54]. In both health and disease, oral bacteria migrate to the gut [55], and certain dysbiotic species are linked to negative, and sometimes life-threatening, health outcomes [56]. These associations suggest that the presence of SARS-CoV-2 in the mouth can prompt oral pathogens to cause infections elsewhere through the oral-lung and oral-gut pathways.

A wide variety of viruses can inhabit different oral niches [57]. Since SARS-CoV-2 can reactivate latent viruses in the mouth, including Epstein-Barr virus, human herpesvirus-6, and adenovirus [58, 59], it is plausible that their concurrent presence with SARS-CoV-2 in the oral cavity could lead to adverse health outcomes (Fig. 21.1).

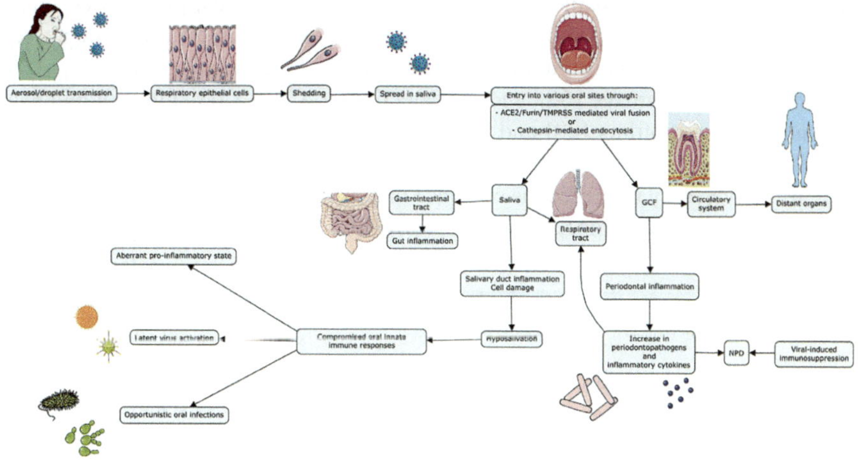

Fig. 21.1 The oral cavity as a reservoir of SARS-CoV-2. (GCF: Gingivocrevicular fluid; NPD: Necrotizing periodontal disease). (Figure prepared using CMapTools (https://cmap.ihmc.us/) with illustrations from Servier Medical Art (https://smart.servier.com), used under CC BY 4.0 license (https://creativecommons.org/licenses/by/4.0/))

21.3 Conclusion/Summary

The widespread presence of ACE2 receptors in oral tissues, efficient aerosol transmission of SARS-CoV-2 via saliva, and its various strategies to infect host cells and oral tissues all contribute to making the oral cavity an effective portal of entry and reservoir for the virus. The connection between the oral mucosa and the respiratory, digestive, lymphatic, and vascular systems allows for the systemic spread of SARS-CoV-2. Aside from the inflammation and dysbiosis resulting from viral migration from the mouth to connected sites, such as the lungs or digestive tract, more complex infection pathways may also occur. For instance, SARS-CoV-2 can transfer from saliva to periodontal pockets, then enter the circulatory system and infect lung tissues [60], while the tonsils and adenoids can also be infected, serving as sites of viral persistence [61].

Saliva provides essential non-specific and specific defense factors to the exposed tissues of the oral mucosa, which can be affected by SARS-CoV-2 infection and the resulting damage to the salivary glands. Salivary glands can serve as short- and long-term reservoirs not only for SARS-CoV-2 but also for other viruses (e.g., cytomegalovirus, Epstein-Barr virus, or hepatitis C virus) [1], with SARS-CoV-2-induced immune impairment possibly facilitating the reactivation of existing or latent viral infections, such as those caused by herpes viruses and adenovirus [59, 62]. SARS-CoV-2 has also been found to decrease histatin-5 levels, a salivary antimicrobial peptide, which may predispose infected patients to opportunistic fungal infections [63]. These factors, together with increased levels of periodontopathogens capable of spreading to other body sites, possible co-infections with opportunistic pathogens, the presence of chronic infections, a depressed immune response, hyperinflammatory states [64], long-standing salivary gland inflammation and damage [65], and the detection of SARS-CoV-2 in supragingival and subgingival biofilms [29] and in salivary tissues months after infection [66], give SARS-CoV-2 the capacity to cause multifaceted and long-lasting effects in the host. Moreover, they reinforce the evidence that the oral cavity is a significant portal of entry and a reservoir for SARS-CoV-2.

References

1. Atyeo N, Perez P, Matuck B, Byrd KM, Warner BM. The mouth as a site of SARS-CoV-2 infection. Curr Oral Health Rep. 2024;11:167–76. https://doi.org/10.1007/s40496-024-00367-2.
2. Tsuchiya H. The oral cavity potentially serving as a reservoir for SARS-CoV-2 but not necessarily facilitating the spread of COVID-19 in dental practice. Eur J Dent. 2023;17:310–8. https://doi.org/10.1055/s-0042-1757909.
3. Jackson CB, Farzan M, Chen B, Choe H. Mechanisms of SARS-CoV-2 entry into cells. Nat Rev Mol Cell Biol. 2022;23:3–20. https://doi.org/10.1038/s41580-021-00418-x.
4. Huang N, Pérez P, Kato T, Mikami Y, Okuda K, Gilmore RC, et al. SARS-CoV-2 infection of the oral cavity and saliva. Nat Med. 2021;27:892–903. https://doi.org/10.1038/s41591-021-01296-8.
5. Drozdzik A, Drozdzik M. Oral pathology in COVID-19 and SARS-CoV-2 infection—molecular aspects. Int J Mol Sci. 2022;23:1431. https://doi.org/10.3390/ijms23031431.
6. Santamaria-Castro I, Leiva-Rebollo R, Marín-Wong S, Jimenez-Guardeño JM, Ortega-Prieto AM. Molecular mechanisms of SARS-CoV-2 entry: implications for biomedical strategies. Microbiol Mol Biol Rev. 2025;89:e0026024. https://doi.org/10.1128/mmbr.00260-24.
7. Lin W, Gao F, Wang X, Qin N, Chen X, Tam KY, et al. The oral manifestations and related mechanisms of COVID-19 caused by SARS-CoV-2 infection. Front Cell Neurosci. 2023;16:1006977. https://doi.org/10.3389/fncel.2022.1006977.
8. Song J, Li Y, Huang X, Chen Z, Li Y, Liu C, et al. Systematic analysis of ACE2 and TMPRSS2 expression in salivary glands reveals underlying transmission mechanism caused by SARS-CoV-2. J Med Virol. 2020;92:2556–66. https://doi.org/10.1002/jmv.26045.
9. Salas Orozco MF, Niño-Martínez N, Martínez-Castañón GA, Patiño Marín N, Sámano Valencia C, Dipp Velázquez FA, et al. Presence of SARS-CoV-2 and its entry factors in oral tissues and cells: a systematic review. Medicina (Kaunas). 2021;57:523. https://doi.org/10.3390/medicina57060523.
10. Galicia JC, Guzzi PH, Giorgi FM, Khan AA. Predicting the response of the dental pulp to SARS-CoV2 infection: a transcriptome-wide effect cross-analysis. Genes Immun. 2020;21:360–3. https://doi.org/10.1038/s41435-020-00112-6.
11. AbdelMassih AF, Ye J, Kamel A, Mishriky F, Ismail HA, Ragab HA, et al. A multicenter consensus: A role of furin in the endothelial tropism in obese patients with COVID-19 infection. Obes Med. 2020;19:100281. https://doi.org/10.1016/j.obmed.2020.100281.
12. Peng J, Sun J, Zhao J, Deng X, Guo F, Chen L. Age and gender differences in ACE2 and TMPRSS2 expressions in oral epithelial cells. J Transl Med. 2021;19:358. https://doi.org/10.1186/s12967-021-03037-4.
13. V'kovski P, Kratzel A, Steiner S, Stalder H, Thiel V. Coronavirus biology and replication: implications for SARS-CoV-2. Nat Rev Microbiol. 2021;19:155–70. https://doi.org/10.1038/s41579-020-00468-6.
14. Gomes SC, Miller LM, Xavier L, Bitencourt FV. The mouth as a reservoir of SARS-CoV-2. Curr Oral Health Rep. 2024;11:144–66. https://doi.org/10.1007/s40496-024-00369-0.

15. Brahim Belhaouari D, Baudoin JP, Lagier JC, Monnet-Corti V, La Scola B, Antezack A. Microscopic observations of SARS-CoV-2 like particles in different oral samples. Eur J Oral Sci. 2022;130:e12903. https://doi.org/10.1111/eos.12903.
16. Sawa Y, Ibaragi S, Okui T, Yamashita J, Ikebe T, Harada H. Expression of SARS-CoV-2 entry factors in human oral tissue. J Anat. 2021;238:1341–54. https://doi.org/10.1111/joa.13391.
17. Zhu F, Zhong Y, Ji H, Ge R, Guo L, Song H, et al. ACE2 and TMPRSS2 in human saliva can adsorb to the oral mucosal epithelium. J Anat. 2022;240:398–409. https://doi.org/10.1111/joa.13560.
18. Matuck BF, Dolhnikoff M, Duarte-Neto AN, Maia G, Gomes SC, Sendyk DI, et al. Salivary glands are a target for SARS-CoV-2: a source for saliva contamination. J Pathol. 2021;254:239–43. https://doi.org/10.1002/path.5679.
19. Guarino P, Chiari F, Caporale CD, Presutti L, Molteni G. Clinical and diagnostic features of salivary glands disease related to COVID-19 infection: a systematic review of the literature. J Oral Maxillofac Surg Med Path. 2025;37:167–74. https://doi.org/10.1016/j.ajoms.2024.08.011.
20. Khoshkalam Z, Soheilifar S, Khoshkalam MH. Does COVID-19 cause xerostomia? A systematic review. Discov Med. 2025;2:94. https://doi.org/10.1007/s44337-025-00288-8.
21. Vila T, Rizk AM, Sultan AS, Jabra-Rizk MA. The power of saliva: antimicrobial and beyond. PLoS Pathog. 2019;15:e1008058. https://doi.org/10.1371/journal.ppat.1008058.
22. Alfaifi AA, Sultan AS, Montelongo-Jauregui D, Meiller TF, Jabra-Rizk MA. Long-term post COVID 19 associated oral inflammatory sequelae. Front Cell Infect Microbiol. 2022;12:831744. https://doi.org/10.3389/fcimb.2022.831744.
23. Baghizadeh FM. Oral saliva and COVID-19. Oral Oncol. 2020;108:104821. https://doi.org/10.1016/j.oraloncology.2020.104821.
24. Kim J, Kim JH. Oral symptomatic manifestations in patients with COVID-19: gustatory and saliva secretion dysfunctions and pathogenetic hypotheses. Int J Oral Biol. 2024;49:61–8. https://doi.org/10.11620/ijob.2024.4.9.3.61.
25. Tsuchiya H. COVID-19 oral sequelae: persistent gustatory and saliva secretory dysfunctions after recovery from COVID-19. Med Princ Pract. 2023;32:166–77. https://doi.org/10.1159/000531373.
26. King KL, Wilson S, Napolitano JM, Sell KJ, Rennert L, Parkinson CL, Dean D. SARS-CoV-2 variants of concern alpha and Delta show increased viral load in saliva. PLoS One. 2022;17:e0267750. https://doi.org/10.1371/journal.pone.0267750.
27. Nagura Ikeda M, Imai K, Tabata S, Miyoshi K, Murahara N, Mizuno T, et al. Clinical evaluation of self-collected saliva by quantitative reverse transcription-PCR (RT-qPCR), direct RT-qPCR, reverse transcription–loop-mediated isothermal amplification, and a rapid antigen test to diagnose COVID-19. J Clin Microbiol. 2020;58:e01438–20. https://doi.org/10.1128/jcm.01438-20.
28. Gomes SC, Fachin S, da Fonseca JG, Angst PDM, Lamers ML, da Silva ISB, Nunes LN. Dental biofilm of symptomatic COVID-19 patients harbours SARS-CoV-2. J Clin Periodontol. 2021;48:880–5. https://doi.org/10.1111/jcpe.13471.
29. Gomes SC, da Fonseca JG, Miller LM, Manenti L, Angst PDM, Lamers ML, et al. SARS-CoV-2 RNA in dental biofilms: Supragingival and subgingival findings from inpatients in a COVID-19 intensive care unit. J Periodontol. 2022;93:1476–85. https://doi.org/10.1002/JPER.21-0623.
30. Silva J, Lucas C, Sundaram M, Israelow B, Wong P, Klein J, et al. Saliva viral load is a dynamic unifying correlate of COVID-19 severity and mortality. medRxiv [PrePrint]. 2021, 2021.01.04.21249236. https://doi.org/10.1101/2021.01.04.21249236.
31. Badran Z, Gaudin A, Struillou X, Amador G, Soueidan A. Periodontal pockets: a potential reservoir for SARS-CoV-2? Med Hypotheses. 2020;143:109907. https://doi.org/10.1016/j.mehy.2020.109907.
32. Wang Y, Deng H, Pan Y, Jin L, Hu R, Lu Y, et al. Periodontal disease increases the host susceptibility to COVID-19 and its severity: a Mendelian randomization study. J Transl Med. 2021;19:528. https://doi.org/10.1186/s12967-021-03198-2.

33. Gupta S, Mohindra R, Chauhan PK, Singla V, Goyal K, Sahni V, et al. SARS-CoV-2 detection in gingival crevicular fluid. J Dent Res. 2021;100:187–93.
34. Matuck BF, Dolhnikoff M, Maia GVA, Sendyk DI, Zarpellon A, Gomes SC, et al. Periodontal tissues are targets for SARS-Cov-2: a post-mortem study. J Oral Microbiol. 2020;13:1848135. https://doi.org/10.1080/20002297.2020.1848135.
35. Marouf N, Cai W, Said KN, Daas H, Diab H, Chinta VR, et al. Association between periodontitis and severity of COVID-19 infection: a case-control study. J Clin Periodontol. 2021;48:483–91. https://doi.org/10.1111/jcpe.13435.
36. Gupta S, Mohindra R, Singla M, Khera S, Sahni V, Kanta P, et al. The clinical association between periodontitis and COVID-19. Clin Oral Investig. 2022;26:1361–74. https://doi.org/10.1007/s00784-021-04111-3.
37. Ting M, Suzuki JB. SARS-CoV-2: overview and its impact on oral health. Biomedicine. 2021;9:1690. https://doi.org/10.3390/biomedicines9111690.
38. Schwartz J, Capistrano KJ, Gluck J, Hezarkhani A, Naqvi AR. SARS-CoV-2, periodontal pathogens, and host factors: the trinity of oral post-acute sequelae of COVID-19. Rev Med Virol. 2024;34:e2543. https://doi.org/10.1002/rmv.2543.
39. Takahashi Y, Watanabe N, Kamio N, Kobayashi R, Iinuma T, Imai K. Aspiration of periodontopathic bacteria due to poor oral hygiene potentially contributes to the aggravation of COVID-19. J Oral Sci. 2020;63:1–3. https://doi.org/10.2334/josnusd.20-0388.
40. Suzuki R, Kamio N, Sugimoto K, Maruoka S, Gon Y, Kaneko T, et al. Periodontopathic bacterium *Fusobacterium nucleatum* affects matrix metalloproteinase-9 expression in human alveolar epithelial cells and mouse lung. In Vivo. 2022;36:649–56. https://doi.org/10.21873/invivo.12749.
41. Mithradas N, Sudhakar U, Rajaram V, Ram S, Ravindran N. Galectin-3 as a biomarker for periodontal disease severity in postcoronavirus disease 2019 patients: a clinical and biochemical investigation. J Indian Soc Periodontol. 2024;28:551–6. https://doi.org/10.4103/jisp.jisp_38_24.
42. Banks JM, Capistrano KJ, Brandini DA, Zaidi F, Thakkar P, Rahat R, et al. Herpesviruses and SARS-CoV-2: viral association with oral inflammatory diseases. Pathogens. 2024;13:58. https://doi.org/10.3390/pathogens13010058.
43. Sanyaolu A, Okorie C, Marinkovic A, Patidar R, Younis K, Desai P, et al. Comorbidity and its impact on patients with COVID-19. SN Compr Clin Med. 2020;2:1069–76. https://doi.org/10.1007/s42399-020-00363-4.
44. Tamimi F, Altigani S, Sanz M. Periodontitis and coronavirus disease 2019. Periodontol. 2000;2022(89):207–14. https://doi.org/10.1111/prd.12434.
45. Shen Z, Xiao Y, Kang L, Ma W, Shi L, Zhang L, et al. Genomic diversity of SARS-CoV-2 in patients with coronavirus disease 2019. Clin Infect Dis. 2020;71:713–20. https://doi.org/10.1093/cid/ciaa203.
46. Shi T, Wang J, Dong J, Hu P, Guo Q. Periodontopathogens *Porphyromonas gingivalis* and *Fusobacterium nucleatum* and their roles in the progression of respiratory diseases. Pathogens. 2023;12:1110. https://doi.org/10.3390/pathogens12091110.
47. Scannapieco FA. Role of oral bacteria in respiratory infection. J Periodontol. 1999;70:793–802. https://doi.org/10.1902/jop.1999.70.7.793.
48. Watanabe N, Yokoe S, Ogata Y, Sato S, Imai K. Exposure to *Porphyromonas gingivalis* induces production of proinflammatory cytokine via TLR2 from human respiratory epithelial cells. J Clin Med. 2020;9:3433. https://doi.org/10.3390/jcm9113433.
49. Hayata M, Watanabe N, Tamura M, Kamio N, Tanaka H, Nodomi K, et al. The periodontopathic bacterium *Fusobacterium nucleatum* induced proinflammatory cytokine production by human respiratory epithelial cell lines and in the lower respiratory organs in mice. Cell Physiol Biochem. 2019;53:49–61. https://doi.org/10.33594/000000120.
50. Gupta A, Bhanushali S, Sanap A, Shekatkar M, Kharat A, Raut C, et al. Oral dysbiosis and its linkage with SARS-CoV-2 infection. Microbiol Res. 2022;261:27055. https://doi.org/10.1016/j.micres.2022.127055.

51. Pathak JL, Yan Y, Zhang Q, Wang L, Ge L. The role of oral microbiome in respiratory health and diseases. Respir Med. 2021;185:106475. https://doi.org/10.1016/j.rmed.2021.106475.
52. Bao L, Zhang C, Dong J, Zhao L, Li Y, Sun J. Oral microbiome and SARS-CoV-2: beware of lung co-infection. Front Microbiol. 1840;2020:11. https://doi.org/10.3389/fmicb.2020.01840.
53. Kitamoto S, Nagao-Kitamoto H, Jiao Y, Gillilland MG 3rd, Hayashi A, Imai J, et al. The intermucosal connection between the mouth and gut in commensal pathobiont-driven colitis. Cell. 2020;182:447–462.e14. https://doi.org/10.1016/j.cell.2020.05.048.
54. Schwartz J, Capistrano K, Hussein H, Hafedi A, Shukla D, Naqvi A. Oral SARS-CoV-2 infection and risk for long Covid. Rev Med Virol. 2025;35:e70029. https://doi.org/10.1002/rmv.70029.
55. Schmidt TS, Hayward MR, Coelho LP, Li SS, Costea PI, Voigt AY, et al. Extensive transmission of microbes along the gastrointestinal tract. elife. 2019;8:e42693. https://doi.org/10.7554/eLife.42693.
56. Xiang Z, Koo H, Chen Q, Zhou X, Liu Y, Simon-Soro A. Potential implications of SARS-CoV-2 oral infection in the host microbiota. J Oral Microbiol. 2020;13:1853451. https://doi.org/10.1080/20002297.2020.1853451.
57. Thakkar P, Banks JM, Rahat R, Brandini DA, Naqvi AR. Viruses of the oral cavity: prevalence, pathobiology and association with oral diseases. Rev Med Virol. 2022;32:e2311. https://doi.org/10.1002/rmv.2311.
58. Davis HE, McCorkell L, Vogel JM, Topol EJ. Long COVID: major findings, mechanisms and recommendations. Nat Rev Microbiol. 2023;21:133–46. https://doi.org/10.1038/s41579-022-00846-2.
59. Hannestad U, Apostolou E, Sjögren P, Bragée B, Polo O, Bertilson BC, et al. Post-COVID sequelae effect in chronic fatigue syndrome: SARS-CoV-2 triggers latent adenovirus in the oral mucosa. Front Med (Lausanne). 2023;10:1208181. https://doi.org/10.3389/fmed.2023.1208181.
60. Lloyd-Jones G, Molayem S, Pontes CC, Chapple I. The COVID-19 pathway: a proposed oral-vascular-pulmonary route of SARS-CoV-2 infection and the importance of oral healthcare measures. J Oral Med Dent Res. 2021;2:1–25. https://doi.org/10.52793/jomdr.2020.2(1)-13.
61. Lima TM, Martins RB, Miura CS, Souza MVO, Cassiano MHA, Rodrigues TS, et al. Tonsils are major sites of persistence of SARS-CoV-2 in children. Microbiol Spectrum. 2023;11:e0134723. https://doi.org/10.1128/spectrum.01347-23.
62. Apostolou E, Rizwan M, Moustardas P, Sjögren P, Bertilson BC, Bragée B, et al. Saliva antibody-fingerprint of reactivated latent viruses after mild/asymptomatic COVID-19 is unique in patients with myalgic-encephalomyelitis/chronic fatigue syndrome. Front Immunol. 2022;13:949787. https://doi.org/10.3389/fimmu.2022.949787.
63. Alfaifi AA, Wang TW, Perez P, Sultan AS, Meiller TF, Rock P, et al. SARS-CoV-2 infection of salivary glands compromises the production of a secreted antifungal peptide with potential implications for development of oral candidiasis. PLoS Pathog. 2024;20:e1012375. https://doi.org/10.1371/journal.ppat.1012375.
64. Brandini DA, Takamiya AS, Thakkar P, Schaller S, Rahat R, Naqvi AR. COVID-19 and oral diseases: crosstalk, synergy or association? Rev Med Virol. 2021;31:e2226. https://doi.org/10.1002/rmv.2226.
65. Shen Y, Voigt A, Goranova L, Abed MA, Kleiner DE, Maldonado JO, et al. Evidence of a Sjögren's disease-like phenotype following COVID-19 in mice and human. JCI Insight. 2023;8:e166540. https://doi.org/10.1172/jci.insight.166540.
66. Stein SR, Ramelli SC, Grazioli A, Chung JY, Singh M, Yinda CK, et al. SARS-CoV-2 infection and persistence in the human body and brain at autopsy. Nature. 2022;612:758–63.

22 COVID-19 Transmission in Dental Settings

Basavaraj Mathapati, Souvik Mitra, and Pronami Gogoi

22.1 Introduction

COVID-19 is the most formidable pandemic to disrupt the global healthcare system in the modern era. The initial outbreak of COVID-19 occurred in Wuhan, China, in December 2019, and the WHO declared it a public health emergency. The primary route of transmission of SARS-CoV-2 from person to person through respiratory droplets, aerosols via sneezing, coughing and contact contamination, including oral, mucosal and nasal contacts and secretions [1].

Within this context, the practice of dentistry and oral surgery entails a close proximity between patients and dental professionals, thereby increasing the risk of COVID-19 transmission. The exposure and transmission of the virus involve the use of rotary dental and surgical instruments, ultrasonic scalers, and air-water syringes that may contain droplets of saliva, water, blood, and microorganisms. The transmission of COVID-19 in dental practice has been widely recognized as a worldwide concern within the dental profession rather than in other occupations [2]. Due to the inherent nature of dental procedures, the virus can readily be transmitted from infected patients to dental professionals and vice versa if appropriate infection control measures are not taken. The oral cavity plays a pivotal role as a reservoir of SARS-CoV-2 virus particles, making dental procedures potential routes for viral transmission [3]. It is crucial to understand the various modes of SARS-CoV-2 transmission due to close patient contact and frequent aerosol generation in dental settings.

To prevent the transmission of SARS-CoV-2, it is important to implement preventive measures among healthcare workers. Pathogens are transmitted from an infected individual to another person without an intermediate host via direct contact. Prolonged or repeated exposure to saliva and blood during treatment is also a

B. Mathapati (✉) · S. Mitra · P. Gogoi
Indian Council of Medical Research (ICMR)-National Institute of Virology (NIV), Pune, Maharashtra, India
e-mail: basavaraj.mathapati@gmail.com

S. R. Prabhu et al. (eds.), *COVID-19 in Dental Practice*,
https://doi.org/10.1007/978-3-032-26000-0_22

risk of transmission. Due to the enclosed room, the aerosol may remain in the air, resulting in high transmission risk. Studies highlighted the transmission of SARS-CoV-2 through different modes, i.e., direct transmission via respiratory droplets and close contact. More transmissible variants (e.g., Delta, Omicron) have shown higher viral loads in the upper respiratory tract, amplifying droplet spread. Aerosol transmission during dental procedures generates aerosol containing saliva, blood, and microorganisms. In poorly ventilated settings, aerosols can remain suspended in the air for extended periods. Fomite transmission (surface contact) through contaminated dental instruments, chairs, countertops, PPE, or gloves may occur [4]. Depending on the material and environmental conditions, the virus can remain viable for hours to days. Saliva and blood-borne transmission is another mode of transmission, as saliva is the main reservoir of SARS-CoV-2, and patients with asymptomatic infection may have high viral loads. Indirect transmission via poor air circulation may increase the risk of viral aerosol spread.

This comprehensive chapter addresses specific transmission modes of SARS-CoV-2 in the dental environment during various dental procedures, evaluates evidence of actual transmission events, and provides infection control measures. Understanding these transmission modes is crucial for developing effective strategies to evidence-based infection protocols, optimizing personal protective equipment, and improving ventilation and disinfection to ensure the safety of both patients and dental professionals.

22.2 Transmission Routes in Dental Settings

22.2.1 Contact Transmission

Dental professionals are always at risk of viral exposure due to frequent direct or indirect contact with infected patients or contaminated dental instruments [5]. Contact transmission in dental settings may occur through direct or indirect mode, direct transmission of the virus from an infected person to another subject without an intermediate object through the mucus membrane, body fluid, or blood [6]. In case of indirect transmission, a person may be infected through pathogen-carrying objects or humans [7]. The specificity of dental procedures increased the risk of exposure due to face-to-face patient communication. Consequently, dental professionals come into direct contact with saliva, blood, or other body fluids, and with oral mucosa, and transmission may occur if proper protection is not implemented. It has been reported that SARS-CoV-2 is consistently detected in saliva which represents the risk of exposure for viral transmission in dentistry [8]. According to earlier studies, SARS-CoV-2 remains viable for hours to days on materials used in dental clinics and increasing the potential for cross-contamination without appropriate disinfection protocols being implemented [9, 10]. Therefore, frequent exposure to the oral cavity increases contact with saliva, oral mucosa, blood, and respiratory secretions, thereby increasing the transmission risk in dental settings. Proper use of personal protective equipment (PPE), surface decontamination, and strict adherence to standard precautions is important to minimize contact contamination [11].

22.2.2 Droplet Transmission

Respiratory droplets serve as vehicles that drive droplet transmission. Large droplets of ≥5–10 μm carrying virus particles represent the primary mode of droplet transmission in dental settings. Droplet transmission is attributed to the patients having respiratory symptoms and a person is in close contact within 1.5 m [12]. During a dental procedure, infectious agents can enter the host through direct or indirect contact with droplets. Droplets are generated during coughing, sneezing, talking, breathing, or airway-related healthcare procedures, and the mucosa, oral cavity, and nasal mucosa act as main entry portals for respiratory viruses [13]. Several studies highlighted that the exhalation air velocity is a critical determinant of droplet dispersion—sneezing (≈50 m/s): droplets may travel >6 m; coughing (≈10 m/s): droplets may travel >2 m; and breathing (≈1 m/s): droplets usually travel <1 m [14–16]. A study found that SARS-CoV-2 can be transmitted through the ocular surface. The virus can reach the eyes through the nasolacrimal ducts from droplets and can then reach the nasal or respiratory system [17].

22.2.3 Airborne Transmission

SARS-CoV-2 transmission via aerosols in dental settings is the most significant concern in clinical practice. Aerosols are typically <5 μm suspended particles in the air and remain airborne for extended periods and travel considerable distances from the source [18]. In dental procedures, drills and ultrasonic devices generate aerosol and splatter, contaminating the air with respiratory pathogens [19]. A study highlighted that dental procedures generated aerosols with the highest volume fraction below 1 μm (d_a), capable of deep respiratory penetration [20]. Another study by Malmgren et al. indicated that the air-water syringe produces the highest number of aerosols from the dental instrument, which can spread virus-containing aerosol throughout the operating room [21]. Although other aerosol-generating instruments used in dentistry, such as ultrasonic scalers and high-speed rotary instruments, generate respirable aerosols and indicate evidence supporting the creation of infectious aerosols and transmission through this mode, this evidence remains weak and inconclusive [22].

22.2.4 Fomite Transmission

Virus-contaminated surfaces, acting as fomites, are an additional transmission mode in dental settings through indirect contact. The transmission can arise via contaminated dental instruments, gloves, chair surfaces, headpieces, or exposed

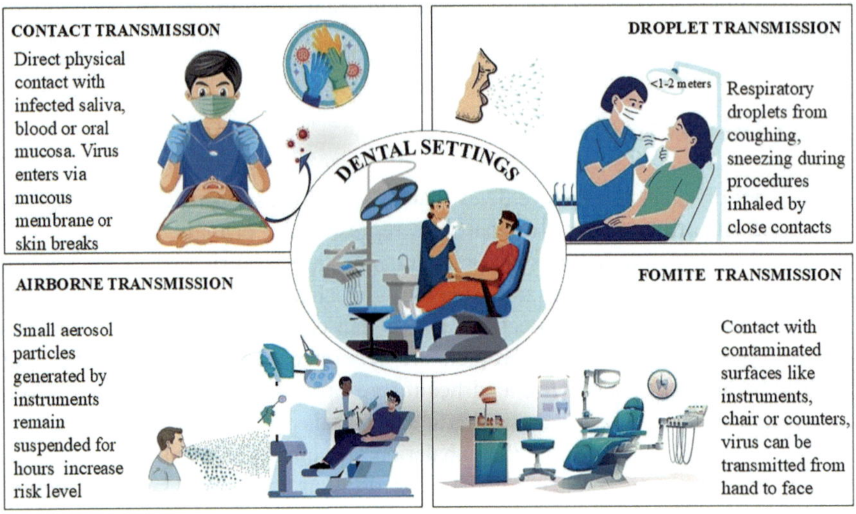

Fig. 22.1 Possible routes of COVID-19 transmission in dental settings. (Source: Created using the pictures and images from freepik.com and shutterstock.com)

environmental surfaces. Contaminated aerosols and splatter produced during various dental procedures by patient or dental unit waterlines (DUWLs) can exist in the fomite form and the viability varies depending on surface type and environmental conditions [13]. According to Ali et al. (2020), fomite transmission risk is exacerbated by frequent contact with multiple instruments and surfaces during a dental procedure. This may create exposure for cross-contamination [23].

The possible route of transmission of SARS-CoV-2 in dental settings is illustrated in Fig. 22.1.

22.3 Risk Factors Associated with Dental Procedures

22.3.1 Aerosol-Generating Procedures

Aerosol-generating procedures (AGPs) in dental practices are considered the highest risk for SARS-CoV-2 transmission. By developing a risk scoring system for SARS-CoV-2 transmission, Bizzoca et al. categorized dental treatments into low (score: 1–3), moderate (score: 4–5), and high (score ≥6) risk categories based on predetermined criteria like aerosol generation, length of the process, direct contact with saliva and blood. High-risk procedures such as crown preparation, cavity preparation with high-speed handpieces, prophylaxis with rotary instruments, ultrasonic scaling, and root canal access procedures were all found to be associated with significant aerosol generation [24].

Although these procedures generate high levels of aerosols containing saliva, blood, and potentially infectious microorganisms, dissemination can be significantly reduced with proper mitigation systems [22]. In fact, during the COVID-19 pandemic, dental infection control practices underwent rapid evolution. During that time, greater emphasis was placed on reducing aerosol generation during AGPs, particularly through measures such as high-volume suction and rubber dam isolation [22, 25].

22.3.2 Proximity and Duration of Exposure During Dental Procedure

The proximity between the patient and the dentist and the duration of the dental procedure are major risk factors for SARS-CoV-2 transmission. Dental procedures require the dentist and staff to work very close to the patient, often within 15–50 cm of the oral cavity, bringing them into direct contact with aerosols and droplets generated during the procedure. The procedures require direct observation during the process, which can only be achieved by staying very close to the patient [1, 26, 27].

The duration of the procedure may also increase the risk of SARS-CoV-2 transmission. Time-consuming, complex dental procedures such as full-mouth rehabilitation, root canal treatments, and periodontal treatments may require hours of close contact to complete. It increases exposure time to droplets and aerosols. Compared to brief medical visits, they significantly increase exposure time and the risk of transmission [24]. To reduce transmission in these scenarios, strict and proper adherence to personal protective equipment is very important, along with other measures described in Table 22.1.

22.3.3 Asymptomatic Transmission Risks

Asymptomatic transmission of SARS-CoV-2 poses a significant challenge for risk assessment. Approximately 75% of COVID-19 patients are asymptomatic, which means that those patients do not show any symptoms but are capable of transmitting the virus and test positive [28]. In many dental clinics, patients commonly wait in a shared area before consultation, which may be a potential site for SARS-CoV-2 transmission. The presence of asymptomatic or presymptomatic individuals further increases the risk of COVID-19 transmission, not only to dental practitioners and clinic staff but also to other patients in the clinic. The incubation period of SARS-CoV-2 is typically 2–14 days, with a median of 5–6 days, that provide a wide window for pre-symptomatic transmission [27, 29]. The risks associated with asymptomatic and presymptomatic transmission of SARS-CoV-2 can be significantly mitigated by enforcing strict rules in the dental clinics—for example, pre-appointment screening by phone or digital questionnaire to assess health status; physical distancing in the waiting area; use of PPE during patient consultation and dental procedures; proper ventilation in the clinic; and other practices. During the COVID-19 pandemic, many preventive measures were implemented to reduce SARS-CoV-2 transmission in dental clinics, but their use has declined

Table 22.1 Control and prevention measures for SARS-CoV-2 transmission in dental settings

Sl. no	Control measures	Protocol and recommendations	References
1	Patient screening	Pre-appointment telephone screening (to assess for fever, cough, shortness of breath, loss of taste or smell, and recent contact with confirmed COVID-19 cases) Temperature checks upon arrival at the clinic Non-emergency dental treatment must be postponed for suspected COVID-19 patients for at least 2 weeks. Emergency dental treatments may be performed, prioritizing infection control strategies	[1, 29]
2	Procedural modification	Pre-procedural mouth rinsing with antimicrobial solutions (solutions containing chlorhexidine, povidone iodine, cetylpyridinium chloride are found to be very effective in inactivating SARS-CoV-2) Using rubber dam isolation during dental procedures and high-volume evacuation systems for reducing aerosol dissemination Clinical practice guidelines recommend strict infection control strategies along with balancing clinical effectiveness and treatment quality	[22, 30]
3	Use of personal protective equipment	Use of PPE in dental practices is common, and its proper use (proper sequencing of donning and doffing) protects the dental practitioner and support staff from infection N95 respirators or FFP-2 masks or above are recommended for use during aerosol-generating procedures Face protector shields may be used in balance with the treatment efficacy Impermeable aprons or gowns, caps, shoe covers, and gloves must be used	[31]
4	Environmental control and ventilation	Effective ventilation systems and portable HEPA filtration units reduce the risk of airborne transmission Surface sterilization using alcohol and hypochlorite-based solutions, both in the chamber and waiting, is recommended	[25]

post-pandemic, even though they remain very relevant. Thus, it is important to strictly follow standard infection prevention and control practices worldwide.

22.4 Prevention and Control

The transmission of SARS-CoV-2 can be prevented with appropriate measures in the dental settings. The general measures of hospital hygiene and infection control, though, are quite adequate for mitigating the transmission of respiratory infections; SARS-CoV-2, with efficient transmission, requires more stringent practices and infection control measures. In dental settings that involve many procedures generating aerosol, extra caution is needed to limit transmission (Table 22.1). These measures can range from improved ventilation in hospital settings to procedural modifications to ensure the safety of health care providers, patients, and accompanying personnel. Adequate signage and displays on general hygiene and COVID-19-specific safety behaviors for visitors' information can help educate them on COVID-19-appropriate practices that can limit the risk of nosocomial infections. Enhanced infection control measures can prevent persons from acquiring and transmitting SARS-CoV-2 in dental settings, safeguarding the health of caregivers and care seekers.

22.5 Future Prospects

Future preparedness in dental healthcare must focus on integrating long-term, evidence-based infection control strategies into routine clinical practice. Further research is required to quantify the actual infectivity of dental aerosols and to better distinguish between viable virus transmission and mere viral detection in clinical environments. Advances in aerosol mitigation technologies, including high-efficiency suction systems, optimized operatory design, and real-time air quality monitoring, hold promise for reducing airborne transmission risks.

The development of standardized risk assessment models tailored to dental procedures will aid in stratifying patient care and guiding infection control decisions. Additionally, continuous training of dental professionals on emerging infectious diseases, proper PPE usage, and updated clinical guidelines is essential. Emphasis should also be placed on improving ventilation standards in small and resource-limited dental clinics, particularly in low- and middle-income countries.

Lessons learned from COVID-19 should inform policies aimed at pandemic preparedness, ensuring that dental care systems remain resilient against future respiratory viral outbreaks. Sustained vigilance, combined with technological innovation and policy support, will be critical in safeguarding dental healthcare settings against emerging infectious threats.

22.6 Conclusion

The COVID-19 pandemic has profoundly reshaped infection prevention and control practices within dental care settings, highlighting the unique vulnerability of dental professionals and patients to SARS-CoV-2 transmission. Owing to close face-to-face interaction, prolonged exposure time, and the routine use of aerosol-generating procedures, dental clinics represent environments with heightened potential for viral spread.

Evidence indicates that aerosol-generating dental procedures, such as ultrasonic scaling and high-speed rotary instrumentation, pose the greatest risk, particularly in poorly ventilated enclosed spaces. The presence of asymptomatic and presymptomatic patients further complicates risk assessment and infection control, as viral shedding may occur in the absence of clinical symptoms. Additionally, prolonged procedure duration and close proximity between dental professionals and patients significantly increase exposure risk.

Despite these challenges, implementing enhanced infection prevention strategies—including pre-appointment screening, appropriate use of personal protective equipment, procedural modifications, surface disinfection, and improved ventilation—has been shown to substantially reduce transmission risk. The experience gained during the COVID-19 pandemic underscores the importance of sustained adherence to standard and transmission-based precautions in dental practice, not only during pandemics but as a routine component of patient care. Strengthening these measures is essential to ensure the safety of dental healthcare workers and patients while maintaining continuity of oral healthcare services.

References

1. Banakar M, Bagheri Lankarani K, Jafarpour D, Moayedi S, Banakar MH, MohammadSadeghi A. COVID-19 transmission risk and protective protocols in dentistry: a systematic review. BMC Oral Health. 2020;20(1):275.
2. Aldahlawi SA, Afifi IK. COVID-19 in dental practice: transmission risk, infection control challenge, and clinical implications. Open Dent J. 2020;14(1):348–54.
3. Alsulami M, Kattan W, Alsamadani L, Alahmari G, Al Juhani W, Almabadi M. An outlook on dental practices to avoid the Oral transmission of COVID-19. Microorganisms. 2023;11(1):146.
4. Dar-Odeh N, Babkair H, Abu-Hammad S, Borzangy S, Abu-Hammad A, Abu-Hammad O. COVID-19: present and future challenges for dental practice. Int J Environ Res Public Health. 2020;17(9):3151.
5. Peng X, Xu X, Li Y, Cheng L, Zhou X, Ren B. Transmission routes of 2019-nCoV and controls in dental practice. Int J Oral Sci. 2020;12(1):9.
6. Otter JA, Donskey C, Yezli S, Douthwaite S, Goldenberg SD, Weber DJ. Transmission of SARS and MERS coronaviruses and influenza virus in healthcare settings: the possible role of dry surface contamination. J Hosp Infect. 2016;92(3):235–50.
7. Mupparapu M, Kothari KRM. Review of surface disinfection protocols in dentistry: a 2019 update. Quintessence Int. 2019;50(1):58–65.
8. To KKW, Tsang OTY, Yip CCY, Chan KH, Wu TC, Chan JMC, et al. Consistent detection of 2019 novel coronavirus in saliva. Clin Infect Dis. 2020;71(15):841–3.
9. Kampf G, Todt D, Pfaender S, Steinmann E. Persistence of coronaviruses on inanimate surfaces and their inactivation with biocidal agents. J Hosp Infect. 2020;104(3):246–51.
10. van Doremalen N, Bushmaker T, Morris DH, Holbrook MG, Gamble A, Williamson BN, et al. Aerosol and surface stability of SARS-CoV-2 as compared with SARS-CoV-1. N Engl J Med. 2020;382(16):1564–7.
11. WHO (World Health Organization). Transmission of SARS-CoV-2: implications for infection prevention precautions (2020). [cited 2026 Jan 15]; Available from: https://www.who.int/news-room/commentaries/detail/transmission-of-sars-cov-2-implications-for-infection-prevention-precautions.
12. Bahl P, Doolan C, de Silva C, Chughtai AA, Bourouiba L, MacIntyre CR. Airborne or droplet precautions for health workers treating coronavirus disease 2019? J Infect Dis. 2022;225(9):1561–8.
13. Amato A, Caggiano M, Amato M, Moccia G, Capunzo M, De Caro F. Infection control in dental practice during the COVID-19 pandemic. Int J Environ Res Public Health. 2020;17(13):4769.
14. Siegel JD, Rhinehart E, Jackson M, Chiarello L. 2007 guideline for isolation precautions: preventing transmission of infectious agents in health care settings. Am J Infect Control. 2007;35(10):S65–164.

15. Xie X, Li Y, Chwang ATY, Ho PL, Seto WH. How far droplets can move in indoor environments? Revisiting the Wells evaporation? Falling curve. Indoor Air. 2007;17(3):211–25.
16. Papineni RS, Rosenthal FS. The size distribution of droplets in the exhaled breath of healthy human subjects. J Aerosol Med. 1997;10(2):105–16.
17. Eissa M, Abdelrazek NA, Saady M. Covid-19 and its relation to the human eye: transmission, infection, and ocular manifestations. Graefes Arch Clin Exp Ophthalmol. 2023;261(7):1771–80.
18. Allison JR, Tiede S, Holliday R, Durham J, Jakubovics NS. Bioaerosols and airborne transmission in the dental clinic. Int Dent J. 2024;74:S418–28.
19. Dave M, Seoudi N, Coulthard P. Urgent dental care for patients during the COVID-19 pandemic. Lancet. 2020;395(10232):1257.
20. Balanta-Melo J, Gutiérrez A, Sinisterra G, del Díaz-Posso M, Gallego D, Villavicencio J, et al. Rubber dam isolation and high-volume suction reduce ultrafine dental aerosol particles: an experiment in a simulated patient. Appl Sci. 2020;10(18):6345.
21. Malmgren R, Välimaa H, Oksanen L, Sanmark E, Nikuri P, Heikkilä P, et al. High-volume evacuation mitigates viral aerosol spread in dental procedures. Sci Rep. 2023;13(1):18984.
22. Vernon JJ, Black EVI, Dennis T, Devine DA, Fletcher L, Wood DJ, et al. Dental mitigation strategies to reduce aerosolization of SARS-CoV-2. J Dent Res. 2021;100(13):1461–7.
23. Ali FM, Patil K, Albashir EI, Alamir AA. Coronavirus disease-19 and dentistry: a review. Open Access Maced J Med Sci. 2020;8(T1):618–21.
24. Bizzoca ME, Campisi G, Lo Muzio L. An innovative risk-scoring system of dental procedures and safety protocols in the COVID-19 era. BMC Oral Health. 2020;20(1):301.
25. Ahmed MA, Alshayeb FR, Alshahry LH, Alshakhs SA, Alshahrani NH, Almutairi AZ, et al. The impact of COVID-19 on infection control practices in dentistry: adaptations and challenges: a literature review. Int J Community Med Public Health. 2024;12(1):570–7.
26. Schwarz KM, Nienhaus A, Diel R. Risk of SARS-CoV-2 infection in dental healthcare workers - a systematic review and meta-analysis. GMS Hyg. Infect Control. 2024;19:Doc09.
27. Kochhar AS, Bhasin R, Kochhar GK, Dadlani H. COVID-19 pandemic and dental practice. Int J Dent. 2020;2020:1–5.
28. Hartig M, Stephens C, Foster A, Fontes D, Kinzel M, García-Godoy F. Stopping the COVID-19 pandemic in dental offices: a review of SARS-CoV-2 transmission and cross-infection prevention. Exp Biol Med. 2021;246(22):2381–90.
29. Tarakji B, Nassani MZ, Alali FM, Alqhtani NR, Nabhan AB, Rafedah AA, et al. The diagnosis and prevention of coronavirus disease in dental clinic – a review article. Open Access Maced J Med Sci. 2021;9(F):171–5.
30. Toschi EM, Mercado LW, Henz SL. Antiviral effect of oral antiseptic solutions commonly used in dentistry practice: a scoping review. Dentistry Review. 2023;3(1):100064.
31. Deana NF, Seiffert A, Aravena-Rivas Y, Alonso-Coello P, Muñoz-Millán P, Espinoza-Espinoza G, et al. Recommendations for safe dental care: a systematic review of clinical practice guidelines in the first year of the COVID-19 pandemic. Int J Environ Res Public Health. 2021;18(19):10059.

The Response of Oral Mucosa and Saliva to COVID-19

23

Oral Mucosa and Saliva in COVID-19: Response Mechanisms and Clinical Implications

Sophie Chen and Devi Atukorallaya

23.1 The Impact of COVID-19 on Oral Health

Coronavirus disease 2019 (COVID-19) is a viral respiratory illness caused by the severe acute respiratory syndrome coronavirus 2 (SARS-CoV-2) [1]. Initial cases emerged in Wuhan, China, in December 2019 [2]. By March 11, 2020, the World Health Organization (WHO) had declared COVID-19 a global pandemic. As of June 15, 2025, more than 778 million confirmed cases and over 7 million deaths have been reported worldwide [3]. In Canada, the first case appeared on February 10, 2020; by the end of 2024, the cumulative tally reached nearly 4.97 million cases and over 60,800 deaths [4]. Following strict public health guidelines, including mask-wearing, physical distancing, and vaccinations, the WHO officially ended the global Public Health Emergency on May 5, 2023 [5].

SARS-CoV-2 is an enveloped, single-stranded RNA virus of the coronavirus family. It encodes four major conserved membrane-associated proteins: spike (S), envelope (E), membrane (M), and nucleoprotein (N). The S protein mediates cell entry via the angiotensin-converting enzyme 2 (ACE2) receptor, while the E, M, and N proteins support virion assembly and contribute to viral pathogenesis [6].

Transmission of SARS-CoV-2 primarily occurs via direct contact with respiratory droplets or aerosols, as well as with bodily fluids such as saliva, tears, feces, urine, and semen. Vertical transmission from mother to child has also been documented. Indirect transmission involves contact with contaminated surfaces, a process known as fomite transmission [7]. The nasal cavity, oral cavity, nasopharynx, and oropharynx are identified as potential replication sites for SARS-CoV-2, with the oral cavity rich in saliva harboring various types of respiratory viruses in its microbiome [8–11].

S. Chen · D. Atukorallaya (✉)
Department of Oral Biology, Dr. Gerald Niznick College of Dentistry, Rady Faculty of Health Sciences, University of Manitoba, Winnipeg, MB, Canada
e-mail: Devi.Atukorallaya@umanitoba.ca

S. R. Prabhu et al. (eds.), *COVID-19 in Dental Practice*,
https://doi.org/10.1007/978-3-032-26000-0_23

Clinically, COVID-19 manifests with respiratory symptoms such as cough and dyspnea, but it also has broad systemic effects [12–14]. Neurological symptoms such as anosmia (loss of smell) and ageusia (loss of taste), along with oral manifestations, including mucosal lesions, as well as cardiovascular, renal, and cerebral complications, have all been documented [13, 15]. The oral manifestations are likely due to the high concentration of ACE2 receptors in the oral epithelium, particularly in the tongue and salivary glands [8, 16–18]. Reported lesions are diverse and include ulcers and erosions, vesiculobullous lesions, and fungal infections such as candidiasis, often presenting as white or red plaques [19–23]. Xerostomia (dry mouth) is another common symptom, thought to be a result of the virus affecting salivary glands [11, 22]. The exact cause of these oral lesions is still under investigation, with theories suggesting direct viral damage to tissue, a hyper-inflammatory "cytokine storm," or microvascular thrombosis as potential mechanisms [24–30]. Considering the diverse clinical features of COVID-19, a comprehensive understanding of the disease's impact on the oral cavity and salivary glands is crucial, particularly for dental clinicians. Therefore, this chapter will examine the effects of COVID-19 on oral mucosa and saliva, exploring the diagnostic and management implications for dental practice.

23.2 Anatomy and Physiology of Oral Mucosa and Saliva: Foundations for Clinical Relevance

The oral mucosa is the moist epithelial lining of the oral cavity, extending from the lips to the pharynx. The oral mucosa plays a critical role in the manifestation of COVID-19-related symptoms due to its complex anatomy, specialized histological features, and region-specific functions. It is composed of stratified squamous epithelium overlying connective tissue (lamina propria) [31]. Functionally, the oral mucosa serves as a barrier, sensory interface, and in some regions, specialized for taste, mastication, and secretion [32]. There are three major types of oral mucosa. The lining mucosa covering the floor of the mouth, cheeks, inner lips, and soft palate is soft, pliable, and nonkeratinized. The masticatory mucosa over the hard palate and alveolar ridges is keratinized and tougher to withstand mechanical forces during mastication. Finally, the specialized mucosa covering the dorsum of the tongue is composed of taste buds embedded in keratinized epithelial papillae (filiform, fungiform, circumvallate, foliate), which also function in mastication [31]. The lips are a special transition zone between the outer skin and inner oral mucosa. They consist of three anatomical areas [37]. As the vermillion approaches the inner oral surfaces, the epithelium gradually becomes non-keratinized, transitioning to lining mucosa associated with seromucous minor salivary glands [38].

In comparison, the skin is a keratinized stratified squamous epithelium overlying the dermis and hypodermis. The connective tissue contains appendages such as hair follicles, sebaceous glands, and sweat glands. The skin functions to excrete waste products, regulate heat, enable touch sensations, and protect against pathogens (Table 23.1) [31].

Table 23.1 Comparative analysis of the structural and functional characteristics of skin and oral mucosa

Feature	Skin	Oral mucosa
Location	Covers external surface of the body	Lines the inside of the mouth
Function	Protection, thermoregulation, sensation	Lubrication, sensation, protection
Epithelial type	Stratified squamous epithelium (keratinized)	Stratified squamous epithelium (keratinized or non-keratinized)
Underlying tissue	Dermis, hypodermis	Lamina propria, submucosa in certain areas
Color	Varies with melanin content	Pink/red Concentration and state of blood vessel dilation Thickness of epithelium Degree of keratinization Amount of melanin pigment in the epithelium
Moisture	Dry surface (except sweat, sebum)	Moist surface (from saliva)
Sensation	Sensitive	Highly sensitive (rich in nerve endings)
Regeneration rate	Slower	Fast
Other structures	Skin appendages: hair, sweat glands, sebaceous glands	Minor salivary glands, taste buds, sebaceous glands (at Fordyce spots)

As the oral cavity is subject to extreme environments, the epithelium has adopted various structural and functional specifications (Table 23.1). Stratification, keratinization, and cell-to-cell interactions are reinforced for barrier integrity in the masticatory mucosa [32]. Epithelial cells also synthesize cytokines, adhesion molecules, growth factors, and chemokines in response to stimuli [33].

The tongue's epithelial functional adaptation features papillae. Filiform papillae are the most abundant, exhibiting a rough texture from keratinized extensions. Fungiform, circumvallate, and foliate papillae house taste buds in their epithelial lining. Taste buds are barrel-shaped structures with ovoid epithelial cells, termed taste receptor cells (TRCs), which contain taste signal transduction proteins. Each taste bud contains 10-14 cells of supporting or sustentacular or basal cells and is innervated by cranial nerves VII, IX, and X [31]. Sour and salty tastes directly activate the specialized membrane channels of TRCs [39, 40], whereas sweet, bitter, and umami taste transduction is mediated through G protein-coupled receptor signaling pathways [41]. New tastes are perceived through the washing out of substances in the epithelium by secretions of Von Ebner glands underlying taste buds [31]. In the context of COVID-19, this intricate taste-sensing system becomes particularly vulnerable. Understanding the structural and functional complexity of the tongue's epithelium is therefore essential for interpreting and managing the gustatory disturbances commonly observed in COVID-19 patients.

Saliva is produced by major (parotid, submandibular, sublingual) and minor salivary glands, composed of serous and mucous acini of epithelial origin. Serous secretions are high in protein and low in carbohydrate, whereas mucous secretions are low in protein and high in carbohydrate [31]. Secreted as a hypotonic solution, saliva is mainly composed of water (94–99%), organic molecules (~0.5%, growth factors, lysozyme, albumin, glucose, lipids, urea, and traces of ammonia), inorganic molecules (0.2%, potassium, sodium chloride, calcium, magnesium, phosphorus, carbonate), enzymes, and immune cells. An average person produces 600mL of saliva per day, with the major salivary glands producing 85-90% of saliva [31, 42]. Typical flow ranges from 0.1 ml/min during sleep and up to 4–5 ml/min during stimulation [43]. Salivary secretion is controlled by neural reflexes during gustatory and masticatory stimulation, as well as oral and pharyngeal pain. Saliva plays a key role in lubrication, digestion, buffering, antimicrobial defense, and tissue protection [31].

The oral cavity hosts a complex and dynamic microbiome composed of bacteria, fungi, and viruses that typically exist in a balanced relationship with the host's immune defenses [34]. Under healthy conditions, this equilibrium supports oral and systemic health, with commensal organisms playing protective and regulatory roles. However, during COVID-19 infection, this balance can be disrupted due to both direct viral effects and systemic immune dysregulation. SARS-CoV-2-induced immunosuppression alters salivary flow, and inflammation can create an environment conducive to the overgrowth of opportunistic pathogens. As a result, patients may experience an increased incidence of oral complications such as dental caries, periodontal disease, oral candidiasis, and secondary viral infections like herpes simplex [35, 36]. These manifestations not only reflect local microbial imbalances but also serve as indicators of broader systemic involvement, underscoring the importance of oral health monitoring in COVID-19 management.

During SARS-CoV-2 infections, the oral mucosa faces heightened stress due to viral invasion, inflammation, and disruption of salivary flow and composition, which can compromise its protective functions [23, 46–48]. However, it counteracts these challenges through a robust innate and adaptive immune response, antimicrobial peptides, rapid epithelial turnover, and the buffering and cleansing actions of saliva [31, 44]. These mechanisms work in concert to maintain mucosal integrity and restore homeostasis, highlighting the oral mucosa's resilience and its critical role in systemic health.

23.3 Oral Mucosal Alterations in COVID-19: Pathophysiology, Clinical Presentation, and Diagnostic Strategies

High levels of SARS-CoV-2 expression and replication have been detected in keratinized oral epithelium, particularly the dorsum of the tongue and hard palate [18]. The virus enters host cells via the ACE2 membrane receptor, leading to cleavage of the S protein by cellular cathepsin L and TMPRSS2 [1, 45]. The nucleocapsid, containing the viral RNA genome, is then released into the cytoplasm, where the virus hijacks the host's translational machinery to begin viral replication and protein synthesis [6, 29]. The replication process triggers a cascade of cellular responses, including inflammation, immune activation, and in some cases, cytopathic effects that contribute to tissue damage. In the oral cavity, this mechanism can lead to symptoms such as xerostomia, dysgeusia, mucosal ulcerations, and other manifestations, reflecting the virus's direct impact on oral epithelial and glandular cells. ACE2 binding also triggers proinflammatory signaling, producing TNFα, cell necrosis, and shedding of the ACE2 ectodomain [46–48]. High ACE2-expressing tissues, including alveolar tissues, oropharyngeal mucosal cells, gastrointestinal tract, kidneys, oral tissues, and endothelial cells, should be considered to be potential high-risk sites for SARS-CoV-2 [9, 18]. Histopathological analyses of oral tissue samples showed altered vascular arrangement, lymphocyte and Langerhans cell infiltration, and keratinocyte apoptosis [19, 20]. Biopsied skin manifestations confirmed vascular ectasia, blood-filled spaces, and perivascular lymphocytic infiltrates [19].

SARS-CoV-2 infection has been associated with diverse oral lesions, including ulcers, erosions, candidiasis, geographic and fissured tongue, keratosis, erythema, white patches, petechiae, and ulcerative necrotic lesions [16, 21–23, 49]. A systematic review reported ulcer prevalence ranging from 16.5% to 42.7%, primarily on lips, tongue, and buccal mucosa, with males (19.4%) more affected than females (14.8%). However, tongue redness was more common in females (7.4% vs. 3.2%). Lesions are more prevalent in adults than in children (20.2%) [23]. Interestingly, a characteristic skin rash can occur in the absence of any other COVID-19 symptoms and should be considered as a key diagnostic sign of the virus [50]. More indirectly, oral lesions may be a consequence of the immune response to COVID-19, as cytokines can cause excessive inflammation that disrupts the oral mucosal integrity [51]. The downregulation of the immune system by medications used to treat COVID-19, such as corticosteroids, antivirals, and antibiotics, can also make individuals susceptible to secondary infections like candidiasis [23].

During the acute phase of the illness, a significant number of patients experience oral and taste disturbances. Xerostomia affects between 45% and 74% of individuals, while dysgeusia (altered taste) is reported in 32% to 59% of cases. Specific taste losses are also common, with 29.3% of patients losing sweet taste perception and 25.9% losing salty taste. Additionally, 20.8% report burning sensations in the mouth, and between 19% and 66% experience ageusia. These symptoms tend to be more prevalent among younger individuals aged 15 and older, as well as those with a lower body mass index [23]. Song et al. reported that loss of taste occurred more (21%) than loss of smell (11%) in hospitalized patients, with loss of taste being associated with severe COVID-19 [52]. Anosmia and dysgeusia were among the longest-lasting symptoms, with ~60% of patients improving within 3 months [23]. Several mechanisms of COVID-19-induced dysgeusia have been proposed [24, 25]: (1) Direct damage to taste buds and epithelium [25–28, 53]; (2) ACE-2 mediated disruption of taste receptor function [54]; (3) neurological injury (olfactory and gustatory pathways) [55, 56]; (4). mechanical obstruction in the olfactory cleft from mucosal type 2 inflammation (edema or nasal polyps) [57]; and (5) salivary gland infection leading to reduced salivation, which reduces the dissolution of food molecules to TRCs and compromises the mucosal barrier, thus increasing the chance of irritation or secondary infections [22, 44, 58]. Xerostomia (subjective experience of oral dryness) and hyposalivation (objective finding of reduced salivary flow) could be aggravated by increased oral breathing from nasal congestion or by impaired salivary gland function [22]. Xerostomia-induced taste loss can be improved by treatment with artificial saliva [59]. Local, direct viral damage to taste bud cells may play a more immediate role in early dysgeusia, whereas central mechanisms in the nervous system could contribute to prolonged or persistent taste alterations. Further research is needed to confirm the dominant mechanisms and their clinical significance [23, 60]. Although oral manifestations and salivary dysfunction are widely reported, the degree of oral lesions and their direct correlation with COVID-19 severity remains uncertain, warranting continued research [22, 23, 61].

Oral lesions typically resolve within 3–28 days. Management options include antimicrobial mouth rinses (chlorhexidine, povidone-iodine), topical or systemic corticosteroids, antibiotics and antivirals [19, 62]. Antiseptic mouthwashes can reduce viral loads in the oral cavity and can be prescribed to patients with mucosal lesions as first line of therapy [63, 64].

While nasal swabs have been the predominant diagnostic method for COVID-19, saliva-based COVID-19 diagnosis has emerged as a promising alternative. SARS-CoV-2 may enter saliva either directly from respiratory tract secretions or from the gingival crevicular fluid [18]. SARS-CoV-2 can also replicate in salivary gland tissues and be released in salivary secretions [65]. Biomarkers in saliva are useful in the diagnosis of several viral infections [42], and it could be a source for early diagnosis of disease prior to respiratory symptoms due to the increased ACE2 expression in minor salivary glands and rapid infection in its epithelial cells [8, 16, 17]. Disease status and severity are correlated with NK cell cytopenia, which is detectable in saliva during early infection, even in ambulatory patients with mild disease, and can be used to identify patients susceptible to severe disease or monitor response to therapies targeting NK cells [66–69]. Furthermore, data have shown that SARS-CoV-2 infection is associated with an increase in proinflammatory mediators positively correlated with viral load [66]. Live virus can be successfully cultivated through saliva samples, with a 92% positive rate of SARS-CoV-2, compared to pooled nasopharyngeal and throat swabs [70, 71]. These characteristics make saliva an accessible, non-invasive tool for COVID-19 diagnosis, monitoring, and public health screening.

23.4 Adapting Dental Practice to COVID-19: A Review of Challenges and Strategic Responses

For dental professionals, the pandemic introduced significant challenges but also opportunities for improvement and innovation. The early months of the pandemic saw widespread treatment deferrals and practice closures. Because SARS-CoV-2 transmits via aerosols and droplets, dentists are at high risk of becoming infected. Dental regulatory bodies were quick to implement guidelines to prevent the spread of disease [72, 73]. Dental health care personnel should continue to be familiar with COVID-19 signs and symptoms to effectively treat the patient or refer to their physician. Patient screening and triage are successful methods to prioritize patients into three categories: triage negative, triage positive, and confirmed COVID-19 cases [71, 73]. In addition to rapid tests, biomarkers in saliva and mucosa are under development to identify asymptomatic carriers [8, 16, 17]. The dental staff should practice infection control to effectively minimize transmission in the dental clinic, including wearing protective equipment, using rubber dams, which reduce aerosol spread by 70% in a 3-foot diameter of the operational field [74], thoroughly disinfecting surfaces, ensuring proper clinic ventilation, and careful disposal of contaminated materials [75]. Studies have also shown that a pre-procedural mouth rinse can significantly reduce microbial load in dental aerosols [76–78]. Vaccines continue to mitigate variant risks and reduce disease severity and transmission. Immunocompromised patients with underlying comorbidities (i.e., diabetes, cancer, cardiovascular disease, hypertension) are at increased risk for COVID-19 and widespread severe oral diseases. Periodontal inflammation interplays with systemic conditions by increasing cytokine production, and disease severity may be increased with COVID-19 infection.[79] It is important to identify such patients and reinforce oral hygiene to prevent further progression of oral diseases.

This chapter highlighted the impact of COVID-19 on clinical dentistry and the relevance of the oral cavity in a SARS-CoV-2 infection. Understanding the oral manifestations associated with SARS-CoV-2 sheds light on the pathogenesis of COVID-19 and opens new avenues for diagnostic approaches using saliva and oral tissue analysis. Ongoing research into the virus's longer-term oral effects, its evolving variants, and refined diagnostic/therapeutic tools ensures dental clinicians remain at the forefront of both oral health and infectious disease control.

References

1. Shi Y, Wang G, Cai XP, Deng JW, Zheng L, Zhu HH, Zheng M, Yang B, Chen Z, et al. An overview of COVID-19. J Zhejiang Univ Sci B. 2020;21(5):343–60. https://doi.org/10.1631/jzus.B2000083.
2. Bchetnia M, Girard C, Duchaine C, Laprise C. The outbreak of the novel severe acute respiratory syndrome coronavirus 2 (SARS-CoV-2): a review of the current global status. J Infect Public Health. 2020;13(11):1601–10. https://doi.org/10.1016/j.jiph.2020.07.011.
3. COVID-19 deaths [Internet]. Geneva: World Health Organization (WHO); c2025 [cited 2025 Aug 6]. Available from: https://data.who.int/dashboards/covid19/deaths?n=o.
4. COVID-19 epidemiology update: Current situation [Internet]. Ottawa: Government of Canada; c2024 [cited 2025 Aug 6]. Available from: https://health-infobase.canada.ca/covid-19/current-situation.html?stat=num&measure=deaths_total&map=pt#a2.
5. Statement on the fifteenth meeting of the IHR (2005) Emergency Committee on the COVID-19 pandemic [Internet]. Geneva: World Health Organization (WHO); 2023 May 5 [cited 2025 Aug 6]. Available from: https://www.who.int/news/item/05-05-2023-statement-on-the-fifteenth-meeting-of-the-international-health-regulations-(2005)-emergency-committee-regarding-the-coronavirusdisease-(covid-19)-pandemic.
6. Neuman BW, Buchmeier MJ. Supramolecular architecture of the Coronavirus particle. Adv Virus Res. 2016;96:1–27. https://doi.org/10.1016/bs.aivir.2016.08.005.
7. Karia R, Gupta I, Khandait H, Yadav A, Yadav A. COVID-19 and its modes of transmission. SN Compr Clin Med. 2020;2(10):1798–801. https://doi.org/10.1007/s42399-020-00498-4.

8. Wang WK, Chen SY, Liu IJ, Chen YC, Chen HL, Yang CF, et al. Detection of SARS-associated coronavirus in throat wash and saliva in early diagnosis. Emerg Infect Dis. 2004;10(7):1213–9. https://doi.org/10.3201/eid1007.031113.
9. Herrera D, Serrano J, Roldán S, Sanz M. Is the oral cavity relevant in SARS-CoV-2 pandemic? Clin Oral Invest. 2020;24(8):2925–30. https://doi.org/10.1007/s00784-020-03413-2.
10. Jeffers L, Webster-Cyriaque JY. Viruses and salivary gland disease (SGD): lessons from HIV SGD. Adv Dent Res. 2011;23(1):79–83. https://doi.org/10.1177/0022034510396882.
11. Santosh ABR, Muddana K. Viral infections of oral cavity. J Family Med Prim Care. 2020;9(1):36–42. https://doi.org/10.4103/jfmpc.jfmpc_807_19.
12. Richardson S, Hirsch JS, Narasimhan M, Crawford JM, McGinn T, Davidson KW, et al. Presenting characteristics, comorbidities, and outcomes among 5700 patients hospitalized with COVID-19 in the New York City Area. JAMA. 2020;323(20):2052–9. https://doi.org/10.1001/jama.2020.6775.
13. Arentz M, Yim E, Klaff L, Lokhandwala S, Riedo FX, Chong M, et al. Characteristics and outcomes of 21 critically Ill patients with COVID-19 in Washington State. JAMA. 2020;323(16):1612–4. https://doi.org/10.1001/jama.2020.4326.
14. Garg S, Kim L, Whitaker M, O'Halloran A, Cummings C, Holstein R, et al. Hospitalization rates and characteristics of patients hospitalized with laboratory-confirmed coronavirus disease 2019 – COVID-NET, 14 States, March 1–30, 2020. MMWR Morb Mortal Wkly Rep. 2020;69(15):458–64. https://doi.org/10.15585/mmwr.mm6915e3.
15. Iranmanesh B, Khalili M, Amiri R, Zartab H, Aflatoonian M. Oral manifestations of COVID-19 disease: a review article. Dermatol Ther. 2020;34(1):e14578. https://doi.org/10.1111/dth.14578.
16. Xu J, Li Y, Gan F, Du Y, Yao Y. Salivary glands: potential reservoirs for COVID-19 asymptomatic infection. J. Dental Res. 2020;99(8):989. https://doi.org/10.1177/0022034520918518.
17. Liu L, Wei Q, Alvarez X, Wang H, Du Y, Zhu H, et al. Epithelial cells lining salivary gland ducts are early target cells of severe acute respiratory syndrome coronavirus infection in the upper respiratory tracts of rhesus macaques. J Virol. 2011;85(8):4025–30. https://doi.org/10.1128/JVI.02292-10.
18. Xu H, Zhong L, Deng J, Peng J, Dan H, Zeng X, et al. High expression of ACE2 receptor of 2019-nCoV on the epithelial cells of oral mucosa. Int J Oral Sci. 2020;12:8. https://doi.org/10.1038/s41368-020-0074-x.
19. Cruz Tapia RO, Peraza Labrador AJ, Guimaraes DM, Matos Valdez LH. Oral mucosal lesions in patients with SARS-CoV-2 infection. Report of four cases. Are they a true sign of COVID-19 disease? Spec Care Dentist. 2020;40(6):555–60. https://doi.org/10.1111/scd.12520.
20. Gianotti R, Zerbi P, Dodiuk-Gad RP. Clinical and histopathological study of skin dermatoses in patients affected by COVID-19 infection in the Northern part of Italy. J Dermatol Sci. 2020;98(2):141–3. https://doi.org/10.1016/j.jdermsci.2020.04.007.
21. Troeltzsch M, Berndt R, Troeltzsch M. Is the oral cavity a reservoir for prolonged SARS-CoV-2 shedding? Med Hypotheses. 2020;146:110419. https://doi.org/10.1016/j.mehy.2020.110419.
22. Brandão TB, Gueiros LA, Melo TS, Prado-Ribeiro ACA, Nesrallah CFA, Prado GVB, et al. Oral lesions in patients with SARS-CoV-2 infection: could the oral cavity be a target organ? Oral Surg Oral Med Oral Pathol Oral Radiol. 2020;131(2):e45–51. https://doi.org/10.1016/j.oooo.2020.07.014.
23. Aliberti A, Gasparro R, Mignogna M, Canfora F, Spagnuolo G, Sammartino G, et al. Unveiling the oral lesions, dysgeusia and osteonecrosis related to COVID-19: a comprehensive systematic review. J Clin Med. 2025;14(4):1267. https://doi.org/10.3390/jcm14041267.
24. Thomas DC, Chablani D, Parekh S, Pichammal RC, Shanmugasundaram K, Pitchumani PK. Dysgeusia: a review in the context of COVID-19. J Am Dent Assoc. 2022;153(3):251–64. https://doi.org/10.1016/j.adaj.2021.08.009.
25. Lozada-Nur F, Chainani-Wu N, Fortuna G, Sroussi H. Dysgeusia in COVID-19: possible mechanisms and implications. Oral Surg Oral Med Oral Pathol Oral Radiol. 2020;130(3):344–6. https://doi.org/10.1016/j.oooo.2020.06.016.

26. Beyerstedt S, Casaro EB, Rangel ÉB. COVID-19: angiotensin-converting enzyme 2 (ACE2) expression and tissue susceptibility to SARS-CoV-2 infection. Eur J Clin Microbiol Infect Dis. 2021;40(5):905–19. https://doi.org/10.1007/s10096-020-04138-6.
27. Wang Z, Zhou J, Marshall B, Rekaya R, Ye K, Liu HX. SARS-CoV-2 receptor ACE2 is enriched in a subpopulation of mouse tongue epithelial cells in nongustatory papillae but not in taste buds or embryonic oral epithelium. ACS Pharmacol Transl Sci. 2020;3(4):749–58. https://doi.org/10.1021/acsptsci.0c00062.
28. Doyle ME, Appleton A, Liu QR, Yao Q, Mazucanti CH, Egan JM. Human taste cells express ACE2: a portal for SARS-CoV-2 infection. bioRxiv [Preprint]. 2021:440680. https://doi.org/10.1101/2021.04.21.440680.
29. Jin Y, Yang H, Ji W, Wu W, Chen S, Zhang W, et al. Virology, epidemiology, pathogenesis, and control of COVID-19. Viruses. 2020;12(4):372. https://doi.org/10.3390/v12040372.
30. Wadowski PP, Panzer B, Józkowicz A, Kopp CW, Gremmel T, Panzer S, et al. Microvascular thrombosis as a critical factor in severe Covid-19. Int J Mol Sci. 2023;24(3):2492. https://doi.org/10.3390/ijms24032492.
31. Chiego DJ. Essentials of oral histology and embryology. 5th ed. St. Louis: Elsevier; 2018.
32. Groeger S, Meyle J. Oral mucosal epithelial cells. Front Immunol. 2019;10:208. https://doi.org/10.3389/fimmu.2019.00208.
33. Groeger SE, Meyle J. Epithelial barrier and oral bacterial infection. Periodontol. 2015;69(1):46–67. https://doi.org/10.1111/prd.12094.
34. Proctor DM, Relman DA. The landscape ecology and microbiota of the human nose, mouth, and throat. Cell Host Microbe. 2017;21(4):421–32. https://doi.org/10.1016/j.chom.2017.03.011.
35. Seneviratne CJ, Jin L, Samaranayake LP. Biofilm lifestyle of Candida: a mini review. Oral Dis. 2008;14(7):582–90. https://doi.org/10.1111/j.1601-0825.2007.01424.x.
36. Aas JA, Paster BJ, Stokes LN, Olsen I, Dewhirst FE. Defining the normal bacterial flora of the oral cavity. J Clin Microbiol. 2005;43(11):5721–32. https://doi.org/10.1128/JCM.43.11.5721-5732.2005.
37. Bindal U, Shajan K, Mitra NK, Priydarshni B. Morphological analysis of Vermilion Border and its forensic applications. Open J. Dent. Oral Med. 2015;3(1):21–8. https://doi.org/10.13189/ojdom.2015.030104.
38. Shang J, Feng X, Chen Y, Gu Z, Liu Y. Human lip vermilion: physiology and age-related changes. J Cosmet Dermatol. 2024;23(8):2676–80. https://doi.org/10.1111/jocd.16317.
39. Horio N, Yoshida R, Yasumatsu K, Yanagawa Y, Ishimaru Y, Matsunami H, et al. Sour taste responses in mice lacking PKD channels. PLoS One. 2011;6(5):e20007. https://doi.org/10.1371/journal.pone.0020007.
40. Zhang Y, Hoon MA, Chandrashekar J, Mueller KL, Cook B, Wu D, et al. Coding of sweet, bitter, and umami tastes: different receptor cells sharing similar signaling pathways. Cell. 2003;112(3):293–301. https://doi.org/10.1016/S0092-8674(03)00071-0.
41. Perez CA, Huang L, Rong M, Kozak JA, Preuss AK, Zhang H, et al. A transient receptor potential channel expressed in taste receptor cells. Nat Neurosci. 2002;5(11):1169–76. https://doi.org/10.1038/nn952.
42. Zhang CZ, Cheng XQ, Li JY, Zhang P, Yi P, Xu X, et al. Saliva in the diagnosis of diseases. Int J Oral Sci. 2016;8(3):133–7. https://doi.org/10.1038/ijos.2016.38.
43. Iorgulescu G. Saliva between normal and pathological. Important factors in determining systemic and oral health. J Med Life. 2009;2(3):303–7.
44. Alfaifi AA, Wang TW, Perez P, Sultan AS, Meiller TF, Rock P, et al. SARS-CoV-2 infection of salivary glands compromises the production of a secreted antifungal peptide with potential implications for development of oral candidiasis. PLoS Pathog. 2024;20(12):e1012375. https://doi.org/10.1371/journal.ppat.1012375.
45. Datta PK, Liu F, Fischer T, Rappaport J, Qin X. SARS-CoV-2 pandemic and research gaps: understanding SARS-CoV-2 interaction with the ACE2 receptor and implications for therapy. Theranostics. 2020;10(16):7448–764. https://doi.org/10.7150/thno.48076.
46. Haga S, Yamamoto N, Nakai-Murakami C, Osawa Y, Tokunaga K, Sata T, et al. Modulation of TNF-alpha-converting enzyme by the spike protein of SARS-CoV and ACE2 induces TNF-alpha

production and facilitates viral entry. Proc Natl Acad Sci USA. 2008;105(22):7809–14. https://doi.org/10.1073/pnas.0711241105.
47. Barlow LA. Progress and renewal in gustation: new insights into taste bud development. Development. 2015;142(21):3620–9. https://doi.org/10.1242/dev.120394.
48. Idriss HT, Naismith JH. TNF alpha and the TNF receptor superfamily: structure-function relationship(s). Microsc Res Tech. 2000;50(3):184–95. https://doi.org/10.1002/1097-0029(20000801)50:3<184::AID-JEMT2>3.0.CO;2-H.
49. Glavina A, Badrov J, Lukenda M, Džaja K, Biočina-Lukenda D, Lugović-Mihić L. COVID-19 and oral lesions: 2020-2024 outpatient case series and literature review. Acta Dermatovenerol Alp Pannonica Adriat. 2024;33(1):41–8.
50. Visconti A, Bataille V, Rossi N, Kluk J, Murphy R, Puig S, et al. Diagnostic value of cutaneous manifestation of SARS-CoV-2 infection. Br J Dermatol. 2021;184(5):880–7. https://doi.org/10.1111/bjd.19807.
51. Saxena S, Kumar S. Understanding the mechanism of commonly occurring COVID-19-associated oral lesions. J Oral Maxillofac Pathol. 2021;25(2):223–5. https://doi.org/10.4103/0973-029X.325118.
52. Song J, Deng Y-K, Wang H, Wang Z-C, Liao B, Ma J, et al. Self-reported taste and smell disorders in patients with COVID-19: distinct features in China. Curr Med Sci. 2021;41(1):14–23. https://doi.org/10.1007/s11596-021-2312-7.
53. Cooper KW, Brann DH, Farruggia MC, Bhutani S, Pellegrino R, Tsukahara T, et al. COVID-19 and the chemical senses: supporting players take center stage. Neuron. 2020;107(2):219–33. https://doi.org/10.1016/j.neuron.2020.06.032.
54. Scotto G, Fazio V, Lo Muzio E, Lo Muzio L, Spirito F. SARS-CoV-2 infection and taste alteration: an overview. Life (Basel). 2022;12(5):690. https://doi.org/10.3390/life12050690.
55. Pacheco-Herrero M, Soto-Rojas LO, Harrington CR, Flores-Martinez YM, Villegas-Rojas MM, León-Aguilar AM, et al. Elucidating the neuropathologic mechanisms of SARS-CoV-2 infection. Front Neurol. 2021;12:660087. https://doi.org/10.3389/fneur.2021.660087.
56. Ahmadirad N, Ghasemi Z. COVID-19 and central nervous system: entry routes and. Basic Clin Neurosci. 2020;11(2):217–24. https://doi.org/10.32598/bcn.11.covid19.2360.1.
57. Mullol J, Mariño-Sánchez F, Valls M, Alobid I, Marin C. The sense of smell in chronic rhinosinusitis. J Allergy Clin Immunol. 2020;145(3):773–6. https://doi.org/10.1016/j.jaci.2020.01.024.
58. Mullol J, Alobid I, Mariño-Sánchez F, Izquierdo-Domínguez A, Marin C, Klimek L, et al. The loss of smell and taste in the COVID-19 outbreak: a tale of many countries. Curr Allergy Asthma Rep. 2020;20(10):61. https://doi.org/10.1007/s11882-020-00961-1.
59. Baghizadeh FM. Oral saliva and COVID-19. Oral Oncol. 2020;108:104821. https://doi.org/10.1016/j.oraloncology.2020.104821.
60. Risso D, Drayna D, Morini G. Alteration, reduction and taste loss: main causes and potential implications on dietary habits. Nutrients. 2020;12(11):3284. https://doi.org/10.3390/nu12113284.
61. Amorim Dos Santos J, Normando AGC, Carvalho da Silva RL, De Paula RM, Cembranel AC, Santos-Silva AR, et al. Oral mucosal lesions in a COVID-19 patient: new signs or secondary manifestations? Int J Infect Dis. 2020;97:326–8. https://doi.org/10.1016/j.ijid.2020.06.012.
62. Carrouel F, Gonçalves LS, Conte MP, Campus G, Fisher J, Fraticelli L, et al. Antiviral activity of reagents in mouth rinses against SARS-CoV-2. J Dent Res. 2021;100(2):124–32. https://doi.org/10.1177/0022034520967933.
63. Yoon JG, Yoon J, Song JY, Yoon SY, Lim CS, Seong H, et al. Clinical significance of a high SARS-CoV-2 viral load in the saliva. J Korean Med Sci. 2020;35(20):e195. https://doi.org/10.3346/jkms.2020.35.e195.
64. Sabino-Silva R, Jardim ACG, Siqueira WL. Coronavirus COVID-19 impacts to dentistry and potential salivary diagnosis. Clin Oral Investig. 2020;24(4):1619–21. https://doi.org/10.1007/s00784-020-03248-x.

65. Graves C, Babikow E, Ghaltakhchyan N, Ngo TQ, Liu C, Wang S, et al. Immune dysregulation in the oral cavity during early SARS-CoV-2 infection. J Dent Res. 2024;103(12):1258–70. https://doi.org/10.1177/00220345241271943.
66. Giamarellos-Bourboulis EJ, Netea MG, Rovina N, Akinosoglou K, Antoniadou A, Antonakos N, et al. Complex immune dysregulation in COVID-19 patients with severe respiratory failure. Cell Host Microbe. 2020;27(6):992–1000.e3. https://doi.org/10.1016/j.chom.2020.04.009.
67. van Eeden C, Khan L, Osman MS, Cohen Tervaert JW. Natural killer cell dysfunction and its role in COVID-19. Int J Mol Sci. 2020;21(17):6351. https://doi.org/10.3390/ijms21176351.
68. Zafarani A, Razizadeh MH, Pashangzadeh S, Amirzargar MR, Taghavi-Farahabadi M, Mahmoudi M. Natural killer cells in COVID-19: from infection, to vaccination and therapy. Future Virol. 2023;18(3):177–91. https://doi.org/10.2217/fvl-2022-0040.
69. Cheng VCC, Wong SC, Chen JHK, Yip CCY, Chuang VWM, Tsang OTY, et al. Escalating infection control response to the rapidly evolving epidemiology of the coronavirus disease 2019 (COVID-19) due to SARS-CoV-2 in Hong Kong. Infect Control Hosp Epidemiol. 2020;41(5):493–8. https://doi.org/10.1017/ice.2020.58.
70. Michailidou E, Poulopoulos A, Tzimagiorgis G. Salivary diagnostics of the novel coronavirus SARS-CoV-2 (COVID-19). Oral Dis. 2020;28(S1):867–77. https://doi.org/10.1111/odi.13729.
71. Spagnuolo G, De Vito D, Rengo S, Tatullo M. COVID-19 outbreak: an overview on dentistry. Int J Environ Res Public Health. 2020;17(6):2094. https://doi.org/10.3390/ijerph17062094.
72. Brian Z, Weintraub JA. Oral health and COVID-19: increasing the need for prevention and access. Prev Chronic Dis. 2020;17:E82. https://doi.org/10.5888/pcd17.200266. Erratum in: Prev Chronic Dis. 2020;17:200266. https://doi.org/10.0.5888/pcd17.200266.
73. Samaranayake LP, Reid J, Evans D. The efficacy of rubber dam isolation in reducing atmospheric bacterial contamination. ASDC J Dent Child. 1989;56(6):442–4.
74. Li Y, Ren B, Peng X, Hu T, Li J, Gong T, et al. Saliva is a non-negligible factor in the spread of COVID-19. Mol Oral Microbiol. 2020;35(4):141–5. https://doi.org/10.1111/omi.12289.
75. Seneviratne CJ, Balan P, Ko KKK, Udawatte NS, Lai D, Ng DHL, et al. Efficacy of commercial mouth-rinses on SARS-CoV-2 viral load in saliva: randomized control trial in Singapore. Infection. 2021;49(2):305–11. https://doi.org/10.1007/s15010-020-01563-9.
76. Marui VC, Souto MLS, Rovai ES, Romito GA, Chambrone L, Pannuti CM. Efficacy of preprocedural mouthrinses in the reduction of microorganisms in aerosol: a systematic review. J Am Dent Assoc. 2019;150(12):1015–1026.e1. https://doi.org/10.1016/j.adaj.2019.06.024.
77. Vergara-Buenaventura A, Castro-Ruiz C. Use of mouthwashes against COVID-19 in dentistry. Br J Oral Maxillofac Surg. 2020;58(8):924–7. https://doi.org/10.1016/j.bjoms.2020.08.016.
78. Pitones-Rubio V, Chávez-Cortez EG, Hurtado-Camarena A, González-Rascón A, Serafín-Higuera N. Is periodontal disease a risk factor for severe COVID-19 illness? Med Hypotheses. 2020;144:109969. https://doi.org/10.1016/j.mehy.2020.109969.

24 Periodontitis and COVID-19: A Hidden Driver of Susceptibility and Severity

Salima Shebbo, Hasna H. Kunhipurayil, Mohammad Abusamak, and Faleh Ahmad Tamimi

24.1 Introduction

As the world struggled with the COVID-19 pandemic, oral health problems such as periodontitis may have silently worsened and contributed to the severity of the illness for millions of people. Periodontitis is a chronic inflammatory disease that is considered the sixth most common condition worldwide, affecting about half of the adult population [1]. As of 2021, according to the Global Burden of Disease Study, there were 1 billion individuals affected by severe periodontal disease globally, making it a significant public health issue [2]. This number is expected to rise to 1.5 billion by 2050 [3]. Understanding the systemic nature of periodontitis is crucial to recognising its impact on infections, especially during a pandemic like COVID-19, which is characterised by systemic immune overactivation.

COVID-19 is the disease caused by SARS-CoV-2, an enveloped beta coronavirus that primarily infects the respiratory tract and can progress to acute respiratory distress syndrome (ARDS), with risk increased in people with comorbidities and older age [4]. The viral genome encodes structural proteins such as spike (S), envelope (E), membrane (M), and nucleocapsid (N) [5]. The S glycoprotein mediates entry by binding to the cell membrane protein angiotensin-converting enzyme 2 (ACE2) and, after protease priming, drives membrane fusion in target airway and

S. Shebbo · H. H. Kunhipurayil
College of Dental Medicine, Qatar University Health, Qatar University, Doha, Qatar
e-mail: salima@qu.edu.qa; hk1512005@student.qu.edu.qa

M. Abusamak
Faculty of Dentistry, Dalhousie University, Halifax, Nova Scotia, Canada
e-mail: mohammad.abusamak@mail.mcgill.ca

F. A. Tamimi (✉)
Faculty of Dental Medicine and Oral Health Sciences, McGill University, Montreal, QC, Canada
e-mail: faleh.tamimimarino@mcgill.ca

S. R. Prabhu et al. (eds.), *COVID-19 in Dental Practice*,
https://doi.org/10.1007/978-3-032-26000-0_24

alveolar epithelial cells [5]. In contrast, the non-structural proteins (nsps) form the replication-transcription complex; notably, nsp12 is the RNA-dependent RNA polymerase (RdRp) that works with nsp7/nsp8 cofactors, while nsp14/nsp10 and nsp16/nsp10 support RNA capping and fidelity [6].

Periodontitis is a chronic inflammatory disease caused by a persistent bacterial infection resulting from a shift in the oral microbiota from a balanced ecosystem (symbiosis) to an imbalanced one (dysbiosis) [7–11]. This leads to damage of the periodontal ligaments, alveolar bone, and surrounding connective tissue, ultimately resulting in tooth loss [7–11]. The disease is not merely a dental issue; it is a global health burden that can worsen the effects of other inflammatory diseases.

Periodontitis is a complex disease primarily influenced by environmental factors, but it may also be polygenic or monogenic in rare, severe cases [8]. Monogenic cases have a clear genetic basis, such as mutations in the ITGB2 gene that impair immune responses and cause severe periodontitis in young individuals. Conversely, polygenic cases involve multiple genes that can either increase susceptibility or offer protection by affecting the host immune response and interaction with the oral microbiota [8]. Important genes involved in this process include IL-1β, IL-6, TNFα, FCGR2A, C5, CD14, and WNT5A, all of which have essential roles in inflammation and immunity [12–14].

Periodontitis involves the systemic spread of bacteria, bacterial components, and pro-inflammatory cytokines into the bloodstream, thereby threatening overall health [15–21]. It is linked to systemic inflammation [35–37] and increased levels of pro-inflammatory cytokines (e.g., interleukin (IL)-6, tumour necrosis factor-alpha (TNF-α), and IL-1β), C-reactive protein (CRP) [7, 8, 38, 39], and neutrophil extracellular traps (NETS) [40], as well as the priming of heightened innate immune responses through the recruitment of peripheral polymorphonuclear leukocytes to both local and distant inflammatory sites [41]. Consequently, this disease is associated with various systemic conditions, including inflammatory bowel disease, type 2 diabetes mellitus, cardiovascular diseases, rheumatoid arthritis, non-alcoholic fatty liver disease, cancer, and pulmonary disorders [8, 22–26]. In fact, emerging evidence supports an oral–lung axis linking periodontitis with pulmonary diseases such as ARDS and pneumonia, through the dissemination of periodontal pathogens (e.g., *Porphyromonas gingivalis* and *Fusobacterium nucleatum*) to the lungs via respiratory and haematogenous routes [27–34].

In COVID-19 cases, disease severity is often driven by a "cytokine storm", an uncontrolled and excessive release of inflammatory mediators including IL-6, TNF-α, IL-1β, IFN-γ, IL-2, granulocyte-macrophage colony-stimulating factor (GM-CSF), monocyte chemoattractant protein-1 (MCP-1), and chemokines such as interferon gamma-induced protein 10 (IP-10 or CXCL10) [42, 43]. This hyperinflammatory state is accompanied by haematological abnormalities, including leukocytosis, leukopenia, anaemia, thrombocytopenia, and elevated D-dimer levels. Furthermore, immune cell infiltration of lung tissue by macrophages, neutrophils, CD4+ T cells, and CD8+ T cells contributes to lung injury. This excessive immune activation can progress to pneumonia, ARDS, multi-organ failure, and mortality [42].

As outlined above, periodontitis and COVID-19 share overlapping inflammatory pathways, as well as genetic factors and medical conditions. Consequently, the

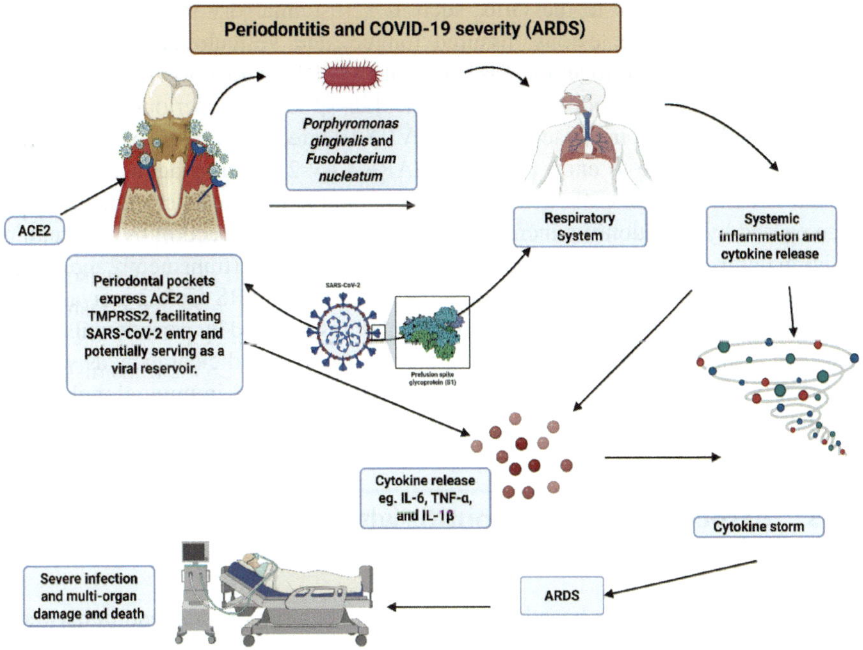

Fig. 24.1 Schematic illustration of the proposed link between periodontitis and COVID-19 severity. Periodontal pockets express ACE2 and TMPRSS2, which facilitate SARS-CoV-2 priming, entry, and replication, potentially acting as viral reservoirs. Periodontal pathogens like *Porphyromonas gingivalis* and *Fusobacterium nucleatum* can contribute to local and systemic inflammation and may affect respiratory health. This can worsen systemic inflammation in COVID-19, leading to the release of cytokines such as IL-6, TNF-α, and IL-1β. Excessive cytokine release can cause widespread tissue damage and may result in acute respiratory distress syndrome (ARDS), severe infection, and death

association of periodontitis with COVID-19 infection and severity has been investigated [44–48]. This chapter explores the potential links between periodontal disease and both the susceptibility to and outcomes of COVID-19. Understanding this relationship will provide new insights for prevention, treatment, and the development of integrated health strategies in response to current and future viral pandemics. Figure 24.1 summarises the potential connection between periodontitis, SARS-CoV-2 infection, and COVID-19 severity.

24.2 Oral Cavity as a Gateway for COVID-19 Infection

The oral cavity is a key site for SARS-CoV-2 infection. In fact, the main protein required for SARS-CoV-2 viral priming and cell entry, angiotensin-converting enzyme receptor-2 (ACE2), is found in oral epithelial cells, especially in the papillae of the tongue, gingiva, periodontal tissues, and oral mucosa, making these cells important entry points for COVID-19. This susceptibility of the oral cavity to SARS-CoV-2 infection may be worsened by existing oral conditions that create an environment favourable to the virus, such as xerostomia (dry mouth), mucositis, haemorrhagic mucosal lesions, fissured tongue, and vesiculobullous eruptions, which have been linked to an increased risk of COVID-19 infection [50–55].

In line with this, periodontitis and interleukin-1β levels in periodontal pockets have been linked to an increased risk of COVID-19 infection [50–55, 57]. The periodontal pockets serve as entry points for SARS-CoV-2 and may act as a reservoir for the virus within the oral cavity [58]. The inflammation and microbiome imbalance caused by periodontitis increase susceptibility to this infection by weakening antiviral defences and boosting the expression of TMPRSS2 (transmembrane serine protease 2) and ACE2, the essential proteins involved in SARS-CoV-2 activation in the gum tissue [49, 56, 58]. Furthermore, metabolites released by periodontal pathogens can further suppress oral mucosal immune defence and clearance, as well as facilitate viral entry by assisting viral attachment to T-cell immunoglobulin-like (TIMs) receptors [49].

24.3 Association of Periodontitis with COVID-19 Infection: Clinical Evidence

Numerous clinical studies have been conducted to explore the connection between COVID-19 infection and periodontitis [8, 35]. A case-control study using a validated questionnaire found that self-reported periodontitis was 3.3 times more common in SARS-CoV-2 positive individuals [59]. Observational studies leveraging real-world registry data from a Florida database confirmed these findings, showing that patients with periodontal disease had higher odds of testing positive for COVID-19 [60, 61]. Additionally, individuals with a genetic predisposition to periodontitis were shown to have an increased risk of infection [57]. In fact, a Mendelian Randomisation (MR) study identified a causal relationship between individuals genetically linked to periodontitis (measured through single nucleotide polymorphisms (SNP) exposure) and susceptibility to COVID-19 infection [62].

24.4 Association of Periodontitis with COVID-19 Severity

Severe COVID-19 is characterised by a cytokine release storm, where an excessive immune response aimed at eliminating and containing the infection backfires and becomes the main cause of uncontrolled systemic inflammation [43, 63, 64]. This leads to ARDS [65], pulmonary embolism [66–68], and ultimately organ failure and death [69–71]. This condition has claimed the lives of millions, prompting scientists to investigate the underlying causes of COVID-19 severity. Beyond comorbidities and immunocompromised conditions that have been linked to severe COVID-19 outcomes, periodontitis has also been studied as a potential contributing factor [38, 72–75].

Survey studies have indicated that self-reported periodontitis is linked to increased severity of COVID-19 [59]. Studies evaluating radiographic signs of periodontal bone loss also identified an association with COVID-19 complications. A case-control study involving 568 patients showed that those with radiographic signs of periodontal bone loss faced a higher risk of severe COVID-19 outcomes, including ICU admission, the need for ventilation, and death [76]. Another case-control study using radiographic signs of periodontitis found a significantly greater risk of severe COVID-19 outcomes, such as requiring mechanical ventilation and ICU admission, among subjects with periodontitis [77].

Studies evaluating clinical signs of periodontitis have also identified similar associations. Case-control studies found a positive relationship between clinically diagnosed periodontitis and the severity and symptoms of COVID-19 [78], including increased hospitalisation, admission to semi-intensive care units, ICU admission, longer ICU stays, greater need for oxygen therapy and ventilation [80, 81], and mortality [81]. Additionally, a cross-sectional study relying on periodontal examinations of hospitalised COVID-19 patients showed a significant association of stage III-IV periodontitis with severe-to-critical COVID-19 and longer hospital stays [79]. Moreover, Clinical attachment loss (CAL) and the gingiva index (GI) were linked to higher odds of adverse events, such as respiratory failure requiring invasive ventilation, transfer to ICU, shock, multiorgan failure, sepsis, coma, or death [79]. These findings underscore the significant role of periodontal health in the progression of COVID-19 disease and highlight the need for targeted oral health care to reduce severe complications. Indeed, a study evaluating the impact of periodontal therapy on COVID-19 outcomes found that patients with periodontitis who received periodontal treatment had a lower risk of COVID-19 complications compared to those with untreated periodontitis [82]. Combining this evidence, it is essential to manage and control periodontitis to prevent the exaggerated inflammatory response in COVID-19 and lessen disease severity.

24.5 Periodontitis and the Cytokine Storm in COVID-19

Periodontitis seems to contribute to the severity of SARS-CoV-2 infections, possibly through the immune response that triggers the cytokine storm and ARDS in COVID-19. Several studies have demonstrated how the impact of periodontitis on systemic inflammation could be driving its link with COVID-19 complications. Research has shown that periodontitis primes the immune system toward an exaggerated systemic inflammatory response that could potentially worsen the clinical outcomes of COVID-19 [25]. In fact, clinical evidence indicates that COVID-19 patients with periodontitis exhibit higher levels of inflammatory biomarkers associated with a poorer COVID-19 prognosis, such as D-dimer and C-reactive protein in serum [76] and IL-6 in saliva [80]. Periodontitis was also linked to increased levels of receptor activator of nuclear factor kappa-B ligand (RANKL) and IL-1β following COVID-19 infection [80]. These findings further suggest a synergistic worsening of COVID-19 systemic inflammation due to periodontitis-induced inflammation.

24.6 Effect of COVID-19 on Oral Health

The connection between COVID-19 and periodontitis appears to be bidirectional; not only can periodontitis influence the progression of COVID-19, but COVID-19 can also impact periodontitis and oral health. SARS-CoV-2 infection and its persistence in the oral cavity can disrupt the balance of the oral microbiome, fostering a pro-inflammatory environment and increasing vulnerability to oral pathogens. This explains why post-acute sequelae of COVID-19 (PASC) include various oral conditions such as dysgeusia, xerostomia, pharyngitis, oral keratoses, pulpitis, and periodontal diseases [83, 84]. This immune dysfunction further raises the risk of additional viral infections and worsens oral conditions like periodontal and endodontic diseases. These ongoing oral health problems can contribute to systemic inflammation, creating a bidirectional relationship between oral and non-oral tissues and potentially leading to post-acute sequelae of COVID-19 (PASC) [85, 86]. Additionally, a case-control study examining patients who had COVID-19 within the previous 3–6 months [87] found that a history of COVID-19 infection was linked to the presence of periodontitis. The study demonstrated that periodontal clinical measurements were significantly higher in the post-COVID-19 group [87].

24.7 Conclusion

Periodontitis is a chronic inflammatory disease that impacts more than just oral health. This condition can worsen infectious diseases, including COVID-19, and increase their severity and long-term effects. The shared inflammatory pathways of these diseases, involving IL-6, TNF-α, and IL-1β, along with the upregulation of proteins essential for viral infection in periodontal disease, provide plausible biological mechanisms for heightened COVID-19 susceptibility and severity. Evidence from various studies—observational, genetic, and mechanistic—indicates a link between periodontitis and a higher risk of COVID-19 infection and poorer outcomes. Therefore, incorporating periodontal health into pandemic preparedness and public health plans is essential, achievable through routine periodontal screening, prompt treatment, and targeted oral hygiene measures. These actions can lower systemic inflammation, strengthen resistance against respiratory pathogens, and reduce severe outcomes in future pandemics.

References

1. Bernabe E, et al. Global, regional, and national levels and trends in burden of oral conditions from 1990 to 2017: a systematic analysis for the global burden of disease 2017 study. J Dent Res. 2020;99(4):362–73.
2. Fu H, et al. Global burden of periodontal diseases among the working-age population from 1990–2021: results from the Global Burden of Disease Study 2021. BMC Public Health. 2025;25(1):1316.

3. Nascimento GG, Alves-Costa S, Romandini M. Burden of severe periodontitis and edentulism in 2021, with projections up to 2050: the global burden of disease 2021 study. J Periodontal Res. 2024;59(5):823–67.
4. Lamers MM, Haagmans BL. SARS-CoV-2 pathogenesis. Nat Rev Microbiol. 2022;20(5):270–84.
5. Jackson CB, et al. Mechanisms of SARS-CoV-2 entry into cells. Nat Rev Mol Cell Biol. 2022;23(1):3–20.
6. Malone B, et al. Structures and functions of coronavirus replication–transcription complexes and their relevance for SARS-CoV-2 drug design. Nat Rev Mol Cell Biol. 2022;23(1):21–39.
7. Martínez-García M, Hernández-Lemus E. Periodontal inflammation and systemic diseases: an overview. Front Physiol. 2021;12:709438.
8. Hajishengallis G. Periodontitis: from microbial immune subversion to systemic inflammation. Nat Rev Immunol. 2015;15(1):30–44.
9. Bhuyan R, et al. Periodontitis and its inflammatory changes linked to various systemic diseases: a review of its underlying mechanisms. Biomedicine. 2022;10(10):2659.
10. Peres MA, et al. Oral diseases: a global public health challenge. Lancet. 2019;394(10194):249–60.
11. Eke PI, et al. Periodontitis in US adults: national health and nutrition examination survey 2009–2014. J Am Dent Assoc. 2018;149(7):576–588.e6.
12. Stabholz A, Soskolne WA, Shapira L. Genetic and environmental risk factors for chronic periodontitis and aggressive periodontitis. Periodontol. 2000;2010(53):138–53.
13. Laine ML, Crielaard W, Loos BG. Genetic susceptibility to periodontitis. Periodontol 2000. 2012;58(1):37–68.
14. Divaris K, et al. Exploring the genetic basis of chronic periodontitis: a genome-wide association study. Hum Mol Genet. 2013;22(11):2312–24.
15. Kitamoto S, et al. The intermucosal connection between the mouth and gut in commensal pathobiont-driven colitis. Cell. 2020;182(2):447–462.e14.
16. Abed J, et al. Fap2 mediates Fusobacterium nucleatum colorectal adenocarcinoma enrichment by binding to tumor-expressed Gal-GalNAc. Cell Host Microbe. 2016;20(2):215–25.
17. Atarashi K, et al. Ectopic colonization of oral bacteria in the intestine drives TH1 cell induction and inflammation. Science. 2017;358(6361):359–65.
18. Blasco-Baque V, et al. Periodontitis induced by Porphyromonas gingivalis drives periodontal microbiota dysbiosis and insulin resistance via an impaired adaptive immune response. Gut. 2017;66(5):872–85.
19. Konig MF, et al. Aggregatibacter actinomycetemcomitans-induced hypercitrullination links periodontal infection to autoimmunity in rheumatoid arthritis. Sci Transl Med. 2016;8(369):369ra176.
20. Sato K, et al. Aggravation of collagen-induced arthritis by orally administered Porphyromonas gingivalis through modulation of the gut microbiota and gut immune system. Sci Rep. 2017;7(1):6955.
21. Hoare A, et al. Chronic inflammation as a link between periodontitis and carcinogenesis. Mediat Inflamm. 2019;2019:1029857.
22. Genco RJ, Sanz M. Clinical and public health implications of periodontal and systemic diseases: an overview. Periodontol 2000. 2020;83(1):7–13.
23. Potempa J, Mydel P, Koziel J. The case for periodontitis in the pathogenesis of rheumatoid arthritis. Nat Rev Rheumatol. 2017;13(10):606–20.
24. Molina A, et al. The association between respiratory diseases and periodontitis: a systematic review and meta-analysis. J Clin Periodontol. 2023;50(6):842–87.
25. Zhang Z, et al. Advances in the relationship between periodontopathogens and respiratory diseases (review). Mol Med Rep. 2024;29(3):42.
26. Brock M, Bahammam S, Sima C. The relationships among periodontitis, pneumonia and COVID-19. Front Oral Health. 2021;2:801815.
27. Shi T, et al. Periodontopathogens Porphyromonas gingivalis and Fusobacterium nucleatum and their roles in the progression of respiratory diseases. Pathogens. 2023;12(9):1110.

28. Suzuki R, et al. Fusobacterium nucleatum exacerbates chronic obstructive pulmonary disease in elastase-induced emphysematous mice. FEBS Open Bio. 2022;12(3):638–48.
29. Li Q, et al. Oral pathogen Fusobacterium nucleatum Coaggregates with Pseudomonas aeruginosa to modulate the inflammatory cytotoxicity of pulmonary epithelial cells. Front Cell Infect Microbiol. 2021;11:643913.
30. Benedyk M, et al. Gingipains: critical factors in the development of aspiration pneumonia caused by Porphyromonas gingivalis. J Innate Immun. 2016;8(2):185–98.
31. Feng N, et al. P. gingivalis alters lung microbiota and aggravates disease severity of COPD rats by up-regulating Hsp90α/MLKL. J Oral Microbiol. 2024;16(1):2334588.
32. Yuanjun Z, et al. Porphyromonas gingivalis-induced hematogenous disseminated severe pneumonia: a case report. J Int Med Res. 2024;52(3):3000605231213760.
33. Chen Y, et al. Porphyromonas gingivalis induced inflammatory responses and promoted apoptosis in lung epithelial cells infected with H1N1 via the Bcl-2/Bax/Caspase-3 signaling pathway. Mol Med Rep. 2018;18(1):97–104.
34. Watanabe N, et al. Exposure to Porphyromonas gingivalis induces production of Proinflammatory cytokine via TLR2 from human respiratory epithelial cells. J Clin Med. 2020;9(11):3433.
35. Hajishengallis G, Chavakis T. Local and systemic mechanisms linking periodontal disease and inflammatory comorbidities. Nat Rev Immunol. 2021;21(7):426–40.
36. Villoria GEM, et al. Periodontal disease: a systemic condition. Periodontol 2000. 2024;96(1):7–19.
37. Bui FQ, et al. Association between periodontal pathogens and systemic disease. Biom J. 2019;42(1):27–35.
38. Tamimi F, Altigani S, Sanz M. Periodontitis and coronavirus disease 2019. Periodontol 2000. 2022;89(1):207–14.
39. Suh JS, et al. Periodontitis-induced systemic inflammation exacerbates atherosclerosis partly via endothelial–mesenchymal transition in mice. Int J Oral Sci. 2019;11(3):21.
40. White PC, et al. Neutrophil extracellular traps in periodontitis: a web of intrigue. J Dent Res. 2016;95(1):26–34.
41. Fine N, et al. Periodontal inflammation primes the systemic innate immune response. J Dent Res. 2021;100(3):318–25.
42. Hiti L, et al. The immunopathogenesis of a cytokine storm: the key mechanisms underlying severe COVID-19. Cytokine Growth Factor Rev. 2025;82:1–17.
43. Zanza C, et al. Cytokine storm in COVID-19: immunopathogenesis and therapy. Medicina. 2022;58:144. https://doi.org/10.3390/medicina58020144.
44. Hoffmann D. The role of the oral cavity in SARS-CoV-2- and other viral infections. Clin Oral Investig. 2023;27(1):15–22.
45. Wadia R. Relevance of oral cavity in COVID. Br Dent J. 2020;229(2):125.
46. Troeltzsch M, Berndt R, Troeltzsch M. Is the oral cavity a reservoir for prolonged SARS-CoV-2 shedding? Med Hypotheses. 2021;146:110419.
47. Coke CJ, et al. SARS-CoV-2 infection and oral health: therapeutic opportunities and challenges. J Clin Med. 2021;10(1):156.
48. Iyer P, Chino T, Ojcius DM. Infection of the oral cavity with SARS-CoV-2 variants: scope of salivary diagnostics. Front Oral Health. 2022;3:1001790.
49. Schwartz J, et al. Oral SARS-CoV-2 infection and risk for long Covid. Rev Med Virol. 2025;35(2):e70029.
50. Herrera D, et al. Is the oral cavity relevant in SARS-CoV-2 pandemic? Clin Oral Investig. 2020;24(8):2925–30.
51. Brandini DA, et al. Covid-19 and oral diseases: crosstalk, synergy or association? Rev Med Virol. 2021;31(6):e2226.
52. Drozdzik A, Drozdzik M. Oral pathology in COVID-19 and SARS-CoV-2 infection-molecular aspects. Int J Mol Sci. 2022;23(3):1431.
53. Bellocchio L, et al. COVID-19 on oral health: a new bilateral connection for the pandemic. Biomedicine. 2023;12(1):60.

54. Farid H, et al. Oral manifestations of Covid-19-a literature review. Rev Med Virol. 2022;32(1):e2248.
55. Martín Carreras-Presas C, et al. Oral vesiculobullous lesions associated with SARS-CoV-2 infection. Oral Dis. 2021;27(Suppl 3):710–2.
56. Ohnishi T, et al. Periodontitis promotes the expression of gingival transmembrane serine protease 2 (TMPRSS2), a priming protease for severe acute respiratory syndrome coronavirus 2 (SARS-CoV-2). J Oral Biosci. 2022;64(2):229–36.
57. Meng Z, et al. Association between periodontitis and COVID-19 infection: a two-sample Mendelian randomization study. PeerJ. 2023;11:e14595.
58. Natto ZS, et al. Can periodontal pockets and caries lesions act as reservoirs for coronavirus? Mol Oral Microbiol. 2022;37(2):77–80.
59. Guardado-Luevanos I, et al. Self-reported periodontal disease and its association with SARS-CoV-2 infection. Int J Environ Res Public Health. 2022;19(16):10306.
60. Katz J, Yue S, Xue W. Dental diseases are associated with increased odds ratio for coronavirus disease 19. Oral Dis. 2022;28(Suppl 1):991–3.
61. Andrews M, et al. Increased odds for COVID-19 infection among individuals with periodontal disease. Clin Oral Investig. 2023;27(10):5925–33.
62. Wang Y, et al. Periodontal disease increases the host susceptibility to COVID-19 and its severity: a Mendelian randomization study. J Transl Med. 2021;19(1):528.
63. Mehta P, et al. COVID-19: consider cytokine storm syndromes and immunosuppression. Lancet. 2020;395(10229):1033–4.
64. Tang Y, et al. Cytokine storm in COVID-19: the current evidence and treatment strategies. Front Immunol. 2020;11:1708.
65. Gibson PG, Qin L, Puah SH. COVID-19 acute respiratory distress syndrome (ARDS): clinical features and differences from typical pre-COVID-19 ARDS. Med J Aust. 2020;213(2):54–56.e1.
66. Doutrelon C, et al. Long-term outcomes of COVID-19-associated pulmonary embolism: a French single-center retrospective study with one-year follow-up. Thrombosis Update. 2024;14:100156.
67. Gul MH, et al. Predictors and outcomes of acute pulmonary embolism in COVID-19; insights from US national COVID cohort collaborative. Respir Res. 2023;24(1):59.
68. Ortega-Paz L, et al. COVID-19-associated pulmonary embolism: review of the pathophysiology, epidemiology, prevention, diagnosis, and treatment. Semin Thromb Hemost. 2023;49(8):816–32.
69. Zaim S, et al. COVID-19 and multiorgan response. Curr Probl Cardiol. 2020;45(8):100618.
70. Wu T, et al. Multi-organ dysfunction in patients with COVID-19: a systematic review and meta-analysis. Aging Dis. 2020;11(4):874–94.
71. Birhanu A, et al. Incidence and predictors of organ failure among COVID-19 hospitalized adult patients in Eastern Ethiopia. Hospital-based retrospective cohort study. BMC Infect Dis. 2022;22(1):412.
72. Lin EC, et al. Unraveling the link between periodontitis and coronavirus disease 2019: exploring pathogenic pathways and clinical implications. Biomedicines. 2023;11(10):2789.
73. Silvestre FJ, Márquez-Arrico CF. COVID-19 and periodontitis: a dangerous association? Front Pharmacol. 2022;12:789681.
74. Al-Maweri SA, et al. The impact of periodontal disease on the clinical outcomes of COVID-19: a systematic review and meta-analysis. BMC Oral Health. 2023;23(1):658.
75. Cai W, et al. Nature of the interplay between periodontal diseases and COVID-19. Frontiers in Dental Medicine. 2021;2:735126.
76. Marouf N, et al. Association between periodontitis and severity of COVID-19 infection: a case-control study. J Clin Periodontol. 2021;48(4):483–91.
77. Marouf N, et al. COVID-19 severity in patients with apical periodontitis: a case control study. Int Dent J. 2024;74(4):736–45.
78. Macherla S, et al. Can periodontitis affect the COVID-19 severity, symptoms, hospital stay, and mortality? A case–control study. Front Public Health. 2024;12:1421380.

79. Moradi Haghgoo J, et al. Association between the severity of periodontitis, COVID-19, C-reactive protein and interleukin-6 levels in hospitalized patients: a case–control study. BMC Oral Health. 2023;23(1):556.
80. Bemquerer LM, et al. Clinical, immunological, and microbiological analysis of the association between periodontitis and COVID-19: a case-control study. Odontology. 2024;112(1):208–20.
81. Gupta S, et al. Compromised periodontal status could increase mortality for patients with COVID-19. Lancet Infect Dis. 2022;22(3):314.
82. Said KN, et al. Association of periodontal therapy, with inflammatory biomarkers and complications in COVID-19 patients: a case control study. Clin Oral Investig. 2022;26(11):6721–32.
83. Roganović J, et al. Post-viral alterations in periodontal health in individuals recovering from COVID-19. Front Oral Health. 2025;6:1654029.
84. Avais LS, et al. Oral manifestations in the post COVID-19 condition: a systematic review with meta-analysis. Rev Med Virol. 2025;35(4):e70057.
85. Isola G, et al. Periodontal health and disease in the context of systemic diseases. Mediat Inflamm. 2023;2023:9720947.
86. Casarin M, et al. Association between sequelae of COVID-19 with periodontal disease and obesity: a cross-sectional study. J Periodontol. 2024;95(7):688–98.
87. Sari A, Dikmen NK, Nibali L. Association between periodontal diseases and COVID-19 infection: a case-control study with a longitudinal arm. Odontology. 2023;111(4):1009–17.

Oral Mucosal Lesions Associated with COVID-19

25

Shankargouda Patil, Shilpa Bhandi, and Frank W. Licari

25.1 Introduction

The coronavirus disease 2019 (COVID-19) emerged in late 2019 and rapidly developed into a global pandemic. It has affected approximately 778 million people worldwide [1]. COVID-19, caused by the severe acute respiratory syndrome coronavirus 2 (SARS-CoV-2), has resulted in widespread mortality and morbidity worldwide. The most common symptoms include fever, cough, fatigue, and loss of smell or taste. In severe cases, patients may develop pneumonia or respiratory failure. While it mainly affects the respiratory tract, other organ systems have also been found to be affected. Among the extrapulmonary manifestations, the oral cavity has garnered increasing attention for its role as both a portal of viral entry and a site of clinical symptoms, including mucosal lesions [2, 3].

Initially, the oral manifestations in COVID-19 patients were often unnoticed and therefore underreported. They were mainly attributed to reactions to medications, secondary infections, or mechanical trauma. However, with an increasing number of COVID-19 patients exhibiting oral mucosal changes, researchers worldwide have emphasized the possibility of direct or indirect viral involvement, suggesting a broader spectrum of clinical implications [4]. A multitude of oral lesions have been reported in COVID-19 patients, namely aphthous-like ulcers, herpetiform lesions, erythema multiforme-like eruptions, desquamative gingivitis, benign migratory glossitis, candidiasis, xerostomia, sialadenitis, altered taste sensation, gingivitis, necrotizing periodontitis, glossitis, white-coated tongue, mucositis, and petechiae. These may manifest as ulcers, erosions, blisters, plaque-like lesions, or maculopapular rashes [4–8].

The oral mucosa is composed of stratified squamous epithelium and functions as a critical protective barrier. It contributes to sensory perception and secretory

S. Patil (✉) · S. Bhandi · F. W. Licari
College of Dental Medicine, Roseman University of Health Sciences, South Jordan, UT, USA
e-mail: spatil@roseman.edu; sbhandi@roseman.edu; flicari@roseman.edu

S. R. Prabhu et al. (eds.), *COVID-19 in Dental Practice*,
https://doi.org/10.1007/978-3-032-26000-0_25

activity while maintaining a complex microbial ecosystem inside the oral cavity. These epithelial cells are metabolically active with the potential to produce cytokines, adhesion molecules, and growth factors in response to various stimuli [3]. This structural and immunological complexity, combined with a diverse microbial environment, makes the oral cavity both a potential entry point for viral pathogens and a reservoir for persistent infections [9].

One of the key factors implicated in COVID-19-associated oral changes is the angiotensin-converting enzyme 2 (ACE2) receptor. SARS-CoV-2, a positive-sense RNA virus with an icosahedral structure, uses its spike (S) proteins to bind to ACE2 receptors on human cells [10]. These receptors are expressed in multiple oral tissues, particularly in the epithelial cells of the tongue and salivary glands [11, 12]. The ACE2 receptor, along with transmembrane protease serine 2 (TMPRSS2), facilitates the entry of SARS-CoV-2 virus into host cells by binding to the S proteins of the virus, thereby enabling them to use the machinery of these host cells to replicate and subsequently destroy these same cells, triggering the oral symptoms and signs [11, 12].

Recent immunohistochemical and transcriptomic studies have shown high levels of ACE2 expression in several regions of the oral mucosa, including the tongue, buccal mucosa, and gingiva, as well as in the ductal and acinar cells of the major and minor salivary glands [11, 12].

The dorsum surface of the tongue, palate, and salivary gland ducts have been reported to demonstrate the highest ACE2 receptor densities, surpassing those of nasal and pharyngeal tissues. Single-cell RNA sequencing has confirmed that ACE2 expression is particularly elevated in these oral tissues, suggesting that the oral cavity is a high-risk site for viral replication [12].

The involvement of the salivary glands is significant, as they can serve as early sites of viral proliferation. Infection of the salivary epithelium can lead to the early release of viral particles into saliva, sometimes even before respiratory symptoms develop. This may help explain cases where oral lesions precede or accompany systemic symptoms in COVID-19 or in patients without significant respiratory involvement, independent of secondary factors such as medication use, trauma, or opportunistic infections [13].

A wide variety of oral mucosal lesions have been reported in individuals with COVID-19. These may appear during the active phase of infection, after recovery, or in association with multisystem inflammatory syndrome in pediatric populations [14]. However, identifying whether these lesions are directly related to SARS-CoV-2 infection can be difficult due to the wide range of contributing factors. Possible causes include stress-related immune suppression, adverse drug reactions, trauma due to mechanical ventilation, and secondary infections [15, 16].

Despite these heterogeneities, increasing evidence emphasizes the need for recognizing oral manifestations associated with COVID-19, which may serve as early diagnostic indicators of severity [17, 18].

Given the diagnostic significance of the oral cavity in systemic illnesses, this chapter provides a comprehensive overview of oral mucosal lesions associated with

COVID-19, exploring their pathogenesis and key considerations for oral healthcare professionals.

25.2 Aphthous-Like Lesions

25.2.1 Definition and Overview

Aphthous-like lesions are painful ulcerations of the oral mucosa clinically resembling recurrent aphthous stomatitis (RAS) but arising in the absence of the classical predisposing factors. Recent studies have reported these lesions in COVID-19 patients across various populations and clinical severities [9, 13]. They typically present as well-defined, painful ulcers. They predominantly affect the non-keratinized mucosa, such as the labial and buccal mucosa, ventral tongue, and floor of the mouth [19, 20].

Unlike classical RAS, which is often linked to genetic factors, trauma, nutritional deficiencies, or immune dysfunction, aphthous-like lesions related to COVID-19 have been observed in individuals without any prior history of recurrent ulcers and often in temporal proximity to SARS-CoV-2 infection [19, 21]. They may occur during the acute viremic phase, as part of the systemic inflammatory cascade, or in the early convalescent period, suggesting a role for ongoing immune dysregulation [21].

In contrast to idiopathic RAS, which tends to recur over time, aphthous-like lesions in COVID-19 are typically acute, self-limiting, and resolve as systemic symptoms improve [7, 22]. While classic RAS normally recurs over months or years following a trigger, several reports suggest that the aphthous-like lesions in COVID-19 cases are acute and self-limiting and may not recur once systemic recovery is achieved [9, 23].

25.2.2 Etiology and Risk Factors

The aphthous-like lesions in COVID-19 have a multifactorial etiology, arising from a complex interplay of direct viral effects, immune dysregulation, vascular pathology, and secondary environmental or iatrogenic factors. This is significantly different from classical recurrent aphthous stomatitis (RAS), which is often linked to genetic predisposition, local trauma, or hematinic deficiencies [13, 19, 20]. A myriad of secondary cofactors further amplifies the risk of aphthous-like lesions in COVID-19, including xerostomia, nutritional deficiencies, and psychological stress. Xerostomia may occur due to salivary gland dysfunction, reducing mucosal lubrication and antimicrobial activity, while nutritional deficiencies (iron, folate, vitamin B12), particularly in debilitated patients, further compromise epithelial integrity of the oral tissues. Further, psychological stress associated with severe infection and prolonged isolation due to the disease may exacerbate immune dysregulation [11, 16, 21]. Moreover, use of varied drugs (antivirals, antibiotics, or immunomodulators) and, sometimes, overuse, can intensify aphthous-like lesions in the oral mucosa. Notably, in hospitalized patients, mechanical trauma from endotracheal intubation additionally predisposes the oral mucosa to breakdown, further leading to ulcerations [6, 24]. Other host factors, such as young age of the patient, no prior history of RAS, and other systemic comorbidities, act as additional risk factors for aphthous-like lesions in the oral cavity [6].

25.2.3 Epidemiology

There is no observed gender predilection in aphthous-like lesions, though a slight female predominance has been noted in some cohorts. This possibly reflects the higher baseline prevalence of idiopathic RAS in women. Additionally, most cases occur in young to middle-aged adults (20–60 years), with pediatric cases being uncommon, possibly due to the milder systemic response in children [6, 13, 19, 20, 24].

25.2.4 Presentation in the Context of COVID-19

Reports have suggested a strong association between aphthous-like lesions and the biological and systemic effects of COVID-19 infection. Studies have shown that SARS-CoV-2 exhibits tropism for oral epithelial cells due to the high expression of ACE2 and TMPRSS2 receptors in the oral mucosa, particularly in non-keratinized areas, such as the tongue, buccal mucosa, and salivary ducts [12]. During the infection, binding of the SARS-CoV-2 virus and its subsequent replication can induce apoptosis of the cells and barrier disruption, thereby leading to ulceration. In addition, immunohistochemical studies have confirmed the presence of SARS-CoV-2 RNA within oral lesions, especially in the epithelial and endothelial cells, further highlighting the direct viral etiology in causing cytopathic injury to oral tissues, leading to these aphthous-like lesions associated with COVID-19 disease [9, 15].

The concept of immune dysregulation and hyperinflammation associated with the aphthous-like lesions in COVID-19 may be attributed to the "cytokine storm," which is characteristic of the infection. This "cytokine storm" causes an increase in the levels of interleukin (IL)-6, tumor necrosis factor (TNF)-α, and IL-1β, which promote apoptosis of the epithelial cells and mucosal breakdown [25]. This immune-mediated epithelial destruction is a plausible explanation for the ulcerative pathology observed in aphthous-like lesions. Moreover, reduced lymphocyte counts (lymphopenia), commonly seen in moderate-to-severe COVID-19, may impair mucosal immune surveillance, predisposing the oral mucosa to ulcerations caused by opportunistic or secondary factors [26].

Studies have shown that COVID-19 is associated with widespread endothelialitis, microvascular injuries, and thrombosis [27]. Furthermore, oral biopsies from patients with ulcerative lesions often reveal edema of endothelial cells, vascular congestion, and microthrombi in subepithelial plexuses, similar to COVID-19 [15]. Local ischemia and necrosis secondary to vascular injury may also have a role in the pathogenesis of these oral ulcers, which often present with intense pain despite their small size, a classic sign also observed in patients with ischemic oral injuries [15]. Clinically, these lesions often appear during the acute or early convalescent phase of infection, sometimes preceding respiratory symptoms, suggesting they may represent an early mucosal indicator of systemic disease. Unlike recurrent aphthous stomatitis, these ulcers are typically acute, self-limiting, and arise in association with SARS-CoV-2 infection, further highlighting their relationship to the pathophysiology of COVID-19 [6, 9, 15, 19, 20].

25.3 Ulcers and Erosion

Oral ulcers and erosions are among the most common mucosal changes observed in patients with COVID-19. Ulcers are defined as discontinuities in the oral epithelium that extend into the underlying connective tissue, often covered by a fibrinous pseudomembrane and surrounded by an erythematous halo. Erosions, on the other hand, are superficial defects confined to the epithelium, usually presenting as shallow, painful, erythematous areas. Both ulcers and erosions are clinically significant as they compromise several oral functions, causing pain and discomfort, and may serve as visible indicators of systemic viral activity [12, 20, 25]. Notably, ulcers and erosions have been reported in the majority of COVID-19 patients, across all disease severities, from mild outpatient cases to critically ill individuals.

25.3.1 Etiology and Risk Factors

The development of ulcers and erosions in COVID-19 has a multifactorial etiology with several risk factors, akin to aphthous-like lesions. The risk factors include immune dysregulation, microvascular injury leading to ischemia, direct epithelial damage by SARS-CoV-2 due to increased ACE2 receptor expression in the oral mucosa, and cytokine release. Additional predisposing factors include xerostomia, poor oral health status, nutritional deficiencies, and opportunistic infections. Candida or herpesviruses are the common opportunistic infections encountered, especially in patients on corticosteroids or broad-spectrum antibiotics, which is quite common during the treatment of COVID-19. Patients with prolonged hospitalization are at heightened risk owing to drug-induced mucositis, trauma from intubation or oxygen devices, and immunocompromised status. In addition, elderly patients with comorbidities and immunosuppression are further predisposed to the development of ulcers and erosions [12, 15, 25–27].

25.3.2 Epidemiology

The reported prevalence of ulcers and erosions ranges from 4% to 20% of infected patients [15, 24]. These lesions have been observed across all age groups but are more frequent in adults, with a female predilection, particularly those with moderate to severe disease or with systemic comorbidities [5, 13].

25.3.3 Presentation in the Context of COVID-19

The COVID-19-associated oral ulcers and erosions are associated with multifaceted pathophysiology. The SARS-CoV-2 virus exhibits tropism for oral epithelial cells and salivary glands due to the abundant expression of ACE2 and TMPRSS2 receptors. This facilitates direct viral entry, leading to apoptosis and mucosal breakdown. In addition, the hyperinflammatory response, characterized by a cytokine storm with elevated IL-6, IL-1β, and TNF-α, causes immune-mediated epithelial necrosis and delays mucosal healing, which is aggravated by the patient's immunocompromised state due to concurrent lymphopenia [4, 9, 10, 12, 25, 27]. In addition, studies have suggested dysfunction of the microvasculature, including endothelialitis, vascular congestion, and microthrombi in oral tissues, which reduces perfusion and produces ischemic necrosis, clinically manifesting as painful ulcerations. These mechanisms are often compounded by nutritional deficiencies, zinc overload, the arbitrary use of high-dose antibiotics and corticosteroids, and other opportunistic infections, such as candidiasis, HSV, and VZV, especially in immunocompromised and long-hospitalized patients. Interestingly, the fact that these ulcers and erosions often appear during the acute or early convalescent phase of COVID-19, sometimes preceding even the systemic symptoms, highlights that these lesions are not incidental but represent both local mucosal damage and systemic disease activity, potentially serving as early indicators of disease severity in COVID-19 [10, 24, 25, 27, 28].

25.4 Vesiculobullous Lesions

Vesiculobullous lesions, though not as common as ulcers and erosions, are another COVID-19-associated oral lesion. They are fluid-filled mucocutaneous lesions characterized by the formation of vesicles (small, <5 mm blisters) and bullae (larger, >5 mm blisters) within or beneath the oral epithelium. These lesions tend to rupture easily, leaving behind shallow, painful erosions or ulcers. They have been reported to occur both in the keratinized and in the non-keratinized oral mucosa, with a predilection for the tongue, palate, lips, and buccal mucosa. These lesions may occur either in isolation or in association with other mucosal alterations such as ulcers, petechiae, or erythematous patches [6, 13].

25.4.1 Etiology and Risk Factors

Vesiculobullous lesions are primarily immune-mediated disorders triggered by viral entry into the body. The SARS-CoV-2 virus causes epithelial injury, weakening the mucosal surface, leading to intraepithelial blister formation. Unlike ulcerative lesions, which are caused by tissue necrosis at a deeper level, vesiculobullous lesions appear to arise from a cytopathic effect at the surface level, often precipitated by localized viral replication or an autoimmune response. Recent studies have also implicated a drug-induced hypersensitivity reaction with presentations similar to erythema multiforme and Stevens-Johnson syndrome, particularly in patients on antivirals, antibiotics, or corticosteroids. Interestingly, these lesions have also been found on individuals after administration of COVID-19 vaccines [29]. Vascular compromise may also be a contributing factor, but more as a secondary aggravating factor than a primary etiological factor [6, 24, 25, 27].

25.4.2 Epidemiology

Vesiculobullous lesions in COVID-19 are relatively uncommon, with studies reporting a prevalence of 1–5% among infected patients [6]. They are more frequently observed in middle-aged and elderly patients with moderate to severe disease, with a slight female prevalence. This is possibly due to the greater tendency of immune-mediated oral conditions in women [13]. However, most systematic reviews emphasize that the occurrence is more closely related to immune status, disease severity, and comorbidities rather than gender differences [15].

25.4.3 Presentation in the Context of COVID-19

The association of vesiculobullous lesions with COVID-19 is a complex interplay of viral, immune, and iatrogenic factors that predispose to intraepithelial blister formation. Unlike ulcerative lesions that predominantly result from necrosis of the epithelial cells and ischemia, vesiculobullous lesions, including pemphigus, pemphigoid, etc., appear to arise from epithelial fragility and tear at the level of epithelium or connective tissue. Oral epithelial cells and keratinocytes in the oral mucosa have a strong affinity for ACE2 and TMPRSS2 receptors and are therefore direct targets of SARS-CoV-2. Viral entry and replication within these cells subsequently disrupt cell–cell adhesion and promote vesicle formation [7, 12, 30]. In addition, the exaggerated immune response and cytokine storm in COVID-19, characterized by elevated IL 6, TNF α, and IFN γ, can induce immune mediated apoptosis of epithe lial cells, leading to epithelial or subepithelial clefting. This creates an ideal environment for vesiculobullous eruptions, which are commonly seen during the disease [25]. Several cases have been linked to drug-induced hypersensitivity reactions, particularly to antivirals, antibiotics, and corticosteroids administered during COVID-19 management. Vaccinations, namely Moderna, Pfizer, AstraZeneca, and

Sinovac vaccines, have also been reported to cause vesicular lesions and papulovesicular lesions in patients infected with the deadly disease [29]. Furthermore, bullous reactions from COVID-19 vaccines have been reported after the first or second dose of the Moderna vaccine. These vesiculobullous reactions could be attributed to immune dysregulation triggered by vaccine-induced cytokine release, which may damage basal keratinocytes and weaken epithelial integrity. This could potentially lead to intra-epithelial separation or separation between epithelium and connective tissue. In some cases, molecular mimicry between SARS-CoV-2 spike proteins and host antigens can precipitate autoimmune blistering diseases, such as pemphigus vulgaris or mucous membrane pemphigoid [25, 32]. Vaccination can also act as a trigger in genetically predisposed individuals, unmasking latent autoimmune disease or causing hypersensitivity to vaccine excipients [7, 30, 31]. These reactions often mimic erythema multiforme or Stevens–Johnson syndrome, with widespread vesiculobullous eruptions affecting both oral and extraoral mucosa [7, 24]. Moreover, vascular alterations secondary to COVID-19, including endothelial damage, microthrombi, and ischemia formation, may act as cofactors that disrupt the basement membrane, facilitating blister development [27]. Opportunistic viral reactivations (notably HSV and VZV) have also been observed in immunosuppressed patients, sometimes presenting as vesiculobullous lesions superimposed on SARS-CoV-2 infection [33, 34].

25.5 Plaques

A plaque is defined as a slightly elevated, flat-topped lesion of the oral mucosa larger than 1 cm in diameter, produced by localized epithelial or connective tissue alterations [35]. Depending on the underlying pathology, plaques may appear white, erythematous, or pigmented, covering a broader surface area. In the oral cavity, plaques are only a clinical manifestation rather than a diagnosis in themselves. They are commonly seen in conditions such as oral lichen planus, leukoplakia, candidiasis, and autoimmune mucocutaneous disorders [35, 36]. In patients with COVID-19, plaques may be found in the oral cavity, possibly reflecting immune reaction to the epithelium, secondary infection, or drug-related mucosal changes. Interestingly, even patients with no apparent symptoms of the disease may develop painful whitish oral plaques, suggesting that even mild or asymptomatic infections may predispose to such mucosal changes [22].

25.5.1 Etiology and Risk Factors

Plaque-type lesions in COVID-19 have varied etiological factors. Opportunistic infections, such as candidiasis, often cause the pseudomembranous curd-type plaques. Several studies have documented oral candidiasis in COVID-19 patients, primarily due to the frequent use of corticosteroids and broad-spectrum antibiotics, immunosuppression, and hyposalivation [6, 13]. Further, “coated” or hairy white tongue plaques are frequently a biofilm phenomenon which commonly arises from salivary gland dysfunction and microbial dysbiosis by the SARS-COV-2 virus, augmented by poor oral hygiene during the illness [19, 22]. Keratotic or lichenoid plaques may reflect post-infectious immune dysregulation or drug-induced mucosal reactions, including those reported after vaccination [15, 37]. Reactivation of latent viruses, such as EBV, can cause hairy (verrucous) leukoplakia-like plaques on the lateral tongue in otherwise immunocompetent hosts [22]. Lastly, in critically ill patients, particularly in the ICU, iatrogenic trauma and dehydration from intubation or oxygen therapy can also lead to necrotic or keratotic plaque formation in the oral cavity [16].

25.5.2 Epidemiology

These are relatively rare lesions among COVID-19 patients but have been documented with a reported frequency of around 2–5% in hospitalized patients with no gender predilection [6, 22]. They appear more commonly in individuals with systemic comorbidities, immunosuppression, or patients on prolonged corticosteroid/antibiotic use [13, 37].

25.5.3 Presentation in the Context of COVID-19

Several studies suggest that plaque-type lesions in COVID-19 arise from a convergence of viral, immune, hematological, and iatrogenic mechanisms. It is well established that SARS-CoV-2 directly infects oral epithelial and salivary acinar cells via the ACE2 receptor, causing epithelial damage and hyposalivation, which facilitates the development of keratotic or coated plaques [12]. In addition, the cytokine storm characteristic of severe infection alters the epithelial turnover and induces lichenoid inflammatory reactions, producing non-scrapable whitish plaques in some patients [25]. Thrombocytopenia and microvascular injury, frequently documented in COVID-19, further produce ischemic changes in the mucosa. Reduced platelet counts, endothelial dysfunction, and fibrin microthrombi impair local tissue healing, favoring necrotic or keratotic plaque formation, particularly in critically ill or ICU-managed patients [16, 38]. *Candida albicans*, an otherwise normal commensal in the oral cavity, is a notorious pathogen that causes secondary opportunistic infections, notably candidiasis, the most frequent plaque-forming etiology. The patients, already in an immunocompromised state with poor oral hygiene, are promptly attacked by this fungus, the effect further escalated by prolonged and intensified COVID treatment protocols, immunosuppression, and xerostomia. These present as curd-like pseudomembranous plaques that are removable, leaving erythematous bases [6, 13]. Interestingly, alterations in the oral microbiome and tongue-coating thickness have been related with disease severity, suggesting that plaque changes may serve as clinical markers of systemic status [19]. Reactivation of latent viruses namely Epstein–Barr virus, can result in hairy leukoplakia-like plaques on the lateral tongue, while trauma during medical procedures and device-related mucosal injury may add to the burden of necrotic plaque formation in hospitalized patients [16, 22]. It is to be noted that such lesions have also been observed in asymptomatic or mildly symptomatic COVID-19 cases, highlighting that oral plaques are not limited to severe disease but represent a broad spectrum COVID-19 manifestation [22].

25.6 Petechiae

Petechiae are defined as small, pinpoint, non-blanching hemorrhagic spots that occur due to extravasation of blood from capillaries into the superficial oral mucosa. They typically measure less than 2 mm in diameter and present as round or irregular reddish to purplish macules that do not disappear on pressure [35]. Unlike erythematous lesions, petechiae imply underlying vascular fragility or platelet dysfunction rather than inflammation. In the oral cavity, petechiae appear as either isolated findings or grouped in clusters, most commonly on the soft palate, buccal mucosa, lips, and tongue. While they are often associated with trauma, systemic infections, or hematologic disorders, their occurrence in COVID-19 has been increasingly documented in several studies. In patients with COVID-19, they are thought to arise from thrombocytopenia, endothelial injury, and microvascular compromise caused by SARS-CoV-2 infection [24, 38]. Thus, oral petechiae may serve as early indicators of systemic coagulopathy or vascular involvement in COVID-19 patients.

25.6.1 Etiology and Risk Factors

Hematologic and vascular changes are widespread in COVID-19 patients, and the formation of oral petechiae can be attributed to the same. Thrombocytopenia is a common finding in moderate to severe forms of the infection and predisposes to capillary bleeding, leading to petechiae [38]. Studies have reported endothelial injury and formation of microthrombi due to SARS-CoV-2–induced vasculitis, which weakens the vessel walls. This subsequently facilitates extravasation of red blood cells [39]. Systemic coagulopathy and platelet dysfunction further contribute to petechial formation in these patients [26].

Furthermore, mechanical trauma from coughing, vomiting, or intubation can accentuate the rupture of mucosal capillaries, serving as potential risk factors [16]. Medications, particularly anticoagulants or corticosteroids used in COVID-19 management, can also increase the bleeding tendency [40]. Further, comorbidities such as diabetes, hypertension, and preexisting hematologic disorders are known to increase the susceptibility to petechiae formation.

25.6.2 Epidemiology

In COVID-19 patients, petechiae is a relatively uncommon oral manifestation. It shows no gender predilection, though some studies indicate a slight male predominance, reflecting a potential higher COVID-19 severity in men. Further, they can occur across age groups but are more common in older adults and severely ill patients [6, 15, 22].

25.6.3 Presentation in the Context of COVID-19

Increasing evidence suggests that petechiae in COVID-19 occur as a consequence of the infection's multifactorial impact on the hematologic and vascular systems. The SARS-CoV-2 virus infects the endothelial cells via ACE2 due to its affinity toward the receptor, causing endothelitis and capillary fragility, predisposing to petechial hemorrhage [39].

Another significant issue, especially reported in moderate to severe COVID-19 patients, is thrombocytopenia. Several studies have associated its presence with poor prognosis in the already deadly infection [38]. This is owing to reduced platelet production due to bone marrow suppression, increased immune-mediated platelet destruction, and widespread microthrombosis [26]. These changes occurring in COVID-19 patients lead to bleeding tendencies that manifest in the oral cavity as petechiae. In addition, the cytokine storm reported in SARS-CoV-2 infection disrupts vascular homeostasis, while disseminated intravascular coagulation (DIC) and altered fibrinolysis increase the risk of microvascular bleeding among patients [41]. Moreover, persistent coughing, vomiting, or endotracheal intubation in critically ill or hospitalized patients can further cause trauma to the already fragile capillaries, leading to petechial lesions [16]. Drug-related factors, particularly anticoagulants used in hospitalized patients, may also increase the frequency of hemorrhagic mucosal changes [39].

25.7 Herpes Simplex Virus Type 1 (HSV-1)

Herpes simplex virus type 1 (HSV-1), known for its rapid replication and neurotropic behavior, is an enveloped, double-stranded DNA virus belonging to the Herpesviridae family. Primary infection typically occurs in childhood, following which it establishes lifelong latency in sensory ganglia, particularly the trigeminal ganglion. Periodic reactivation may occur under conditions of immunosuppression, stress, fever, or systemic illness, resulting in a myriad of clinical presentations, including primary herpetic gingivostomatitis, recurrent intraoral herpes, and herpes labialis [35, 42].

HSV-1 reactivation is a common presentation in COVID-19 patients and has been increasingly observed among patients with moderate to severe forms of the disease or those on corticosteroids and immunomodulators. The underlying mechanism involves immune dysregulation, with lymphopenia and cytokine storm, predisposing to uncontrolled viral proliferation, with hypoxia, prolonged hospitalization, and mechanical ventilation serving as further risk factors. Apart from mucocutaneous lesions, the DNA of the HSV-1 virus has been detected in respiratory and blood samples, highlighting the possibility of systemic involvement [42–45].

25.7.1 Etiology and Risk Factors

The primary infection by HSV-1 usually occurs in childhood, while reactivation is caused by triggers such as immune dysregulation due to COVID-19, marked by lymphopenia, depleted T-cells, and cytokine storm. The common treatment modalities for these patients, including corticosteroids and immunomodulators, further suppress cell-mediated immunity, leading to uncontrolled viral proliferation. Critical patients in the ICU or prolonged hospitalization may suffer sepsis, hypoxia, mechanical iatrogenic trauma with intense physiologic stress, acting as classic triggers. Local factors, including mucosal dryness from salivary dysfunction or oxygen therapy, may facilitate replication of HSVs [42–45].

25.7.2 Epidemiology

In COVID-19, herpes simplex infection has been documented in 2–12% patients, particularly among hospitalized and critically ill individuals [43, 44]. Reactivation occurs more often in vulnerable individuals with severe systemic compromise, immunosuppression, or prolonged ICU stay. There is no gender predilection, although middle-aged and older adults appear more susceptible [6, 42, 45].

25.7.3 Presentation in the Context of COVID-19

Herpes simplex virus type 1 (HSV-1) reactivation has been increasingly reported during the COVID-19 pandemic, particularly in patients with a more severe disease and those requiring intensive care. The association is primarily attributed to COVID-19-induced immune dysregulation. SARS-CoV-2 infection leads to lymphopenia, impaired $CD4^+$ and $CD8^+$ T-cell responses, and elevated inflammatory cytokines. This collectively compromises the viral immune surveillance by the host, facilitating HSV-1 to emerge from latency [43, 44].

In addition, risk factors such as mechanical ventilation, prolonged hospitalization, hypoxia, and treatment using systemic corticosteroid or immunomodulatory therapy in critically ill COVID-19 patients further exacerbate HSV-1 reactivation [44–46]. A study by Le Balc'h et al. in 2020 reported frequent reactivation of HSV-1 and CMV among ICU patients with COVID-19, suggesting that viral activation is indeed a feature of critically ill patients [45]. Another study by Giacobbe et al. (2022) emphasized can either present as mucocutaneous lesions in COVID-19 patients or be detected in respiratory secretions, thereby implying a potential contribution to pulmonary injury in these individuals [44].

Apart from these, HSV-1 lesions have also been observed in milder COVID-19 infections. Shanshal and Ahmed (2021) documented oral HSV lesions in COVID-19 patients, later confirmed by PCR. This finding further highlighted that reactivation of the virus is not just limited to ICU populations but may appear as painful vesiculoulcerative lesions on the oral mucosa of even mildly infected COVID patients [43]. Katz et al. (2021) further noted that both HSV and varicella-zoster virus (VZV) reactivation occurred in COVID-19 patients across different severities, reinforcing the concept that herpesviruses are opportunistic pathogens that take advantage of the immunocompromised state caused due to SARS-CoV-2–virus infection [47]. Thus, it is safe to say that oral HSV lesions may serve as a clinical indicator of systemic immune compromise in COVID patients, serving as a potential marker of disease severity.

25.8 Angina Bullosa Hemorrhagica

Angina bullosa hemorrhagica (ABH) is a benign, acquired oral mucosal disorder characterized by the sudden appearance of blood-filled subepithelial blisters. It is commonly found on the soft palate, but also reported on the buccal mucosa, lateral tongue, and pharyngeal wall. These blisters rupture spontaneously within 24–48 h, leaving superficial erosions that heal without scarring [48]. Notably, ABH is distinct from autoimmune vesiculobullous disorders and systemic bleeding diatheses, as it presents without associated hematologic, immunologic, or dermatologic diseases [49]. ABH has been frequently reported during the COVID-19 pandemic. Several studies have suggested that the immune dysregulation in COVID-19 patients, corticosteroid therapy, associated diabetes, hypertension, and the endothelial fragility due to the infection, may predispose patients to ABH-like lesions [48, 50, 51]. While ABH is self-limiting and generally not life-threatening, its clinical similarity to autoimmune vesiculobullous disorders underscores the need for careful recognition, especially in COVID-19 patients, to avoid misdiagnosis and unnecessary interventions.

25.8.1 Etiology and Risk Factors

The exact cause of ABH remains unclear; however, it is thought to arise from mucosal tear and rupture of superficial capillaries at the epithelial-connective tissue junction. It has often been linked to arterial hypertension, diabetes mellitus, age-related mucosal atrophy, chronic respiratory conditions, and the long-term use of inhaled steroids [52]. Trauma to the mucosa due to mastication, ingestion of hot food, dental procedures, or endoscopy is a common etiological factor. Associations with endocrine disorders, particularly diabetes, suggest that microvascular changes may contribute to lesion development [49].

25.8.2 Epidemiology

Although ABH is a rare oral lesion, it has been increasingly reported in COVID-19 patients. Described more frequently in middle-aged to elderly patients with comorbidities and those receiving corticosteroid therapy, there is no evidence of a clear gender predilection [50, 53].

25.8.3 Presentation in the Context of COVID-19

The association of angina bullosa hemorrhagica (ABH) with COVID-19 is attributed to a myriad of factors. A combination of renin–angiotensin system (RAS) imbalance, immune dysregulation, and systemic comorbidities is thought to contribute to the formation of ABH. The deadly virus is also responsible for downregulating ACE2 receptors, which reduces angiotensin-(1–7) and increases angiotensin II. This subsequently results in enhanced inflammation, impaired mucosal repair, and loss of mucosal protection [54]. Concurrently, viral replication and pyroptosis release damage-associated molecular patterns (DAMPs), driving a cascade of pro-inflammatory cytokines such as IL-6, IP-10, MIP-1α, and MCP-1, thereby amplifying local and systemic inflammation [55, 56]. Exaggerated Th1 responses and potential cross-reactivity of SARS-CoV-2-specific T cells with oral mucosal antigens may further contribute to epithelial fragility and injury [55]. In addition, diabetes, hypertension, asthma, chronic kidney disease, and long-term corticosteroid use exacerbate mucosal fragility and vascular instability in COVID-19, further leading to the formation of these blood-filled blisters in the oral mucosa [50, 52, 57].

25.9 Kawasaki-Like Disease

25.9.1 Definition and Overview

Kawasaki-like disease (KLD), also known as multisystem inflammatory syndrome (MIS), is a hyperinflammatory condition that resembles classic Kawasaki disease (KD) but is associated with SARS-CoV-2 infection. It is an acute, systemic vasculitis of medium-sized vessels, characterized by persistent fever, lymphadenopathy, conjunctival injection, mucocutaneous inflammation, gastrointestinal symptoms, and cardiovascular involvement, often including myocarditis, pericarditis, and coronary artery abnormalities [58–62]. Unlike classic KD, which predominantly affects children under 5 years, COVID-19-associated KLD has been reported in older children, adolescents, and even adults [71, 72]. Several studies have revealed that compared to classic KD, COVID-19-related KLD tends to present with more severe systemic inflammation, a higher incidence of shock, and requires intensive care [58–63]. Pathogenetically, the disease is thought to result from a compromised immune response to SARS-CoV-2, leading to cytokine storm and widespread vascular inflammation [58, 59]. KLD is increasingly recognized as a distinct clinical entity within the spectrum of COVID-19-related hyperinflammatory disorders.

25.9.2 Etiology and Risk Factors

The definite etiology of Kawasaki-like disease associated with COVID-19 remains unclear. However, a review of the existing literature suggests a multifactorial interplay of viral triggers, immune dysregulation, and host susceptibility. Infectious triggers have been proposed in the etiology owing to an epidemic pattern and marked seasonality [64]. Various infectious agents, including bacteria such as *Streptococcus pyogenes*, *Staphylococcus aureus*, and *Yersinia pseudotuberculosis*, and viruses such as adenovirus, enteroviruses, Epstein–Barr virus, and coronavirus (New Haven coronavirus/HCoVNH) have been implicated in the etiology of KD [65, 66]. Furthermore, single nucleotide polymorphisms (SNPs) in multiple genes have been associated with increased susceptibility to KD, including inositol 1,4,5 triphosphate kinase-C (ITPKC), caspase-3 (CASP3), FCGR2A, B-cell lymphoid kinase (BLK), CD40, ORAI1, MBL, HLA class II [64, 67].

In COVID-19 patients, SARS-CoV-2 infection is believed to act as an immunological trigger, leading to overproduction of cytokines, injury of endothelial cells, and systemic vasculitis [58, 59]. Hyperactivation and dysregulation of innate and adaptive immune pathways, including Th1/Th17 polarization, macrophage activation, and T-cell expansion, contribute to the hyperinflammatory state seen in Kawasaki-like disease [60, 62]. Several clinical risk factors have also been identified and reported. Unlike classic Kawasaki disease, which usually affects children <5 years, COVID-19-associated KLD more often occurs in older children, adolescents, and even adults, and tends to present with more severe cardiovascular involvement, shock, and need for ICU admission [59, 61, 63]. Comorbidities such as obesity, asthma, and preexisting cardiovascular disease have also been reported as potential aggravating factors [59, 62]. Genetic and ethnic factors appear to contribute to KD susceptibility, as evidenced by the disproportionately elevated incidence observed among Asian children, as well as those of African and Hispanic descent.

25.9.3 Epidemiology

The Kawasaki-like disease has emerged as a rare but significant complication of COVID 19, with an estimated prevalence of 0.14 0.6% among the population [59, 60]. It predominantly affects children and adolescents, with a slight male predominance, and has been associated with certain ethnicities such as African, Hispanic, and South Asian descent [61–63].

25.9.4 Presentation in the Context of COVID-19

Unlike classic Kawasaki disease, which is thought to result from unidentified infectious triggers, COVID-19-related KLD represents a post-viral hyperinflammatory response that develops several weeks after exposure to SARS-CoV-2 [60, 62]. The primary role may be attributed to the dysregulated innate and adaptive immunity in COVID patients, leading to viral endocytosis and replication, promoting pyroptotic cell death, releasing damage-associated molecular patterns (DAMPs) that trigger excessive production of pro-inflammatory cytokines such as IL-6, IL-1β, TNF-α, and interferon-γ. This, in turn, results in a cytokine storm, characterized by systemic vasculitis, endothelial dysfunction, and multi-organ inflammation as seen in COVID patients [58–60]. In addition, studies have also suggested a Th1/Th17 polarization and an increase in cytotoxic T cells, with cross-reactivity between SARS-CoV-2 antigens and host vascular/mucosal antigens, leading to immune-mediated tissue injury [59, 63]. In addition, SARS-CoV-2 downregulates ACE2 expression, leading to increased angiotensin II levels and promoting vasoconstriction, oxidative stress, and endothelial inflammation [59]. This endothelial injury is in line with the coronary artery involvement frequently observed in affected patients. Further, post-infectious immune phenomenon is also suggested because clusters of KLD lesions appeared 2–6 weeks after COVID-19 peaks in several regions, with most affected patients testing positive for SARS-CoV-2 antibodies [59, 61, 62].

25.10 Gingival Lesions

25.10.1 Definition and Overview

Gingival lesions in COVID-19 patients encompass a wide range of inflammatory and ulcerative conditions affecting the gingival tissues, from erythematous or edematous changes to severe necrotizing periodontal involvement. These lesions caused by SARS-CoV-2 infection may present either as primary viral-associated changes or as secondary complications due to secondary infections, immune dysregulation, and poor oral hygiene of the COVID patients [68, 69]. Several studies report COVID-19-related gingival involvement in a myriad of forms. Some cases present as viral enanthema, characterized by erythematous patches, petechiae, and gingival ulcerations that may mimic other viral exanthematous diseases [70]. In more severe forms, patients may develop necrotizing periodontal disease, including necrotizing gingivitis and periodontitis, which manifests as painful ulceration, spontaneous bleeding, and rapid destruction of gingival tissues. This may be associated with systemic immunosuppression and increased microbial load [68]. Additionally, rare presentations such as gingival recession triggered by herpes simplex virus (HSV) reactivation in COVID-19 patients have also been documented, highlighting the role of viral coinfection and altered immune response involved in gingival pathology [71].

25.10.2 Etiology and Risk Factors

Gingival lesions in COVID-19 are multifactorial, involving a complex interaction between viral, microbial, and host-related factors. The oral mucosa and the endothelial cells expressing ACE2 receptors are targeted by the virus, leading to inflammation of the vessels and mucosal disruption. On the other hand, viral reactivation, namely herpes simplex virus, has been linked to gingival recession and ulceration [70, 71]. Secondary bacterial infections and microbial dysbiosis in the oral environment, worsened by poor oral hygiene and immunosuppression status, predispose patients to necrotizing periodontal diseases [68]. Systemic comorbidities such as diabetes, hypertension, obesity, and smoking increase susceptibility to gingival diseases by impairing vascular and immune responses. While therapeutic interventions, such as corticosteroids or broad-spectrum antibiotics, may suppress local immunity and delay wound healing, they may also predispose individuals to secondary oral infections, thereby causing mucosal atrophy. Behavioral factors, including stress, dehydration, and poor oral care during illness or hospitalization, further increase the risk, making gingival lesions in COVID-19 a consequence of both local and systemic disease processes [23, 69, 70].

25.10.3 Epidemiology

Gingival lesions in COVID-19 have been reported in 2–6% of affected patients, mostly in those with poor oral hygiene status, systemic comorbidities, or immunosuppression. They occur across all age groups, but are more common in adults, with an increased severity of the disease [68, 70, 71].

25.10.4 Presentation in the Context of COVID-19

Similar to other oral lesions associated with COVID-19, gingival lesions are also caused when the SARS-CoV-2 virus targets the abundant ACE2 receptors in the epithelial and endothelial cells of the oral mucosa. This further leads to endothelial injury, microvascular damage, and increased mucosal atrophy [70]. The dysregulated inflammatory response, characterized by excessive cytokine release (IL-6, TNF-α, IL-1β), further disrupts the local tissue homeostasis, predisposing patients to gingival inflammation, ulceration, and bleeding. Additionally, the immune suppression and lymphopenia present in COVID-19 patients often reduce the host's defense, increasing susceptibility to opportunistic infections. Further, the local factors, especially the oral hygiene status of the individuals, particularly in critically ill or hospitalized patients, facilitate the onset of necrotizing periodontal disease, a severe manifestation marked by rapid gingival tissue destruction [68]. Reactivation, particularly of herpes simplex virus, has also been implicated in localized gingival recession and ulcerative lesions in COVID-19 cases [71]. Comorbidities, including diabetes, hypertension, and obesity, if present, further aggravate gingival vulnerability by impairing vascular supply and altering immune responses. Corticosteroids and broad-spectrum antibiotics are the standard treatment modalities in COVID patients, which may further contribute to oral dysbiosis and mucosal thinning, worsening gingival lesions.

25.11 Lichen Planus

25.11.1 Definition and Overview

Oral lichen planus (OLP) is a chronic, immune-mediated inflammatory disorder of the oral mucosa characterized by aberrant T-cell responses against basal keratinocytes, resulting in a range of mucocutaneous lesions. Affecting 1–2% of the population, lichen planus has a predilection for middle-aged adults, particularly women, commonly affecting the gingiva, buccal mucosa, and tongue [72]. Clinically, OLP manifests as bilateral, often symmetrical lesions that may present in one of the following subtypes, namely reticular, erosive, atrophic, plaque-like, papular, or bullous forms. Patients commonly complain of burning sensations, especially after consuming spicy food, mucosal sensitivity, and significant pain in an erosive form [73]. Though generally benign, OLP is considered a potentially malignant disorder, with a reported malignant transformation rate ranging between 0.5% and 2% [73, 74].

During the COVID-19 pandemic, several cases of new-onset OLP or exacerbation of preexisting lesions have been reported among COVID-19 patients. This is possibly linked to increased psychological stress due to the illness and prolonged hospitalization, virus-induced immune dysregulation, and widespread use of COVID medications, sometimes inadvertently [74, 75].

25.11.2 Etiology and Risk Factors

The oral lichen planus is an autoimmune mucocutaneous disorder with the exact cause being unknown. However, it is established that OLP is a T-cell-mediated autoimmune response triggered in genetically susceptible individuals by factors such as viral infections, certain medications (like NSAIDs, beta-blockers, and antimalarials), and contact with allergens, including dental materials. The pathophysiology involves a cell-mediated autoimmune response, wherein CD8+ T lymphocytes target the basal keratinocytes, presenting altered self-antigens, thereby leading to apoptosis and chronic inflammation [72, 75]. Genetic predisposition, particularly associations with HLA subtypes, may enhance susceptibility to the immune dysregulation seen in these patients [76]. The risk factors include psychological stress and anxiety which have been shown to exacerbate the disease through dysregulated hypothalamic–pituitary–adrenal (HPA) axis responses [77]. A shared inflammatory and autoimmune pathway has been suggested in several studies that revealed that OLP patients show a greater prevalence of systemic comorbidities such as diabetes mellitus, hypertension, metabolic syndrome, and autoimmune thyroid disorders

[78]. Lifestyle factors, including use of tobacco and alcohol consumption, have been associated with more severe clinical presentations and increased malignant transformation risk [73].

During the COVID-19 pandemic, additional risk factors include ACE2 receptor-mediated epithelial injury, immune hyperactivation, and cytokine release, which promote chronic mucosal inflammation [79]. Furthermore, COVID-19 vaccination has been reported to trigger lichenoid reactions in susceptible individuals, likely through molecular mimicry and cross-reactivity of the T-cells [80]. Long-term use of various drugs during COVID-19 management has also been reported to induce oral lichenoid drug reactions, clinically and histologically resembling OLP [81].

25.11.3 Epidemiology

Oral lichen planus has been reported sporadically in COVID-19 patients, with an estimated prevalence of <2% among reported oral manifestations. It appears more frequently in middle-aged to older adults, with a female predominance, consistent with the general epidemiology of OLP [37, 74].

25.11.4 Presentation in the Context of COVID-19

The association of Oral lichen planus and COVID-19 is largely attributed to immune dysregulation in the COVID-19 patients. The cytokine storm that occurs due to SARS-CoV-2 infection leads to elevated levels of IL-6, TNF-α, IL-17, and IFN-γ, which overlap with OLP pathogenesis [72, 73, 75] The virus directly targets the abundant ACE2 receptors found on oral keratinocytes, thereby further promoting epithelial injury and antigen exposure, which initiates lichenoid immune responses [76]. In addition, the remarkable psychological stress during the pandemic has been recognized as an essential precipitating factor among the vulnerable population [77]. Additionally, the aberrant use of broad-spectrum antibiotics, antivirals, and corticosteroids in COVID-19 treatment has been implicated in oral lichenoid drug reactions, mimicking idiopathic OLP [79]. Interestingly, the vaccines that were designed to combat the virus caused lichenoid responses in people, possibly due to T-cell activation and molecular mimicry [80]. These mechanisms thus highlight COVID-19 as both a direct immunological trigger and an indirect modulator of OLP expression.

25.12 Summary

Oral mucosal lesions associated with COVID-19 encompass a wide range of presentations, including nonspecific ulcers, petechiae, and aphthous-like lesions, which often appear in moderate to severe cases and sometimes persist in post-COVID conditions. These lesions may result from direct viral effects, immune responses, secondary infections, or treatment-related trauma, with the expression of the ACE2 receptor in oral tissues possibly contributing to their pathogenesis. While the exact link between SARS-CoV-2 and its oral manifestations remains uncertain due to study heterogeneity and bias, clinicians should remain vigilant, as oral manifestations may serve as early indicators of systemic involvement and warrant integrated care.

References

1. Organization WH. Coronavirus (2022). Available at: https://www.who.int/health-topics/coronavirus#tab=tab_3.
2. Xu H, Zhong L, Deng J, et al. High expression of ACE2 receptor of 2019-nCoV on the epithelial cells of oral mucosa. Int J Oral Sci. 2020;12(1):1–5. https://doi.org/10.1038/s41368-020-0074-x.
3. Amorim Dos Santos J, Normando AG, Carvalho da Silva RL, Acevedo AC, De Luca Canto G, Sugaya N, Santos-Silva AR, Guerra EN. Oral manifestations in patients with COVID-19: a living systematic review. J Dent Res. 2021;100(2):141–54.
4. Farid H, Khan M, Jamal S, Ghafoor R. Oral manifestations of Covid-19-a literature review. Rev Med Virol. 2021;32(1):e2248. https://doi.org/10.1002/RMV.2248.
5. Fidan V, Koyuncu H, Akin O. Oral lesions in Covid 19 positive patients. Am J Otolaryngol. 2021;42(3):102905. https://doi.org/10.1016/J.AMJOTO.2021.102905.
6. Riad A, Kassem I, Hockova B, Badrah M, Klugar M. Tongue ulcers associated with SARS-CoV-2 infection: a case series. Oral Dis. 2022;28(S1):988–90. https://doi.org/10.1111/ODI.13635.
7. Martín Carreras-Presas C, Amaro Sánchez J, López-Sánchez AF, Jané-Salas E, Somacarrera Pérez ML. Oral vesiculobullous lesions associated with SARS-CoV-2 infection. Oral Dis. 2020;27(Suppl 3):710. https://doi.org/10.1111/ODI.13382.
8. Sekar R, Bottu K, Protyusha GB, Ramasamy J, Venkatesalu B. Comparative analysis of candidal carriage rates in long-term and short-term COVID-19 patients: an RT-PCR study. J Oral Biol Craniofacial Res. 2025;15(4):899. https://doi.org/10.1016/J.JOBCR.2025.06.014.
9. Favia G, Tempesta A, Barile G, et al. COVID-19 symptomatic patients with oral lesions: clinical and histopathological study on 123 cases of the university hospital policlinic of bari with a purpose of a new classification. J Clin Med. 2021;10(4):1–10. https://doi.org/10.3390/JCM10040757.
10. Gutierrez-Camacho JR, Avila-Carrasco L, Martinez-Vazquez MC, et al. Oral lesions associated with COVID-19 and the participation of the buccal cavity as a key player for establishment of immunity against SARS-CoV-2. Int J Environ Res Public Health. 2022;19(18):11383. https://doi.org/10.3390/IJERPH191811383.
11. Pascolo L, Zupin L, Melato M, Tricarico PM, Crovella S. TMPRSS2 and ACE2 coexpression in SARS-CoV-2 salivary glands infection. J Dent Res. 2020;99(10):1120–1. https://doi.org/10.1177/0022034520933589.
12. Sakaguchi W, Kubota N, Shimizu T, et al. Existence of SARS-CoV-2 entry molecules in the oral cavity. Int J Mol Sci. 2020;21(17):1–16. https://doi.org/10.3390/IJMS21176000.
13. Iranmanesh B, Khalili M, Amiri R, Zartab H, Aflatoonian M. Oral manifestations of COVID-19 disease: a review article. Dermatol Ther. 2021;34(1):e14578. https://doi.org/10.1111/DTH.14578.
14. Zaheer K, Sanikop R, Cant A, Bhujel N, Singh RP. Oral lesions in paediatric patients with COVID-19 and paediatric inflammatory multisystem syndrome: a review. Adv Oral Maxillofac Surg. 2021;5:100213. https://doi.org/10.1016/J.ADOMS.2021.100213.

15. Brandão TB, Gueiros LA, Melo TS, et al. Oral lesions in patients with SARS-CoV-2 infection: could the oral cavity be a target organ? Oral Surg Oral Med Oral Pathol Oral Radiol. 2021;131(2):e45–51. https://doi.org/10.1016/j.oooo.2020.07.014.
16. Dziedzic A, Wojtyczka R. The impact of coronavirus infectious disease 19 (COVID-19) on oral health. Oral Dis. 2021;27(S3):703–6. https://doi.org/10.1111/ODI.13359.
17. Marouf N, Cai W, Said KN, et al. Association between periodontitis and severity of COVID-19 infection: a case–control study. J Clin Periodontol. 2021;48(4):483–91. https://doi.org/10.1111/JCPE.13435.
18. Gupta S, Mohindra R, Chauhan PK, et al. SARS-CoV-2 detection in gingival crevicular fluid. J Dent Res. 2021;100(2):187–93. https://doi.org/10.1177/0022034520970536.
19. Wu YH, Wu YC, Lang MJ, Lee YP, Jin YT, Chiang CP. Review of oral ulcerative lesions in COVID-19 patients: a comprehensive study of 51 cases. J Dent Sci. 2021;16(4):1066–73. https://doi.org/10.1016/j.jds.2021.07.001.
20. Dominguez-Santas M, Diaz-Guimaraens B, Fernandez-Nieto D, Jimenez-Cauhe J, Ortega-Quijano D, Suarez-Valle A. Minor aphthae associated with SARS-CoV-2 infection. Int J Dermatol. 2020;59(8):1022. https://doi.org/10.1111/IJD.15004.
21. Chiang CP, Yu-Fong Chang J, Wang YP, Wu YH, Wu YC, Sun A. Recurrent aphthous stomatitis—etiology, serum autoantibodies, anemia, hematinic deficiencies, and management. J Formos Med Assoc. 2019;118(9):1279–89. https://doi.org/10.1016/j.jfma.2018.10.023.
22. Corchuelo J, Ulloa FC. Oral manifestations in a patient with a history of asymptomatic COVID-19: case report. Int J Infect Dis. 2020;100:154–7. https://doi.org/10.1016/j.ijid.2020.08.071.
23. Sarasati A, Agustina D, Surboyo MDC. The oral lesion in the COVID-19 patient: is it true oral manifestation or not? Infect Drug Resist. 2023;16:4357. https://doi.org/10.2147/IDR.S411615.
24. Amorim dos Santos J, Normando AGC, Carvalho da Silva RL, et al. Oral manifestations in patients with COVID-19: a living systematic review. J Dent Res. 2021;100(2):141–54. https://doi.org/10.1177/0022034520957289.
25. Tay MZ, Poh CM, Rénia L, MacAry PA, Ng LFP. The trinity of COVID-19: immunity, inflammation and intervention. Nat Rev Immunol. 2020;20(6):363–74. https://doi.org/10.1038/S41577-020-0311-8.
26. Terpos E, Ntanasis-Stathopoulos I, Elalamy I, et al. Hematological findings and complications of COVID-19. Am J Hematol. 2020;95(7):834–47. https://doi.org/10.1002/AJH.25829.
27. Ackermann M, Verleden SE, Kuehnel M, et al. Pulmonary vascular endothelialitis, thrombosis, and angiogenesis in Covid-19. N Engl J Med. 2020;383(2):120–8. https://doi.org/10.1056/NEJMOA2015432.
28. Protyusha GB, Kavitha B, Sivapathasundharam B, et al. Accidental finding of COVID-associated mucormycosis (CAM) in a patient presenting as toothache: a case report and review of literature. Clin Case Reports. 2023;11(5):e7292. https://doi.org/10.1002/CCR3.7292.
29. Mahmood F, Cyr J, Li A, Lipson J, Pratt M, Beecker J. Vesiculobullous and other cutaneous manifestations of COVID-19 vaccines: a scoping and narrative review. J Cutan Med Surg. 2023;27(3):260. https://doi.org/10.1177/12034754231156561.
30. Palaia G, Pernice E, Pergolini D, et al. Erythema multiforme as early manifestation of COVID-19: a case report. Pathogens. 2022;11(6):654. https://doi.org/10.3390/PATHOGENS11060654.
31. Etaee F, Eftekharian M, Naguib T, Daveluy S. Erythema multiforme in COVID-19 patients and following COVID-19 vaccination: manifestations, associations and outcomes. J Eur Acad Dermatol Venereol. 2022;36(7):e524 30. https://doi.org/10.1111/JDV.18063.
32. Torrelo A, Andina D, Santonja C, et al. Erythema multiforme-like lesions in children and COVID-19. Pediatr Dermatol. 2020;37(3):442–6. https://doi.org/10.1111/PDE.14246.
33. Amorim dos Santos J, Normando AGC, Carvalho da Silva RL, et al. Oral mucosal lesions in a COVID-19 patient: new signs or secondary manifestations? Int J Infect Dis. 2020;97:326–8. https://doi.org/10.1016/J.IJID.2020.06.012.

34. Jimenez-Cauhe J, Ortega-Quijano D, Carretero-Barrio I, et al. Erythema multiforme-like eruption in patients with COVID-19 infection: clinical and histological findings. Clin Exp Dermatol. 2020;45(7):892–5. https://doi.org/10.1111/CED.14281.
35. Neville BW, Damm DD, Allen CM, Neville BW, Damm DD, Allen CM, Chi AC. Oral and Maxillofacial Pathology. 4th ed. St. Louis: Elsevier; 2016.
36. Warnakulasuriya S, Kujan O, Aguirre-Urizar JM, et al. Oral potentially malignant disorders: a consensus report from an international seminar on nomenclature and classification, convened by the WHO Collaborating Centre for Oral Cancer. Oral Dis. 2021;27(8):1862–80. https://doi.org/10.1111/ODI.13704.
37. Aragoneses J, Suárez A, Algar J, Rodríguez C, López-Valverde N, Aragoneses JM. Oral manifestations of COVID-19: updated systematic review with meta-analysis. Front Med. 2021;8:726753. https://doi.org/10.3389/FMED.2021.726753/FULL.
38. Lippi G, Plebani M, Henry BM. Thrombocytopenia is associated with severe coronavirus disease 2019 (COVID-19) infections: a meta-analysis. Clin Chim Acta. 2020;506:145–8. https://doi.org/10.1016/J.CCA.2020.03.022.
39. Varga Z, Flammer AJ, Steiger P, et al. Endothelial cell infection and endotheliitis in COVID-19. Lancet. 2020;395(10234):1417–8. https://doi.org/10.1016/S0140-6736(20)30937-5.
40. Nijakowski K, Wyzga S, Singh N, Podgórski F, Surdacka A. Oral manifestations in SARS-CoV-2 positive patients: a systematic review. J Clin Med. 2022;11(8):2202. https://doi.org/10.3390/JCM11082202.
41. Ciccarese G, Drago F, Boatti M, Porro A, Muzic SI, Parodi A. Oral erosions and petechiae during SARS-CoV-2 infection. J Med Virol. 2021;93(1):129–32. https://doi.org/10.1002/JMV.26221.
42. Katz J, Yue S, Xue W. Herpes simplex and herpes zoster viruses in COVID-19 patients. Ir J Med Sci. 2022;191(3):1093–7. https://doi.org/10.1007/S11845-021-02714-Z.
43. Shanshal M, Ahmed HS. COVID-19 and herpes simplex virus infection: a cross-sectional study. Cureus. 2021;13(9):e18022. https://doi.org/10.7759/CUREUS.18022.
44. Giacobbe DR, Di Bella S, Lovecchio A, et al. Herpes simplex virus 1 (HSV-1) reactivation in critically ill COVID-19 patients: a brief narrative review. Infect Dis Ther. 2022;11(5):1779. https://doi.org/10.1007/S40121-022-00674-0.
45. Le Balc'h P, Pinceaux K, Pronier C, Seguin P, Tadié JM, Reizine F. Herpes simplex virus and cytomegalovirus reactivations among severe COVID-19 patients. Crit Care. 2020;24(1):530. https://doi.org/10.1186/S13054-020-03252-3.
46. Sivapathasundharam B. Shafers textbook of oral pathology. 10th ed. Elsevier; 2024.
47. Balasopoulou A, Kokkinos P, Pagoulatos D, et al. Symposium recent advances and challenges in the management of retinoblastoma globe - saving treatments. BMC Ophthalmol. 2017;17(1):1. https://doi.org/10.4103/ijo.IJO.
48. Kurban M, Kibbi AG, Ghosn S. Expanding the histologic spectrum of angina bullosa hemorrhagica: report of one case. Am J Dermatopathol. 2007;29(5):477–9. https://doi.org/10.1097/DAD.0B013E3181492BEB.
49. Hopkins R, Walker DM. Oral blood blisters: angina bullosa haemorrhagica. Br J Oral Maxillofac Surg. 1985;23(1):9–16. https://doi.org/10.1016/0266-4356(85)90073-7.
50. Nayak P, Gupta S, Pathak VK, Kalra R. Angina bullosa haemorrhagica in COVID 19: a diagnostic conundrum. Case report and review of literature. Indian J Otolaryngol Head Neck Surg. 2023;75(3):2650–6. https://doi.org/10.1007/S12070-023-03584-W.
51. Sharma A, Goel A. Mucormycosis: risk factors, diagnosis, treatments, and challenges during COVID-19 pandemic. Folia Microbiol (Praha). 2022;67(3):363–87. https://doi.org/10.1007/s12223-021-00934-5.
52. Okobi OE, Evbayekha EO, Ebili U, Ogbonna UO, Ogundiran F, Ebong IL. Angina bullosa hemorrhagica: a rare and interesting presentation. Cureus. 2022;14(3):e23335. https://doi.org/10.7759/CUREUS.23335.
53. Goel S, Gupta S, Bhalla K, Maheshwari I. Angina bullosa hemorrhagica in five Covid-19-positive patients: a concomitance or an important oral manifestation. Indian Dermatol Online J. 2022;14(1):88. https://doi.org/10.4103/IDOJ.IDOJ_231_22.

54. Bourgonje AR, Abdulle AE, Timens W, et al. Angiotensin-converting enzyme 2 (ACE2), SARS-CoV-2 and the pathophysiology of coronavirus disease 2019 (COVID-19). J Pathol. 2020;251(3):228–48. https://doi.org/10.1002/PATH.5471.
55. Blanco-Melo D, Nilsson-Payant BE, Liu WC, et al. Imbalanced host response to SARS-CoV-2 drives development of COVID-19. Cell. 2020;181(5):1036–1045.e9. https://doi.org/10.1016/j.cell.2020.04.026.
56. Vabret N, Britton GJ, Gruber C, et al. Immunology of COVID-19: current state of the science. Immunity. 2020;52(6):910–41. https://doi.org/10.1016/j.immuni.2020.05.002.
57. Edwards S, Wilkinson JD, Wojnarowska F. Angina bullosa haemorrhagica—a report of three cases and review of the literature. Clin Exp Dermatol. 1990;15(6):422–4. https://doi.org/10.1111/J.1365-2230.1990.TB02135.X.
58. Viner RM, Whittaker E. Kawasaki-like disease: emerging complication during the COVID-19 pandemic. Lancet. 2020;395(10239):1741–3. https://doi.org/10.1016/S0140-6736(20)31129-6.
59. Gkoutzourelas A, Bogdanos DP, Sakkas LI. Kawasaki disease and COVID-19. Mediterr J Rheumatol. 2020;31(3 Supplement 2):268–74. https://doi.org/10.31138/MJR.31.3.268.
60. Toubiana J, Poirault C, Corsia A, et al. Kawasaki-like multisystem inflammatory syndrome in children during the covid-19 pandemic in Paris, France: prospective observational study. BMJ. 2020;369:m2094. https://doi.org/10.1136/BMJ.M2094.
61. Sokolovsky S, Soni P, Hoffman T, Kahn P, Scheers-Masters J. COVID-19 associated Kawasaki-like multisystem inflammatory disease in an adult. Am J Emerg Med. 2021;39:253.e1–2. https://doi.org/10.1016/j.ajem.2020.06.053.
62. Mardi P, Esmaeili M, Iravani P, Abdar ME, Pourrostami K, Qorbani M. Characteristics of children with Kawasaki disease-like signs in COVID-19 pandemic: a systematic review. Front Pediatr. 2021;9:625377. https://doi.org/10.3389/FPED.2021.625377.
63. Akca UK, Kesici S, Ozsurekci Y, et al. Kawasaki-like disease in children with COVID-19. Rheumatol Int. 2020;40(12):2105–15. https://doi.org/10.1007/S00296-020-04701-6.
64. Noval Rivas M, Arditi M. Kawasaki disease: pathophysiology and insights from mouse models. Nat Rev Rheumatol. 2020;16(7):391. https://doi.org/10.1038/S41584-020-0426-0.
65. Matsubara T, Ichiyama T, Furukawa S. Immunological profile of peripheral blood lymphocytes and monocytes/macrophages in Kawasaki disease. Clin Exp Immunol. 2005;141(3):381–7. https://doi.org/10.1111/J.1365-2249.2005.02821.X.
66. Kottek A, Shimizu C, Burns JC. Kawasaki disease in monozygotic twins. Pediatr Infect Dis J. 2011;30(12):1114. https://doi.org/10.1097/INF.0B013E31822AC4FF.
67. McCrindle BW, Rowley AH, Newburger JW, et al. Diagnosis, treatment, and long-term management of Kawasaki disease: a scientific statement for health professionals from the American Heart Association. Circulation. 2017;135(17):e927–99. https://doi.org/10.1161/CIR.0000000000000484.
68. Patel J, Woolley J. Necrotizing periodontal disease: oral manifestation of COVID-19. Oral Dis. 2021;27(S3):768–9. https://doi.org/10.1111/ODI.13462.
69. Tan L, Zhong MM, Liu Q, et al. Potential interaction between the oral microbiota and COVID-19: a meta-analysis and bioinformatics prediction. Front Cell Infect Microbiol. 2023;13:1193340. https://doi.org/10.3389/FCIMB.2023.1193340/FULL.
70. Rocha BA, Souto GR, de Grossmann SMC, et al. Viral enanthema in oral mucosa: a possible diagnostic challenge in the COVID-19 pandemic. Oral Dis. 2020;27(Suppl 3):776. https://doi.org/10.1111/ODI.13473.
71. Franceschi D, Di Gianfilippo R, Rubino I, Serni L, Prato GPP. Gingival recessions caused by herpes simplex virus in a patient with COVID-19 infection. Clin Case Reports. 2022;10(8) https://doi.org/10.1002/ccr3.6056.
72. Lavanya N, Jayanthi P, Rao U, Ranganathan K. Oral lichen planus: an update on pathogenesis and treatment. J Oral Maxillofac Pathol. 2011;15(2):127–32. https://doi.org/10.4103/0973-029X.84474.

73. González-Moles MÁ, Warnakulasuriya S, González-Ruiz I, et al. Worldwide prevalence of oral lichen planus: a systematic review and meta-analysis. Oral Dis. 2021;27(4):813–28. https://doi.org/10.1111/ODI.13323.
74. Saleh W, SHawky E, Halim GA, Ata F. Oral lichen planus after COVID-19, a case report. Ann Med Surg. 2021;72:103051. https://doi.org/10.1016/J.AMSU.2021.103051.
75. Srinivas K, Aravinda K, Ratnakar P, Nigam N, Gupta S. Oral lichen planus - review on etiopathogenesis. Natl J Maxillofac Surg. 2011;2(1):15. https://doi.org/10.4103/0975-5950.85847.
76. Scully C, Carrozzo M. Oral mucosal disease: lichen planus. Br J Oral Maxillofac Surg. 2008;46(1):15–21. https://doi.org/10.1016/J.BJOMS.2007.07.199.
77. Chaudhary S. Psychosocial stressors in oral lichen planus. Aust Dent J. 2004;49(4):192–5. https://doi.org/10.1111/J.1834-7819.2004.TB00072.X.
78. López-Jornet P, Camacho-Alonso F, Rodríguez-Martnes MA. Alterations in serum lipid profile patterns in oral lichen planus: a cross-sectional study. Am J Clin Dermatol. 2012;13(6):399–404. https://doi.org/10.2165/11633600-000000000-00000.
79. Eisen D, Carrozzo M, Sebastian JVB, Thongprasom K, Number V. Oral lichen planus: clinical features and management. Oral Dis. 2005;11(6):338–49. https://doi.org/10.1111/j.1601-0825.2005.01142.x.
80. Sapadin YK, Mermelstein E, Phelps RG, Basler CF, Tufariello JAM, Lebwohl MG. COVID-19 vaccine-induced lichenoid eruptions—clinical and histopathologic Spectrum in a case series of fifteen patients with review of the literature. Vaccine. 2023;11(2):438. https://doi.org/10.3390/VACCINES11020438.
81. Farhi D, Dupin N. Pathophysiology, etiologic factors, and clinical management of oral lichen planus, part I: facts and controversies. Clin Dermatol. 2010;28(1):100–8. https://doi.org/10.1016/j.clindermatol.2009.03.004.

Burning Mouth Syndrome (BMS) Associated with COVID-19

26

Shankargouda Patil, Shilpa Bhandi, and Frank W. Licari

26.1 Introduction

26.1.1 Definition and Overview

Burning mouth syndrome (BMS) is a chronic neuropathic condition that affects the nerves, causing a burning or scalding sensation in the mouth. It occurs in about 1.73% of the general population and up to 7.72% of patients seen in clinical settings [1]. It is usually classified as idiopathic, with the exact cause still unclear. The symptoms include a persistent burning, tingling, or hot sensation, often without any visible changes in the mouth. BMS mostly affects middle-aged and older women. This condition primarily affects the tongue, lips, palate, or sometimes the entire oral cavity, often lasting for months to years [2]. It typically presents without any corresponding clinical or laboratory presentation or histopathological findings [2]. While the tongue is the most frequently involved site (63.6%), it may also affect the gingiva (61.9%) or palate (45.3%). Many patients also report changes in taste (dysgeusia) and a dry mouth sensation (xerostomia), even though their salivary flow remains normal [3]. Although mostly idiopathic, approximately one-third of cases occur after dental procedures, systemic illnesses, or medication use, with recent studies revealing a potential complex interaction between peripheral nerve dysfunction and central pain processing mechanisms [2]. The chronic nature of the condition, absence of an identifiable etiology, and resistance to conventional therapies make it a challenging condition for both diagnosis and management. With the advent of the COVID-19 pandemic, BMS has drawn renewed attention. BMS has been reported as a possible symptom or long-term effect in patients infected with SARS-CoV-2 [4–6].

S. Patil (✉) · S. Bhandi · F. W. Licari
College of Dental Medicine, Roseman University of Health Sciences, South Jordan, UT, USA
e-mail: spatil@roseman.edu

S. R. Prabhu et al. (eds.), *COVID-19 in Dental Practice*,
https://doi.org/10.1007/978-3-032-26000-0_26

In general, "neuropathic pain" refers to any pain arising directly from a lesion or disease affecting the somatosensory system, often leading to abnormal pain responses such as spontaneous burning, tingling, or electric shock-like sensations [7]. BMS, which is considered a chronic neuropathic condition, involves mechanisms suggestive of damage to the trigeminal nerve, tiny unmyelinated C fibers, and thinly myelinated Aδ fibers. These small fibers are part of the peripheral nervous system and are especially responsible for the transmission of thermal and pain sensations in the body [8]. C fibers conduct impulses slowly and are usually linked to dull, aching, and poorly localized pain. In contrast, Aδ fibers carry signals more quickly and are responsible for sharp, well-defined pain [9]. In BMS, there is often damage or dysfunction in these small nerve fibers. This leads to symptoms consistent with small fiber neuropathy. Trigeminal neuropathy, on the other hand, may involve damage anywhere along the trigeminal nerve pathway, including both peripheral and central parts [10]. This is different from nociceptive pain, which is usually caused by tissue damage or inflammation, such as in the case of dental caries or trauma. A specific stimulus typically triggers nociceptive pain [11]. In BMS, pain is often chronic, spontaneous, and felt on both sides of the mouth. It usually occurs without any visible clinical signs, which makes diagnosis more challenging. As a result, BMS is considered a diagnosis of exclusion, meaning other possible conditions must be ruled out first. Table 26.1 lists conditions that can mimic BMS and should be considered during diagnosis [11, 12]. Furthermore, tongue biopsies from patients with BMS reveal histopathological pictures showing reduced intraepithelial nerve fiber density. This supports the theory that BMS has a neuropathic cause [8]. It is therefore imperative to distinguish neuropathic BMS from nociceptive oral pain, as the treatment strategies differ significantly. Neuropathic pain often requires centrally acting medications, such as tricyclic antidepressants or gabapentinoids. In contrast, nociceptive pain usually responds well to common painkillers or anti-inflammatory drugs [13].

Table 26.1 Potential differential diagnoses of burning mouth syndrome

Trauma	Geographic tongue
Parafunctional habits	Autoimmune reactions
Drug-related side effects	Contact hypersensitivity
Xerostomia	Hormonal disturbances
Candidiasis	Parkinson's disease
Lichen planus	Local nerve damage
Vesiculoulcerative lesions	Nutritional deficiencies: B1, B2, B12, folate, iron, zinc

26.2 Biomarkers and COVID-19-Related Factors in BMS

Recent literature reviews highlight biological markers in BMS, which further help understand its pathophysiology. Elevated levels of pro-inflammatory cytokines, such as interleukin-6 (IL-6) and tumor necrosis factor-alpha (TNF-α), have been reported in some BMS patients. These findings suggest that inflammation may play a role in the condition. There is also evidence of a possible link between BMS and autoimmune susceptibility. For example, some patients show lower levels of CD28, a molecule involved in immune system function. This could indicate a tendency toward an immune system imbalance in specific individuals [16]. Neuropeptides like calcitonin gene-related peptide (CGRP) are also believed to be involved in BMS. CGRP plays a role in transmitting pain and promoting inflammation in the nervous system. Its presence may contribute to both peripheral and central sensitization—processes that make the nervous system more responsive to pain [16, 17].

Apart from the above-mentioned etiologies of BMS, the advent of the COVID-19 pandemic has led to widespread use of a range of medications, including antivirals, systemic corticosteroids, and antibiotics, for the treatment of patients. Likely, these medications alone or in combination with the psychological distress of the patients could have contributed to oral dysbiosis and dysgeusia, possibly triggering BMS-like symptoms in those patients. Notably, several patients required long-term hospitalization during the pandemic, especially in the ICU, leading to stress, depression, and anxiety in these patients. This may have potentially increased their vulnerability to the condition or even exacerbated the symptoms, especially in individuals already predisposed to neuropathic or psychogenic pain conditions [9–11].

26.3 Burning Mouth Syndrome and Its Association with COVID-19

Since the emergence of the COVID-19 pandemic, an expanding spectrum of systemic and oral manifestations has been documented in the literature. Among these, burning mouth sensation or symptoms consistent with burning mouth syndrome (BMS) have been increasingly reported, either during the acute phase or as part of post-acute sequelae, commonly referred to as "long COVID" [21, 22]. This association has prompted a growing interest in the underlying mechanisms, clinical presentation, and management of BMS-like symptoms in the context of SARS-CoV-2 infection.

One possible explanation is the development of post-viral neuropathy. Viral infections such as COVID-19 may cause lasting changes in the peripheral or central nervous systems, leading to chronic pain or altered sensations. In BMS, studies have found a reduction in the number of nerve fibers in the mouth's epithelial tissue. Changes in the levels of specific neuropeptides, such as substance P and calcitonin gene-related peptide (CGRP), have also been reported. This suggests small-fiber neuropathy of viral origin in some cases of BMS [23].

This pathophysiological mechanism appears closely related to postherpetic neuralgia (PHN). In PHN, reactivation of the varicella-zoster virus leads to irreversible nerve damage and persistent neuropathic pain [23]. Both BMS and PHN involve the trigeminal nerve and are associated with spontaneous pain and abnormal sensations (dysesthesia). However, PHN usually follows a known viral infection and presents with pain in a specific nerve distribution (dermatomal pattern). In contrast, BMS typically has no clear cause and produces a more widespread burning sensation in the mouth [3].

The importance of viral neuropathy has become more evident in the context of COVID-19. SARS-CoV-2 has been shown to affect cranial nerves and oral tissues, leading to symptoms such as altered taste, burning sensations, and nerve-related pain. These symptoms closely resemble those seen in BMS and support the theory that some cases may follow a post-viral pattern [24]. Additionally, BMS patients may exhibit altered thermal and mechanical pain thresholds, which suggests the involvement of central sensitization. This is also observed in conditions like PHN. Because of these similarities, treatments used in PHN, such as gabapentinoids and topical capsaicin, may also be helpful in managing BMS symptoms [25]. However, unlike PHN, definitive viral markers in BMS remain elusive, necessitating further research into neurotropic viral triggers and immune-mediated nerve damage in the oral mucosa.

Recent studies have also pointed to neuroinflammation and glial cell activation as possible contributors to long-term post-viral pain [26]. In particular, SARS-CoV-2 has been associated with the activation of microglia and astrocytes—cells that play a role in brain and nerve inflammation. These activated cells release inflammatory cytokines such as interleukin-6 (IL-6) and tumor necrosis factor-alpha (TNF-α), as well as other substances that increase nerve sensitivity. These are the potential pathways responsible for sensitizing nociceptive pathways [27]. These mechanisms may therefore be attributed to the pathogenesis of chronic orofacial pain, including BMS. They may also help explain why some patients continue to experience symptoms despite no detectable peripheral nerve damage [27].

Another significant post-COVID-19 development is the occurrence of SARS-CoV-2-related neuropathies, particularly their role in causing dysautonomia. Studies have reported that COVID-19 can lead to small fiber neuropathy, which presents with burning pain, tingling sensations (paresthesia), and symptoms related to autonomic nervous system dysfunction. These symptoms are parallel to those seen in BMS [28]. Additionally, postural orthostatic tachycardia syndrome (POTS), another form of autonomic dysfunction, has been increasingly identified in patients recovering from COVID-19. POTS is associated with symptoms such as dry mouth (xerostomia), altered taste (dysgeusia), dizziness, and chronic fatigue. These symptoms share significant overlap with the clinical features of BMS [29]. This similarity is especially relevant in cases of long COVID. In such patients, it is essential to conduct a detailed evaluation to differentiate between primary BMS and symptoms caused by small fiber or autonomic neuropathy. Diagnostic tests may include quantitative sensory testing (QST), skin biopsy to assess nerve fiber density, or autonomic function tests. These assessments can help ensure accurate diagnosis and guide appropriate management [30, 31].

26.4 COVID-19 and Neuropathic Mechanisms in BMS

One of the main theories linking COVID-19 to burning mouth syndrome (BMS) is that the virus affects the nervous system. SARS-CoV-2 has been shown to impact both the central and peripheral nervous systems. This can lead to a variety of neurological symptoms, including loss of smell (anosmia), loss of taste (ageusia), nerve-related pain, and burning sensations in the mouth [16, 23]. This effect on the nervous system, known as neurotropism, is believed to be mediated by the angiotensin-converting enzyme 2 (ACE2) receptor. These receptors are highly expressed in oral mucosal epithelial cells, salivary glands, taste buds, and neuronal tissue [24, 32].

Entry of SARS-CoV-2 into these cells may result in direct damage to sensory neurons or disruption of taste pathways, leading to symptoms akin to BMS [32].

Neuropathic pain conditions like BMS are believed to involve changes in how small nerve fibers function, along with a process called central sensitization. Both of these mechanisms can be triggered or worsened by viral infections [33]. A recent study by Díaz Rodríguez et al. reported persistent oral burning and dysgeusia in a subset of COVID-19 patients. These symptoms suggest possible involvement of the trigeminal nerve or its processing centers in the brain [33]. These findings align with known pathophysiologic theories of primary BMS, which include peripheral nerve dysfunction (particularly of the chorda tympani or lingual nerve) and altered pain modulation within the central nervous system [34].

26.5 Taste Disturbances and Oral Dysesthesia

Taste disorders such as dysgeusia (distorted taste), ageusia (loss of taste), and parageusia (altered taste perception) are among the most common oral symptoms reported in COVID-19. These taste disturbances often occur alongside burning sensations in the mouth, suggesting a shared underlying mechanism involving nerve dysfunction. A systematic review by Amorim Dos Santos et al. found that 15% of COVID-19 patients with oral symptoms experienced burning mouth sensations, which were frequently accompanied by dysgeusia and dry mouth [18]. Given the strong association between taste alterations and BMS, this overlap is clinically significant.

Several studies suggest that damage to taste buds or the nerves responsible for taste can indirectly trigger pain signals from the trigeminal nerve. This process can lead to the burning sensations typically seen in BMS [35]. This concept, known as the "disinhibition theory," may explain the onset of BMS-like symptoms in COVID-19 patients who develop loss of taste perception [23].

Taste and pain signals are processed in shared brain regions. Both pathways converge in the nucleus of the solitary tract (NTS) and parabrachial nucleus. Any disruption in taste input can lead to enhanced activity in trigeminal nociceptors, resulting in burning sensations [36].

At the molecular level, taste is detected by Type II taste receptor cells. These cells are responsible for sensing sweet, bitter, and umami flavors through G-protein-coupled receptors (GPCRs). The T1R receptor family (T1R1, T1R2, T1R3) is involved in sweet and umami taste, while T2R receptors detect bitter taste [37]. Changes or loss of function in these receptors can impair taste and also disturb normal sensory regulation in the mouth. This may be accompanied by abnormal afferent signaling, often perceived as burning or dysesthesia.

Type II taste cells do not form conventional synapses. Instead, they release ATP through specific channels known as CALHM1. This ATP then activates nearby gustatory nerves. When ATP signaling is disrupted, sensory balance in the mouth may be affected, possibly leading to BMS-like symptoms [38].

26.6 Salivary Gland Involvement and Xerostomia

Salivary gland dysfunction has been observed in many COVID-19 patients and is believed to contribute to xerostomia, or dry mouth, a common symptom of burning mouth syndrome (BMS). The salivary glands contain a high number of ACE2 receptors, which are the entry point for SARS-CoV-2. The presence of the virus in saliva suggests that it may replicate in or damage the salivary tissues directly [23, 36]. A reduction in saliva flow or changes in the composition of saliva can cause oral dryness, discomfort, increased risk of dental caries, and sensitivity of the oral mucosa. These effects can lead to a burning sensation in the mouth, particularly in patients recovering from COVID-19.

In a study by Favia et al., 45% of hospitalized COVID-19 patients reported xerostomia. Many also experienced a burning mouth sensation and changes in taste [36]. Xerostomia is a well-recognized factor in secondary BMS. When saliva levels are low, the oral tissues become less lubricated, increasing friction and irritation and worsening the burning sensation [20].

The differences in symptom severity among patients may be due to variations in ACE2 receptor density in different parts of the mouth and salivary glands. Areas with more receptors may be more vulnerable to viral invasion and inflammation. This supports the neuroinvasive model that SARS-CoV-2 may contribute to both local glandular dysfunction and nerve-related symptoms. Through either direct viral damage or immune-mediated processes, the virus may play a role in triggering or worsening burning mouth symptoms [39].

26.7 Psychological Stress and Central Sensitization

The COVID-19 pandemic has brought significant psychological challenges. Fear of illness, social isolation, financial instability, and grief have contributed to a rise in anxiety, depression, and stress-related disorders. These psychological issues are all well-recognized risk factors for BMS, which has a significant impact on the quality of life of these patients [20, 40, 41]. Functional neuroimaging studies in BMS patients have shown increased activity in brain regions responsible for pain processing and emotional control. These findings suggest that central nervous system changes and emotional stress may play a role in the development and persistence of BMS symptoms [14].

A cross-sectional study by López-Jornet et al. during the pandemic revealed a significant correlation between perceived stress levels and oral burning symptoms, even in COVID-negative individuals, suggesting a psychogenic component to symptom onset [15]. In patients who have recovered from COVID-19, conditions such as post-traumatic stress disorder (PTSD) and chronic fatigue have also been linked to ongoing physical symptoms, including oral burning. These patterns are consistent with post-viral nerve damage or somatoform pain disorders [15]. Together, these findings suggest that psychological distress may directly contribute to the onset or worsening of BMS, especially in the context of COVID-19. Addressing emotional health may therefore be an essential part of managing this condition.

26.8 Drug-Induced BMS-Like Symptoms

Treatment regimens for COVID-19 often include medications known to cause adverse oral effects. Drugs such as antivirals (e.g., lopinavir/ritonavir), corticosteroids, antibiotics, and antimalarials (e.g., hydroxychloroquine) have been associated with changes in taste, mucous membrane desquamation, and burning sensations [42]. These iatrogenic effects can mimic or precipitate BMS in patients with COVID-19 even after their recovery. Corticosteroids can thin the oral mucosa and affect the perception of pain. Antibiotics may disrupt the natural balance of bacteria in the mouth, increasing the risk of fungal infections such as oral candidiasis or causing inflammation. These changes may lead to greater sensitivity and discomfort in the mouth [43].

Prolonged and unintended use of these drugs can interfere with voltage-gated sodium channels (Na_V) in peripheral nerves. This may alter nociceptive signal transduction and result in dysesthesia or burning sensation as seen in BMS [44]. In addition, medications like antidepressants, corticosteroids, and antivirals, commonly given to COVID-19 patients, can influence central nervous system pathways that involve serotonin and dopamine. These neurotransmitters play an important role in pain regulation and taste perception [44]. Some of these drugs also exert cytotoxic or inflammatory effects on taste receptor cells, leading to receptor damage and disrupted taste transduction [45]. Given the trend of polypharmacy, which is common in COVID-19 management, distinguishing drug-induced symptoms from true BMS becomes extremely pivotal and clinically significant.

26.9 Post-acute COVID-19 Syndrome and Chronicity of Symptoms

One of the major findings in recent research is the recognition of long COVID, also called post-acute COVID-19 syndrome. This condition is defined by symptoms that continue for more than 12 weeks after the initial infection [46]. Burning mouth symptoms, fatigue, brain fog, and myalgia are increasingly recognized components of this syndrome. A meta-analysis by Lopez-Leon et al. identified oral pain and dysgeusia among over 50 long-term effects of COVID-19, highlighting the potential chronicity of these symptoms among the patients [19].

New evidence also suggests that SARS-CoV-2 may affect the vagus nerve. This could occur through direct viral invasion, inflammation, or disturbances in autonomic nervous system regulation [46]. The vagus nerve plays a key role in many functions, including the control of facial sensations, saliva production, and the body's inflammatory responses [47]. Damage or dysfunction in this nerve may upset the balance between trigeminal and vagal inputs, leading to ongoing oral burning or dysesthesia. Reduced vagal tone has also been implicated in impaired anti-inflammatory responses, leading to a feed-forward loop of neuroinflammation and peripheral sensitization, similar to the mechanisms suggested for primary BMS [48].

Symptoms such as oral burning, altered taste, and mucosal discomfort in long COVID are very similar to those seen in BMS. Many researchers now understand long COVID as a post-viral neuropathic pain condition. It may be driven by chronic inflammation, ongoing viral presence in tissues, autoimmune activity, and changes in how the nervous system processes pain. These exact mechanisms have also been proposed in BMS and other chronic pain syndromes [49]. As a result, patients with persistent burning symptoms after COVID-19 may benefit from multidisciplinary care involving dental specialists, neurologists, and pain management teams. Proper diagnosis and individualized treatment are essential to managing these long-lasting symptoms.

26.10 Pathophysiology

The pathophysiology of burning mouth syndrome, particularly in post-COVID-19 patients, is a complex interplay between peripheral neuropathy, central sensitization, and autonomic dysfunction. At the peripheral level, SARS-CoV-2 is believed to damage small unmyelinated C-fibers and Aδ fibers via direct viral neurotropism or immune-mediated responses, thereby altering thermal and nociceptive signaling [28, 50, 51]. This is supported by findings from quantitative sensory testing (QST) and skin biopsies in long COVID patients showing small fiber neuropathy (SFN) [52]. Additionally, viral interference with voltage-gated sodium channels ($Na_v1.7/1.8$) and transient receptor potential (TRP) channels has been proposed to enhance neuronal hyperexcitability and pain transmission [44].

At the central level, inflammation in the nervous system (neuroinflammation) may play a key role. This involves the activation of glial cells and an increase in pro-inflammatory cytokines such as interleukin-6 (IL-6) and tumor necrosis factor-alpha (TNF-α). Disruption in serotonin and dopamine pathways may also contribute to abnormal pain processing and prolonged discomfort [53]. Brain imaging studies in BMS patients have shown changes in activity in several brain areas involved in pain perception, including the anterior cingulate cortex, insula, and thalamus. These areas are commonly associated with other chronic pain conditions as well [54].

Autonomic dysfunction has also been observed in some long COVID patients. Reduced vagal tone and brainstem involvement may affect functions such as salivary production, taste perception, and facial pain regulation. These factors further support the idea that BMS symptoms in post-COVID individuals may result from the disruption of the autonomic nervous system [46–48]. Overall, the combination of peripheral nerve injury, changes in brain function, and autonomic imbalance suggests that burning mouth symptoms seen after COVID-19 could represent a form of post-viral neuropathic pain, with both peripheral and central components involved.

26.11 Clinical Implications and Future Directions

Healthcare providers should consider burning mouth syndrome (BMS) in patients recovering from COVID-19 who report oral burning sensations, especially when these are accompanied by altered taste (dysgeusia) or dry mouth (xerostomia). A detailed medical history is essential and should include recent or past COVID-19 infection, current or past medications, and the patient's psychological condition. A multidisciplinary approach involving dental specialists, neurologists, psychologists, and pain management experts may be warranted in complex cases. Given the evolving understanding of COVID-19-related neuropathies, further research is needed to elucidate the precise mechanisms by which SARS-CoV-2 induces BMS-like symptoms. Well-designed longitudinal studies are essential for determining the duration, prognosis, and optimal treatment strategies for affected individuals.

References

1. Wu S, Zhang W, Yan J, Noma N, Young A, Yan Z. Worldwide prevalence estimates of burning mouth syndrome: a systematic review and meta-analysis. Oral Dis. 2022;28:1431–40. https://doi.org/10.1111/odi.13868.
2. Lin X, Jin R, Huang W, Ye Y, Jin J, Zhu W. Trends of burning mouth syndrome: a bibliometric study. Front Neurol. 2024;15:1443817. https://doi.org/10.3389/fneur.2024.1443817.
3. Scala A, et al. Burning mouth syndrome: a diagnostic and therapeutic dilemma. J Oral Rehabil. 2012;39(7):547–52. https://doi.org/10.1111/j.1365-2842.2012.02308.x.
4. Dos Santos JA, Normando AGC, Carvalho da Silva RL, et al. Oral manifestations in patients with COVID-19: a living systematic review. J Dent Res. 2021;100(2):141–54.
5. Nuno-Gonzalez A, Martin-Carrillo P, Magaletsky K, et al. Prevalence of mucocutaneous manifestations in 666 patients with COVID-19. Br J Dermatol. 2021;184(1):184–5.

6. Dziedzic A, Wojtyczka R. The impact of coronavirus infectious disease 19 (COVID-19) on oral health. Oral Dis. 2021;27(Suppl 3):703–6. https://doi.org/10.1111/odi.13359.
7. Treede RD, Jensen TS, Campbell JN, et al. Neuropathic pain: redefinition and a grading system for clinical and research purposes. Neurology. 2008;70(18):1630–5. https://doi.org/10.1212/01.wnl.0000282763.29778.59.
8. Lauria G, Majorana A, Borgna M, et al. Trigeminal small-fiber sensory neuropathy causes burning mouth syndrome. Pain. 2005;115(3):332–7. https://doi.org/10.1016/j.pain.2005.03.028.
9. Zakrzewska JM. Differential diagnosis of facial pain and guidelines for management. Br J Anaesth. 2013;111(1):95–104. https://doi.org/10.1093/bja/aet125.
10. Benoliel R, Eliav E. Neuropathic orofacial pain. Oral Maxillofac Surg Clin North Am. 2008;20(2):237–54. https://doi.org/10.1016/j.coms.2007.12.001.
11. Klasser GD, Fischer DJ, Epstein JB. Burning mouth syndrome: recognition, understanding, and management. Oral Maxillofac Surg Clin North Am. 2008;20(2):255–71. https://doi.org/10.1016/j.coms.2007.12.012.
12. Zakrzewska JM, Forssell H, Glenny AM. Interventions for the treatment of burning mouth syndrome. Cochrane Database Syst Rev. 2005;3:CD002779. https://doi.org/10.1002/14651858.CD002779.
13. Alsabbagh R, Ouanounou A. Burning mouth syndrome: etiology, clinical presentations, and treatment alternatives. Dent Rev. 2022;2(1):100036.
14. Hagelberg N, Forssell H, Aalto S, et al. Altered dopamine D2 receptor binding in atypical facial pain. Pain. 2003;106(1–2):43–8. https://doi.org/10.1016/s0304-3959(03)00275.
15. López-Jornet P, Camacho-Alonso F. The efficacy of a cognitive-behavioral therapy technique in the treatment of burning mouth syndrome. J Oral Pathol Med. 2010;39(9):702–8.
16. Pekiner FN, Demirel GY, Gümrü B, Ozbayrak S. Serum cytokine and T regulatory cell levels in patients with burning mouth syndrome. J Oral Pathol Med. 2008;37(9):528–34. https://doi.org/10.1111/j.1600-0714.2008.00668.
17. Schou WS, Ashina S, Amin FM, et al. Calcitonin gene-related peptide and pain: a systematic review. J Headache Pain. 2017;18(1):34. https://doi.org/10.1186/s10194-017-0741-2.
18. Grushka M, Epstein JB, Gorsky M. Burning mouth syndrome. Am Fam Physician. 2002;65(4):615–20.
19. Lopez-Leon S, Wegman-Ostrosky T, Perelman C, et al. More than 50 long-term effects of COVID-19: a systematic review and meta-analysis. Sci Rep. 2021;11(1):16144.
20. López-Jornet P, Camacho-Alonso F, Lucero-Berdugo M. Quality of life in patients with burning mouth syndrome. J Oral Pathol Med. 2008;37(7):389–94. https://doi.org/10.1111/j.1600-0714.2008.00672.x.
21. Cuevas-Gonzalez MV, Espinosa-Cristóbal LF, Donohue-Cornejo A, et al. COVID-19 and its manifestations in the oral cavity: a systematic review. Medicine (Baltimore). 2021;100(51):e28327. https://doi.org/10.1097/MD.0000000000028327.
22. Mao L, Jin H, Wang M, et al. Neurologic manifestations of hospitalized patients with coronavirus disease 2019 in Wuhan, China. JAMA Neurol. 2020;77(6):683–90.
23. Xu H, Zhong L, Deng J, et al. High expression of ACE2 receptor of 2019-nCoV on the epithelial cells of oral mucosa. Int J Oral Sci. 2020;12(1):8. https://doi.org/10.1038/s41368-020-0074-x.
24. Grace PM, Hutchinson MR, Maier SF, Watkins LR. Pathological pain and the neuroimmune interface. Nat Rev Immunol. 2014;14(4):217–31. https://doi.org/10.1038/nri3621.
25. Doceda MV, Gavriiloglou M, Petit C, Huck O. Oral health implications of SARS-CoV-2/COVID-19: a systematic review. Oral Health Prev Dent. 2022;20:b2960801.
26. Kanazi GE, Johnson RW, Dworkin RH. Treatment of postherpetic neuralgia: an update. Drugs. 2000;59(5):1113–26. https://doi.org/10.2165/00003495-200059050-00007.
27. Orliaguet M, Misery L. Neuropathic and psychogenic components of burning mouth syndrome: a systematic review. Biomolecules. 2021;11(8):1237. https://doi.org/10.3390/biom11081237.
28. Oaklander AL, Mills AJ, Kelley M, et al. Peripheral neuropathy evaluations of patients with prolonged long COVID. Neurol Neuroimmunol Neuroinflamm. 2022;9(2):e1146. https://doi.org/10.1212/NXI.0000000000001146.

29. Abrams RMC, Simpson DM, Navis A, Jette N, Zhou L, Shin SC. Small fiber neuropathy associated with SARS-CoV-2 infection. Muscle Nerve. 2022;65(4):440–3. https://doi.org/10.1002/mus.27458. Epub 2021 Nov 22. PMID: 34766365; PMCID: PMC8661991.
30. Ponirakis G, Odriozola A, Ortega L, et al. Quantitative sensory testing defines the trajectory of sensory neuropathy after severe COVID-19. Diabetes Res Clin Pract. 2024;207:111029. https://doi.org/10.1016/j.diabres.2023.111029.
31. Kouri M, Adamo D, Vardas E, Georgaki M, Canfora F, Mignogna MD, Nikitakis N. Small fiber neuropathy in burning mouth syndrome: a systematic review. Int J Mol Sci. 2024;25(21):11442. https://doi.org/10.3390/ijms252111442.
32. Ni W, Yang X, Yang D, et al. Role of angiotensin-converting enzyme 2 (ACE2) in COVID-19. Crit Care. 2020;24:422. https://doi.org/10.1186/s13054-020-03120-0.
33. Iranmanesh B, Khalili M, Amiri R, Zartab H, Aflatoonian M. Oral manifestations of COVID-19 disease: a review article. Dermatol Ther. 2021;34(1):e14578.
34. Díaz Rodríguez M, Jimenez Romera A, Villarroel M. Oral manifestations associated with COVID-19. Oral Dis. 2022;28(S1):960–3.
35. Breslin PA. An evolutionary perspective on food and human taste. Curr Biol. 2013;23(9):R409–18. https://doi.org/10.1016/j.cub.2013.04.010.
36. Favia G, Tempesta A, Barile G, et al. COVID-19 symptomatic patients with oral lesions: clinical and histopathological study. Int J Environ Res Public Health. 2021;18(12):6011.
37. Chaudhari N, Roper SD. The cell biology of taste. J Cell Biol. 2010;190(3):285–96. https://doi.org/10.1083/jcb.201003144.
38. Taruno A, Vingtdeux V, Ohmoto M, et al. CALHM1 ion channel mediates purinergic neurotransmission of sweet, bitter and umami tastes. Nature. 2013;495(7440):223–6. https://doi.org/10.1038/nature11906.
39. Sakaguchi W, Kubota N, Shimizu T, et al. Existence of SARS-CoV-2 entry molecules in the oral cavity. Int J Mol Sci. 2020;21(17):6000. https://doi.org/10.3390/ijms21176000.
40. Xiong J, Lipsitz O, Nasri F, et al. Impact of COVID-19 pandemic on mental health: a systematic review. J Affect Disord. 2020;277:55–64.
41. Pereira JV, Normando AGC, Rodrigues-Fernandes CI, Rivera C, Santos-Silva AR, Lopes MA. The impact on quality of life in patients with burning mouth syndrome: a systematic review and meta-analysis. Oral Surg Oral Med Oral Pathol Oral Radiol. 2021;131(2):186–94. https://doi.org/10.1016/j.oooo.2020.11.019.
42. Cirillo N. COVID-19 outbreak: succinct advice for dentists and oral healthcare professionals. Clin Oral Investig. 2020;24(7):2529–35.
43. Femiano F, Scully C. Burning mouth syndrome (BMS): double blind controlled study of alpha-lipoic acid (thioctic acid) therapy. J Oral Pathol Med. 2002;31(5):267–9.
44. Li C, Liu S, Lu X, Tao F. Role of descending dopaminergic pathways in pain modulation. Curr Neuropharmacol. 2019;17(12):1176–82. https://doi.org/10.2174/1570159X17666190430102531. PMID: 31182003; PMCID: PMC7057207.
45. Bartoshuk LM. Comparing sensory experiences across individuals: recent psychophysical advances illuminate genetic variation in taste perception. Chem Senses. 2000;25(4):447–60. https://doi.org/10.1093/chemse/25.4.447.
46. Nalbandian A, Sehgal K, Gupta A, et al. Post-acute COVID-19 syndrome. Nat Med. 2021;27(4):601–15. https://doi.org/10.1038/s41591-021-01283-z.
47. Arnold LM, Bennett RM, Crofford LJ, et al. AAPT diagnostic criteria for fibromyalgia. J Pain. 2019;20(6):611–28. https://doi.org/10.1016/j.jpain.2018.10.008.
48. Yong SJ. Persistent brainstem dysfunction in long-COVID: a hypothesis. ACS Chem Neurosci. 2021;12(4):573–80. https://doi.org/10.1021/acschemneuro.0c00793.
49. Woo MS, Shafiq M, Fitzek A, Dottermusch M, Altmeppen H, Mohammadi B, Mayer C, Bal LC, Raich L, Matschke J, Krasemann S, Pfefferle S, Brehm TT, Lütgehetmann M, Schädler J, Addo MM, Schulze Zur Wiesch J, Ondruschka B, Friese MA, Glatzel M. Vagus nerve inflammation contributes to dysautonomia in COVID-19. Acta Neuropathol. 2023;146(3):387–94. https://doi.org/10.1007/s00401-023-02612-x. Epub 2023 Jul 15. PMID: 37452829; PMCID: PMC10412500.

50. Shiers S, Ray PR, Wangzhou A, et al. ACE2 and SCARF expression in human dorsal root ganglia: implications for SARS-CoV-2 neurological effects. Pain. 2020;161(11):2494–501. https://doi.org/10.1097/j.pain.0000000000002050.
51. Sene D. Small fiber neuropathy: diagnosis, causes, and treatment. Joint Bone Spine. 2018;85(5):553–9. https://doi.org/10.1016/j.jbspin.2017.08.001.
52. Bandinelli F, Di Carlo M, Colantuono VA, et al. Post-COVID-19 small fiber neuropathy as a new emerging quality of life-threatening disease: a systematic review. Microorganisms. 2025;13(2):328. https://doi.org/10.3390/microorganisms13020328.
53. Brooks JCW, Nurmikko TJ, Bimson WE, Singh KD, Roberts N. fMRI of thermal pain: effects of stimulus laterality and attention. NeuroImage. 2002;15(2):293–301. https://doi.org/10.1006/nimg.2001.0982.
54. Lin CS. Brain signature of chronic orofacial pain: a systematic review and meta-analysis on neuroimaging research of trigeminal neuropathic pain and temporomandibular joint disorders. PLoS One. 2014;9(4):e94300. https://doi.org/10.1371/journal.pone.0094300. PMID: 24759798; PMCID: PMC3997345.

Chemosensory Dysfunction in COVID-19

27

Ruwan Duminda Jayasinghe, Rasika Manori Jayasinghe, and Lakshman Samaranayake

27.1 Introduction

The COVID-19 pandemic emerged unexpectedly in 2020, resulting in significant mortality and morbidity, with thousands succumbing to the disease. However, the causative agent is a respiratory pathogen, and the disease presents with many extra-pulmonary, protean manifestations, including those of mucocutaneous tissues.

Dermatologists were among the first to recognise the mucocutaneous manifestations of COVID-19 [1, 2], noting that they were very similar to cutaneous manifestations (exanthems) of common viral diseases. However, some of these lesions, observed in the skin and oral mucosa, may have been adverse drug reactions to COVID-19 treatments rather than direct manifestations of the infection [3].

One of the earliest and most pathognomonic oral manifestations of COVID-19 is taste disturbance, including complete loss of taste (ageusia, Greek geusis—taste) or altered taste (dysgeusia). These symptoms were often associated with anosmia (loss of smell). This duality of manifestations in both taste and smell is also referred to as chemosensory dysfunction.

R. D. Jayasinghe (✉)
Department of Oral Medicine and Periodontology, Faculty of Dental Sciences, University of Peradeniya, Peradeniya, Sri Lanka
e-mail: ruwanja@dental.pdn.ac.lk

R. M. Jayasinghe
Department of Prosthetic Dentistry, Faculty of Dental Sciences, University of Peradeniya, Peradeniya, Sri Lanka

Department of Prosthetic Dentistry, Mahsa International college (Penang), Butter worth, Malaysia
e-mail: manorija@dental.pdn.ac.lk

L. Samaranayake
Professor Emeritus & Former Dean of Dentistry, University of Hong Kong, Hong Kong, Hong Kong
e-mail: lakshman@hku.hk

S. R. Prabhu et al. (eds.), *COVID-19 in Dental Practice*,
https://doi.org/10.1007/978-3-032-26000-0_27

Chemosensory dysfunction, the ability of organisms to detect and respond to chemical stimuli, particularly through the senses of taste (gustation) and smell (olfaction), is often observed during the pre-symptomatic or early symptomatic phase of the disease. While many patients commonly exhibit a combination of both taste and smell disturbances, some display an isolated impairment [4]. The reported prevalence of these chemosensory changes varies, with early studies indicating around 50% affected [5] and others reporting rates as high as 80% [6]. However, these figures should be interpreted with caution, as they often rely on self-reporting, which may be subject to inaccuracies.

Fortunately, taste dysfunction improves significantly for most patients and is uncommon after a year of exposure to COVID-19. The average duration of anosmia is about 7 days and usually resolves within 28 days [5]. However, some loss of smell may persist in roughly one-third of patients. For many post-COVID patients, taste complaints might actually result from this ongoing olfactory loss rather than a genuine gustatory impairment [7]. A small number of patients may experience these changes for years. Boscolo-Rizzo et al. (2023) [8] reported a 3-year prevalence of smell or taste alteration of 5%, with a 92% recovery rate.

Persistent symptoms like anosmia and dysgeusia are hallmark features of "Long COVID," a chronic condition with prolonged complications affecting multiple organ systems.

27.2 Aetiology of Dysgeusia

Although not life-threatening, taste alterations can cause sufficient discomfort and result in loss of appetite, changes in eating patterns, and potentially affect quality of life. Taste alterations can be due to multiple etiological agents, including genetic and environmental factors, such as ageing, chemical exposure to the tongue, drugs, trauma, high alcohol consumption, cigarette smoking, poor oral health, and viral infections, including COVID-19. A complete list of conditions that may cause dysgeusia is given in Table 27.1.

Table 27.1 Conditions that may cause dysgeusia or ageusia

Category	Factors
Genetics	Genetic variations affect sensitivity to flavours
Age	Taste perception can decline with age
Infections	Infections such as COVID-19 can temporarily change taste perception
Physiological	Affection of gustatory nerve pathways Abnormal zinc homeostasis
Psychological	Emotional State: Mood affects food choices and taste perception
Dietary	New Diets: Switching diets alters taste preferences
Iatrogenic	Oral Surgical procedures involving the tongue, gums, or palate can damage taste buds or nerves, leading to altered taste.
Life style	Smoking, poor oral health, heavy alcohol consumption
Metabolic	Abnormal zinc homeostasis

27.3 Epidemiology of Dysgeusia

COVID-19 is a disease with protean manifestations. Although the infective agent SARS-CoV-2 was not known to cause multi-organ disease, it became clear that the infection is a multisystem disease with almost all organs involved, including the oral cavity. Among the many oral symptoms and signs of COVID-19 infection, one of the most typical and well-recognised manifestations is chemosensory dysfunction, resulting in alterations of taste (dysgeusia) and smell (anosmia).

Dysgeusia is recognised as a pathognomonic symptom of the disease [9]. In a meta-analysis, Dos Santos et al. (2021) [10] reported a global prevalence of taste disorders in 45% of COVID-19 patients, with 24% experiencing ageusia, 35% experiencing hypogeusia, and 38% experiencing dysgeusia. They also found, with moderate certainty, that taste disorders are associated with COVID-19 positivity, mild-to-moderate severity, and female sex. Some workers have evaluated the specific loss of different flavours in COVID-19-related dysgeusia [4]. The salt taste was the least affected, while the umami taste was more severely affected than the other taste variants, including sweet, sour, and bitter.

27.4 Prevalence of Dysgeusia and Anosmia

Several reviews are currently available on the prevalence and related characteristics of both dysgeusia and anosmia in COVID-19 [9, 11]. In general, a review of data from over a dozen studies across various regions of the world suggests that both dysgeusia and anosmia are present as prodromal, subclinical, or clinical manifestations in up to two-fifths to three-quarters of ambulatory COVID-19 patients [9, 11].

Several reviewers have paid particular attention to evaluating the association between olfactory and gustatory dysfunction in COVID-19, with a focus on the temporal presentation of these symptoms, i.e., whether the gustatory and olfactory symptoms occur simultaneously or sequentially and, if so, which precedes the other. Anosmia and dysgeusia can present either in isolation or together. Whether anosmia precedes dysgeusia or vice versa is unclear based on the available data. However, the current data are far from complete due to methodological limitations, the retrospective nature of most studies, and low response rates resulting from patient noncompliance.

Suppose dysgeusia and anosmia are indeed present during the early prodrome of the disease or in otherwise asymptomatic patients harbouring the virus. In that case, this raises the intriguing possibility of identifying patients in the early prodromal and/or pre-symptomatic phase of the disease, either through self-assessment or telediagnosis. In particular, dental practitioners are ideally placed to make an early diagnosis of COVID-19, as they can forewarn the patient of the possibility and take necessary interventional measures to prevent further spread of the disease among the patient's family members and the community. Although the threat of a recurrent COVID-19 epidemic has abated due to the wide availability of efficacious vaccines, dental practitioners should be cognisant of this cause of dysgeusia when managing patients.

Reports indicate that most patients with COVID-19 experience significant olfactory impairment rather than taste impairment, and the latter is significantly correlated with symptom onset and hospitalisation [12].

Marked geographic differences of patients with taste and smell disturbances in COVID-19 have also been observed. European studies often reported higher prevalence (up to 70%) than East Asian cohorts (10–20%). Gustatory alterations were most prevalent in American studies compared to European, Middle Eastern, or East Asian studies [13]. Such heterogeneity in dysgeusia incidence could be due to genetic differences, variations in viral strains, and methodological differences in symptom reporting and recording, including both subjective and objective confounders.

27.5 Anatomy and Pathophysiology of Ageusia/Dysgeusia

Taste is considered a special sensation associated with eating and nutrition. Traditionally, five basic taste types have been identified in humans: sour, salty, sweet, bitter, and umami. More recently, additional taste types, such as metallic, fatty, and calcium, have also been included in this repertoire [14].

The functional unit of taste sensation is the taste bud, which is located in numerous clusters on the various tongue papillae. While specific anatomical locations were once thought to correspond to particular tastes, current findings suggest that all areas of the tongue are equally responsible for all types of taste. In addition to the tongue, taste buds are present on other oral sites, including the palate, pharynx, epiglottis, and oesophagus.

Taste buds contain receptors responsible for impulse generation (Fig. 27.1). They act as biological transducers, converting chemical energy from the taste-provoking chemical molecules (tastants) into electrical energy. This conversion facilitates the transmission of generated taste impulses. Taste signals are then transmitted to the brain stem via cranial nerves, namely, facial (VIIth), glossopharyngeal (IXth,) and vagus (Xth).

The orbitofrontal cortex (secondary taste cortex) of the brain is responsible for the identification of taste. Abnormalities in this pathway can lead to taste disorders (Table 27.2). These abnormalities include changes in transport (the inability of the tastant in the oral cavity to reach the taste receptor), abnormalities of peripheral sensory organs (gustatory units), and abnormalities of the neuronal unit due to damage to the peripheral or central nervous system. Depending on the severity of the taste abnormality, it can lead to dysgeusia or ageusia.

Gustatory receptors can be exposed to pathologies (such as inflammation), drugs, or artificial restorative dental materials (such as acrylic), thus affecting gustation. Genetic mutations in the genes responsible for gustatory receptors (e.g. ENaC, T1R, T2R, TAS2R, and TRPV1) can rarely result in a taste disorder. Ageing is also a factor in reducing taste sensation [14] (Table 27.2). It is essential to note that taste

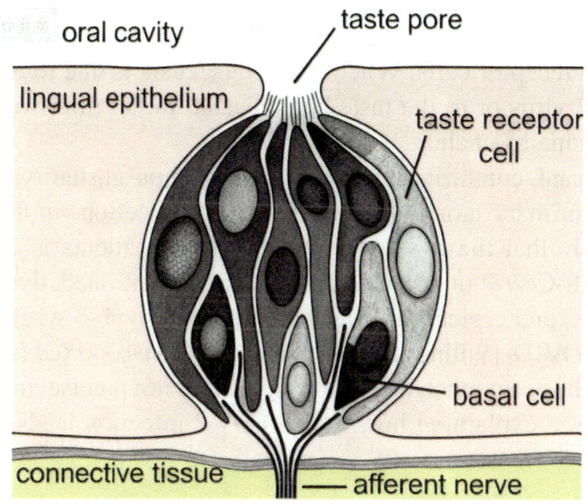

Fig. 27.1 AI-generated anatomy of a taste bud, indicating the supporting basal cells that are infected by SARS-CoV-2

Table 27.2 Risk factors for gustatory and olfactory alterations

Category	Smell (Olfaction)	Taste (Gustation)
Neurological conditions	Parkinson's disease, Alzheimer's disease, Head trauma, Multiple sclerosis	Stroke, Bell's palsy, Alzheimer's disease, Parkinson's disease
Infections	Upper respiratory infections, COVID-19, Sinusitis	Oral infections, COVID-19—Poor dental hygiene
Medical conditions	Chronic sinusitis, Nasal polyps, Allergic rhinitis	Diabetes, Xerostomia (dry mouth) Nutrient deficiencies (zinc, B12)
Medications & treatments	Chemotherapy, Radiation to head/ neck, Nasal decongestants	Antibiotics (e.g. metronidazole), Antidepressants, Chemotherapy
Environmental & lifestyle	Smoking, alcohol abuse, Chemical exposure (solvents, metals)	Smoking, Alcohol, and Poor oral hygiene
Age related decline	Common in adults >60 years due to olfactory nerve decline	Common in older adults due to taste bud atrophy or reduced saliva
Congenital/genetic factors	Congenital anosmia (e.g. Kallmann syndrome; rare)	Congenital taste disorders (rare)

always acts in conjunction with smell (olfaction). Some of the commonest gustatory dysfunctions (such as dysgeusia) are the result of impaired smell (olfaction) rather than loss of taste (gustation).

The causes of taste loss in COVID-19 are unclear. Angiotensin-converting enzyme 2 (ACE2) receptors, found in all human cells, including those in the taste buds, have been identified as the main host cell receptor of the coronavirus. These ACE2 receptors play a crucial role in the virus's entry into the cell, leading to COVID-19 infection. Indeed, ACE2 is highly enriched in epithelial cells of the tongue [15]. Some speculate that the increased number of ACE-2 receptors on the tongue's keratinocytes, along with the associated cell death and desquamation that block the taste buds, may adversely affect taste perception. The virus can infect basal progenitor cells in the taste buds (Fig. 27.1), which are responsible for regenerating new taste receptor cells. Whether the dysgeusia is due to direct damage by the SARS-CoV-2 virus or to the taste buds located in the filiform, fungiform, and vallate papillae remains unclear.

On the other hand, contrarians have reported that non-gustatory papillary epithelial cells are the primary target cells in COVID-19 infections in the tongue; therefore, it is unlikely that the dysgeusia in COVID-19 patients is caused by direct infection of SARS-CoV-2 in taste bud cells [16]. As mentioned, dysgeusia is almost always temporary, and typical taste sensation returns by 4–6 weeks after recovery from the acute COVID-19 illness. Only a very few have reported long-term effects.

Even though the exact mechanism of dysgeusia is not precise, multiple pathways have been proposed explaining how SARS-CoV-2 infection leads to dysgeusia, as outlined below:

1. As ACE2 receptors for SARS-CoV-2 are also abundant in the salivary glandular tissues. Hence, it is likely that human salivary glands may be targeted in the presymptomatic phase of the infection, resulting in salivary gland dysfunction. The resultant impairment of salivary flow and its effects on both the quality and quantity of saliva may manifest as dysgeusia.
2. A neurologic pathway, where it has been hypothesised that, as dysgeusia and anosmia are closely linked, impairment of the olfactory system with an abundance of ACE2 receptors for the virus may have an indirect impact on taste sensation, leading to dysgeusia.
3. The infection could directly damage peripheral taste neurosensory chemoreceptors through the cranial nerves responsible for gustation and, in particular, the chorda tympani (VII) nerve. It has been posited that the virus could access the chorda tympani by first travelling from the nasopharynx to the eustachian tube, then colonising the middle ear, from which it could access the chorda tympani, eventually causing dysgeusia.
4. Inflammatory response pathway has been proposed wherein the SARS-CoV-2 virus enters ACE2-expressing epithelial cells of the taste buds, triggering an inflammatory response, which in turn may lead to cellular and genetic changes that could alter taste. Pro-inflammatory cytokines, such as TNF-α, IFN-γ, and IL-6, generated during inflammation, can interfere with stem cell proliferation. Inflammation may also reduce the lifespan of mature taste bud receptors and cells. Furthermore, in COVID-19 patients, high levels of TNF-α, IFN-γ, and IL-6 have been observed, and it has been speculated that these cytokines may lead to dysgeusia by interfering with short to medium-term cellular regeneration of taste buds. Indeed, others have proposed that, as the severity of COVID-19 infection is proportional to levels of these pro-inflammatory cytokines, the quality and severity of dysgeusia may help identify mild, moderate, and severe cases [14, 17].
5. Abnormal zinc homeostasis can cause dysgeusia by disrupting the structure and function of taste buds, as zinc is essential for their maintenance and regeneration.

Zinc deficiency impairs the ability of taste cells to respond to tastants and alters saliva composition, both of which are crucial for taste perception. Additionally, zinc plays a vital role in neuronal function, and irregular zinc levels can disrupt the transmission of taste signals from taste buds to the brain. Furthermore, zinc modulates inflammation, and its imbalance may exacerbate inflammatory processes, further contributing to altered taste perception [14].

27.6 Pathophysiology of Anosmia

The pathophysiology of anosmia appears to be less complex than that of dysgeusia. While anosmia may result from direct infection and disruption of the olfactory nerve by the SARS-CoV-2 virus, studies show that angiotensin-converting enzyme II (ACE2)—COVID-19 receptor on host cells—and Transmembrane serine protease 2 (TMPRSS2), a key protease implicated in viral infection, are not significantly expressed in mature olfactory sensory neurons. Instead, these receptors are predominantly found in sustentacular cells, which support olfactory neurons, and to a lesser extent in olfactory stem cells. Therefore, it is believed that infection of these support cells and regenerative stem cells, rather than direct infection and damage to the olfactory nerve itself, is the primary cause of anosmia. Eventually, the loss of significant quantities of supporting cells surrounding olfactory neurons appears to inhibit their function. Studies conducted in murine models have demonstrated that juveniles express lower levels of ACE2 and TMPRSS2 than adults, which explains the variable disease severity observed in humans.

Notably, coronaviruses are known to infect the central nervous system (CNS) via the cribriform plate of the skull, triggering an inflammatory response that can further impair olfactory function [17]. The pathogenesis of anosmia also involves the participation of inflammatory cytokines, which, in turn, alter neuronal signalling and contribute to the loss of smell experienced by patients.

Variants of SARS-CoV-2 are genetically distinct from the original virus due to mutations in their spike proteins, resulting in different symptom profiles, including anosmia and dysgeusia [18]. As described above, dysgeusia often presents alongside anosmia in COVID-19 patients, possibly due to the peripheral neurotropism of SARS-CoV-2 or direct toxicity to taste buds or the olfactory epithelium [18].

27.7 Risk Factors for Gustatory and Olfactory Alterations

Although numerous demographic and clinical variables have been linked to gustatory and/or olfactory dysfunctions (Table 27.2), this section focuses specifically on those associated with COVID-19-related smell and taste loss only. Evidence indicates that individuals experiencing these symptoms were typically younger, female and more likely to report cough, chest pain, headache, or a history of chronic obstructive pulmonary disease (COPD) but with minimal high-risk comorbidities [19].

In addition, genetic factors, especially the UGT2A1/UGT2A2 locus, have been implicated in COVID-19-related loss of anosmia or ageusia [20]. Other associated risk factors with a higher odd of reporting a loss of smell included the use of e-cigarettes, ethnicity, and a higher BMI [21].

27.8 Metrics of Taste and Smell

In the absence of a universally standardised measurement index for either gustatory or olfactory impairment, most studies have relied on subjective, self-reported assessments to evaluate these sensory functions. This reliance on patient perception introduces procedural biases, as many are unable to accurately assess their own sense of taste and, more notably, their sense of smell. Perceptual accuracy can be influenced by various factors, further complicating the reliability of self-reported data. Indeed, studies using objective measures of smell have shown that self-reporting surveys may even underestimate the prevalence of anosmia in COVID-19 patients.

There are multiple objective methods available for assessing disturbances in taste and smell, which can enhance diagnostic accuracy and improve our understanding of sensory impairments associated with viral infections, such as COVID-19. These methods are briefly outlined below.

27.8.1 The Visual Analogue Scale (VAS)

The VAS scale has been used as a diagnostic tool for evaluating olfactory and gustatory dysfunction (OGD) in many studies. It has also proven effective for COVID-19 [22]. Notably, the European Position Paper on Rhinosinusitis and Nasal Polyps (EPOS) guidelines proposed a classification for sinonasal symptoms, using a VAS. According to the EPOS guidelines, all olfactory and gustatory symptoms can be classified into mild (VAS: 0–3), moderate (VAS > 3–7) and severe (VAS > 7–10) degrees of disease [23].

27.8.2 The Connecticut Chemosensory Clinical Research Centre (CCCRC) Test and the University of Pennsylvania Smell Identification Test (UPSIT)

The CCCRC has been reported in the literature as a standard test for olfactory function. The CCCRC test consists of two components: an odour threshold component and an odour identification component. These two components are combined for a composite score.

For the threshold test, one nostril is closed, and the subject is presented with a solution of dilute butanol or water. The subject must identify which solution contains something other than water in four consecutive trials; if the subject guesses incorrectly, a higher concentration of butanol is then used. For the identification test, seven scents are used, and the identification score is based on the number of correct identifications. The University of Pennsylvania Smell Identification Test (UPSIT) requires the identification of 40 different smells [17].

27.8.3 The Odour Stick Identification Test for Japanese (OSIT-J)

The OSIT-J utilises disposable aromatic sticks that are easy to use. It is easy to use, faster, works well with novice clinicians and has been demonstrated to work well across cultural divides.

Apart from the above, there are several gustatory tests described in the literature that attempt to evaluate taste sensation, and these include.

27.8.4 The Gustatory Test

The gustatory test evaluates taste, in which patients rate the intensity of standardised salty, sweet, sour, and bitter solutions on a scorecard. The Connecticut Chemosensory Clinical Research Centre (CCCRC) has been used to evaluate anosmia and dysgeusia in patients with COVID-19 [17].

27.8.5 The Electrogustometry Method

Electrogustometry tests the taste sensory nerves by measuring the electrical taste threshold in the soft tissue areas supplied by specific sensory nerves [14].

27.8.6 The Filter Paper Disk Method

Here, test discs soaked in solutions representing different taste qualities (e.g., sweet, salty, sour, bitter, and umami) are placed on specific regions of the oral cavity. These discs contain graded concentrations of the test solutions, starting with the lowest. The procedure continues sequentially until the participant can correctly identify the taste quality, thereby determining the taste detection threshold for each taste modality [14].

27.8.7 The Whole Mouth Method

This method tests for taste threshold. Here, the participants are asked to rinse their mouths with multiple taste solutions with various molarities of the solutes and are then required to identify the taste [14].

27.8.8 The Taste Strip Method

This test uses filter paper strips embedded with the four basic tastes. They are placed in successive graded concentrations at the centre of the anterior one-third of the tongue when the tongue is protruded, and the participants are required to identify the taste [14].

27.8.9 The E-tongue Method

This is not a test used in routine clinical practice but mostly in pharmaceutical research, and it uses an analytical instrument that helps interpret the data from a sensor that records electrical signals from the taste fibres [14].

27.9 Management of Anosmia and Dysgeusia in Patients with COVID-19

The abrupt onset of dysgeusia and anosmia, even in the absence of other symptoms, may be an early sign of SARS-CoV-2 infection. Such cases warrant further investigation to confirm or exclude the diagnosis of COVID-19. The majority of patients with anosmia and dysgeusia spontaneously recover, but a small proportion of patients take a longer period. Therefore, early intervention is necessary to prevent the chronicity of these conditions. However, due to the unclear pathophysiology, there is currently no standardised, evidence-based management protocol for the condition.

For anosmia, a combination of olfactory therapy and budesonide nasal irrigation has shown promising results in accelerating and enhancing recovery. Additional therapeutic options include saline irrigation, nasal corticosteroids, non-corticoid decongestants, and vitamin supplementation.

On the other hand, dysgeusia management in COVID-19 patients may be more challenging. Most patients with unspecified dysgeusia are treated with 0.5–1 mg of oral clonazepam once a day. Gustatory dysfunction can also be treated with L-carnitine and vitamin supplements. As these neurologic symptoms recover spontaneously in the majority of patients, supportive and symptomatic care is considered appropriate [18].

27.10 Conclusions and Future Directions

Chemosensory dysfunction, particularly anosmia and dysgeusia, has emerged as one of the most distinctive and early clinical features of COVID-19. These symptoms often precede classic respiratory signs and may serve as critical diagnostic clues, especially in individuals who are asymptomatic or mildly symptomatic. Despite their transient nature in most cases, a significant subset of patients experiences prolonged or even permanent loss of taste and smell, contributing to the burden of long COVID.

The pathophysiology of these dysfunctions is multifactorial, involving viral entry via ACE2 receptors in epithelial cells, inflammatory damage, neuronal disruption, and possibly genetic susceptibility through loci such as UGT2A1/UGT2A2. While subjective self-reporting has been the mainstay of diagnosis, objective assessments are crucial for accurately quantifying chemosensory deficits. Management remains supportive, mainly, with olfactory training and pharmacological interventions showing some benefit.

Given the high prevalence and impact of these symptoms, both dental and medical professionals must stay vigilant. Early detection, patient education, and the incorporation of chemosensory screening into clinical practice can assist in prompt diagnosis and isolation, thereby reducing the spread of the disease. Ultimately, understanding the mechanisms behind COVID-19-induced chemosensory dysfunction will guide both treatment strategies and preparedness for future viral pandemics.

References

1. Galván Casas C, Català A, Carretero Hernández G, Rodríguez-Jiménez P, Fernández-Nieto D, Rodríguez-Villa Lario A, Navarro Fernández I, Ruiz-Villaverde R, Falkenhain-López D, Llamas Velasco M, García-Gavín J, Baniandrés O, González-Cruz C, Morillas-Lahuerta V, Cubiró X, Figueras Nart I, Selda-Enriquez G, Romaní J, Fustà-Novell X, Melian-Olivera A, Roncero Riesco M, Burgos-Blasco P, Sola Ortigosa J, Feito Rodriguez M, García-Doval I. Classification of the cutaneous manifestations of COVID-19: a rapid prospective nationwide consensus study in Spain with 375 cases. Br J Dermatol. 2020;183:71–7. https://doi.org/10.1111/bjd.19163.
2. Recalcati S. Cutaneous manifestations in COVID-19: a first perspective. J Eur Acad Dermatol Venereol. 2020;34:e212–3. https://doi.org/10.1111/jdv.16387.
3. Skroza N, Bernardini N, Balduzzi V, Mambrin A, Marchesiello A, Michelini S, Tolino E, Proietti I, Di Cristofano C, Petrozza V, Potenza C. A late-onset widespread skin rash in a previous COVID-19-infected patient: viral or multidrug effect? J Eur Acad Dermatol Venereol. 2020;34:e438–9. https://doi.org/10.1111/jdv.16633.
4. Catton G, Gardner A. COVID-19 induced taste dysfunction and recovery: association with smell dysfunction and oral health behaviour. Medicina (Kaunas). 2022;58(6):715. https://doi.org/10.3390/medicina58060715.
5. Klopfenstein T, Zahra H, Kadiane-Oussou NJ, Lepiller Q, Royer PY, Toko L, Gendrin V, Zayet S. New loss of smell and taste: uncommon symptoms in COVID-19 patients on Nord Franche-Comte cluster, France. Int J Infect Dis. 2020;100:117–22. https://doi.org/10.1016/j.ijid.2020.08.012. Epub 2020 Aug 7
6. Cooper KW, Brann DH, Farruggia MC, Bhutani S, Pellegrino R, Tsukahara T, Weinreb C, Joseph PV, Larson ED, Parma V, et al. COVID-19 and the chemical senses: supporting players take center stage. Neuron. 2020;107:219–33. https://doi.org/10.1016/j.neuron.2020.06.032.
7. Sharetts R, Moein ST, Khan R, Doty RL. Long-term taste and smell outcomes after COVID-19. JAMA Netw Open. 2024;7(4):e247818. https://doi.org/10.1001/jamanetworkopen.2024.7818.

8. Boscolo-Rizzo P, Spinato G, Hopkins C, Marzolino R, Cavicchia A, Zucchini S, Borsetto D, Lechien JR, Vaira LA, Tirelli G. Evaluating long-term smell or taste dysfunction in mildly symptomatic COVID-19 patients: a 3-year follow-up study. Eur Arch Otorrinolaringol. 2023;280(12):5625–30. https://doi.org/10.1007/s00405-023-08227-y. Epub 2023 Sep 16
9. Samaranayake L, Sadir Fakhruddin K, Panduwawala C. Loss of taste and smell. Br Dent J. 2020;228:813. https://doi.org/10.1038/s41415-020-1732-2.
10. Amorim Dos Santos J, Normando AGC, Carvalho da Silva RL, Acevedo AC, De Luca CG, Sugaya N, Santos-Silva AR, Guerra ENS. Oral manifestations in patients with COVID-19: a living systematic review. J Dent Res. 2021;100(2):141–54. https://doi.org/10.1177/0022034520957289. Epub 2020 Sep 11
11. Carrillo-Larco RM, Altez-Fernandez C. Anosmia and dysgeusia in COVID-19: a systematic review. Wellcome Open Res. 2020;5:94. https://doi.org/10.12688/wellcomeopenres.15917.1.
12. Mazzatenta A, Neri G, D'Ardes D, De Luca C, Marinari S, Porreca E, Cipollone F, Vecchiet J, Falcicchia C, Panichi V, Origlia N, Di Giulio C. Smell and taste in severe CoViD-19: self-reported vs. esting. Front Med. 2020;7:589409. https://doi.org/10.3389/fmed.2020.589409.
13. Cirillo N. Taste alteration in COVID-19: significant geographical differences exist in the prevalence of the symptom. J Infect Public Health. 2021;14(8):1099–105. https://doi.org/10.1016/j.jiph.2021.07.002. Epub 2021 Jul 9
14. Thomas DC, Chablani D, Parekh S, Pichammal RC, Shanmugasundaram K, Pitchumani PK. Dysgeusia a review in the context of COVID-19. JADA. 2022;153(3):251–64. https://doi.org/10.1016/j.adaj.2021.08.009.
15. Xu H, Zhong L, Deng J, et al. High expression of ACE2 receptor of 2019-nCoV on the epithelial cells of oral mucosa. Int J Oral Sci. 2020;12:8. https://doi.org/10.1038/s41368-020-0074-x.
16. Wang Z, Zhou J, Marshall B, Rekaya R, Ye K, Liu HX. SARS-CoV-2 receptor *ACE2* is enriched in a subpopulation of mouse tongue epithelial cells in nongustatory papillae but not in taste buds or embryonic oral epithelium. ACS Pharmacol Transl Sci. 2020;3(4):749–58. https://doi.org/10.1021/acsptsci.0c00062.
17. Eshraghi AA, Mirsaeidi M, Davies C, Telischi FF, Chaudhari N, Mittal R. Potential mechanisms for COVID-19 induced anosmia and dysgeusia. Front Physiol. 2020;11:1039. https://doi.org/10.3389/fphys.2020.01039.
18. Krishnakumar HN, Momtaz DA, Sherwani A, Mhapankar A, Gonuguntla RK, Maleki A, Abbas A, Ghali AN, Al Afif A. Pathogenesis and progression of anosmia and dysgeusia during the COVID-19 pandemic. Eur Arch Otorrinolaringol. 2023;280(2):505–9. https://doi.org/10.1007/s00405-022-07689-w. Epub 2022 Oct 9
19. Johnson BJ, Salonen B, O'Byrne TJ, Choby G, Ganesh R, Stokken JK, O'Brien EK. Patient factors associated with COVID-19 loss of taste or smell patient factors in smell/taste loss COVID-19. Laryngoscope Investig Otolaryngol. 2022;7(6):1688–94. https://doi.org/10.1002/lio2.911.
20. Shelton JF, Shastri AJ, Fletez-Brant K, et al. The *UGT2A1/UGT2A2* locus is associated with COVID-19-related loss of smell or taste. Nat Genet. 2022;54:121–4. https://doi.org/10.1038/s41588-021-00986-w.
21. Razura DE, Badash I, Wrobel B, Hur K. Factors associated with loss and recovery of smell and taste after COVID-19 infection. Laryngoscope Investig Otolaryngol. 2024;9(5):e70014. https://doi.org/10.1002/lio2.70014.
22. Zarachi A, Lianou AD, Pezoulas V, et al. Visual analogue scale for the evaluation of olfactory and gustatory dysfunction of COVID-19 patients in northwestern Greece. Cureus. 2023;15(3):e36413. https://doi.org/10.7759/cureus.36413.
23. Fokkens WJ, Lund VJ, Hopkins C, Hellings PW, Kern R, Reitsma S, et al. European position paper on rhinosinusitis and nasal polyps 2020. Rhinology. 2020;58(Suppl s29):1–464.

Dry Mouth in COVID-19

28

Joseph Katz and Jane C. Atkinson

28.1 Introduction

Oral discomfort associated with COVID-19 is frequently reported, including subjective patient complaints and objective assessments by healthcare providers. During pandemic periods, more than 50% of patients developed oral complications according to one study [1]. The incidence of reported xerostomia (dry mouth) ranged from 20% to 74% [1, 2] and was the most common oral manifestation [3]. The prevalence of dry mouth increased to 74% when SARS-CoV-2 infection was studied under mechanical non-invasive ventilation [4]. Among the 301 participants, 54.8% were females [4]. The prevalence of xerostomia in participants with active COVID-19 was 39.53%, and after recovery, 34.88% [5]. In one study using Electronic Health Records (EHR), the odds ratio for COVID-19 with a complaint of dry mouth was 5.15 [6].

Dry mouth is a condition that can result from various causes, including auto immune, endocrine, and neurological conditions, as well as the use of certain medications. In addition, intensive medical therapies, especially those in intensive care units, can significantly contribute to subjective and objective dry mouth symptoms.

The wide range of dry mouth prevalence associated with COVID-19 disease could be attributed to confusion in reporting both xerostomia, a subjective complaint that presents as a qualitative outcome, and hyposalivation, an objective, quantitative diagnosis made by a healthcare professional. Additionally, because the time

J. Katz (✉)
Department of Oral Diagnostic Sciences, University of Florida College of Dentistry, Gainesville, FL, USA
e-mail: jkatz@dental.ufl.edu

J. C. Atkinson
(Retired) National Institutes of Health, Bethesda, MD, USA

S. R. Prabhu et al. (eds.), *COVID-19 in Dental Practice*,
https://doi.org/10.1007/978-3-032-26000-0_28

from infection to recovery may vary significantly among individuals, the prevalence of dry mouth in both the acute phase and the post-recovery period may also vary. Differences in race, gender and geographic location should also be considered.

28.2 Mechanisms of SARS-CoV-2–Induced Dry Mouth

How does the SARS-CoV-2 virus cause dry mouth and xerostomia in COVID-19 patients? Three potential mechanisms have been suggested.

1. The virus has a direct effect on the salivary gland tissue that may result in diminished secretion of the saliva.
2. There is a neurotrophic effect of the virus on the nerve fibres innervating the salivary glands.
3. There is an autoimmune response to the viral infection that induces a Sjogren's-like disease, destroying acinar and ductal components of the salivary glands.

The oral cavity is an important site of SARS-CoV-2 infection, and investigations implicate saliva as a potential route of SARS-CoV-2 transmission. Saliva from SARS-CoV-2-infected individuals harboured epithelial cells exhibiting ACE-2, a receptor through which SARS-CoV-2 enters cells, and TMPRSS expression and sustained SARS-CoV-2 infection. Acellular and cellular salivary fractions from asymptomatic individuals were found to transmit SARS-CoV-2 ex vivo [7].

The ACE-2 receptor is abundantly expressed on the epithelial cells of the salivary glands, and when infected by SARS-CoV-2, these receptors are overexpressed [1]. It is speculated that the signalling of the ACE-2 receptor by the virus triggers a cascade of inflammatory processes, culminating in acute and chronic sialadenitis, which disrupts salivary secretion and causes dry mouth [2, 3]. It was hypothesised that the reported xerostomia is caused by fibrosis repairment [4] or by the neuroinvasive and neurotropic potential of SARS-CoV-2 [8].

A few investigators have suggested that SARS-CoV-2 binds to ACE-2 receptors on the epithelium of the salivary glands, replicates, causes cell lysis, and propagates chronic sialadenitis, characterised by discomfort, inflammation, and pain in the major salivary glands [2, 3]. The dry mouth may also result from the neurotoxic effects of the virus on target organs, with an impact on the CNS [4].

28.3 Autoimmunity and the Development of Sjogren-Like Disease

Infection with SARS-CoV-2 and the accompanying hyperinflammation can lead to clinical features in some patients that resemble those of known autoimmune diseases, including Sjögren's syndrome (Sjögren's disease), type 1 diabetes, lupus, and inflammatory rheumatoid arthritis [9, 10]. The new onset of an autoimmune disease is now recognised as one of the sequelae of acute COVID-19 [9, 10]. The current

National Academies of Sciences, Engineering, and Medicine Committee on Examining the Working Definition for Long COVID includes the presentation of autoimmune disorders such as lupus, rheumatoid arthritis, and Sjögren's syndrome (Sjögren's disease) for at least 3 months after SARS-CoV-2 infection as a component of long COVID [10].

Several suggested mechanisms for the development of autoimmune diseases, including Sjögren's disease, have been proposed, including post-acute COVID-19 [11]. In recent years, acute infections have been linked to the development of chronic diseases such as chronic fatigue syndrome, multiple sclerosis and post-treatment Lyme disease. This class of conditions is known as infection-associated chronic conditions [12]. The development of immune-mediated events after infection with SARS-CoV-2 is hypothesised to be the result of antiviral host defence mechanisms in combination with pathways that the virus uses to evade destruction in a genetically susceptible host [13]. The resulting release of pro-inflammatory cytokines and the development of severe COVID-19 in some patients are accompanied by a pathological hyperinflammatory response [14].

One mechanism that may contribute to the progression of long COVID is the development of persistent autoantibodies in some patients following COVID-19. These autoantibodies include those targeting components of the immune system, cardiovascular system, and hypothalamic-pituitary-thyroid axis and autoantibodies associated with rheumatic diseases such as Sjögren's disease [15]. They may be produced secondary to the polyclonal activation of B-lymphocytes that occurs during infection with SARS-CoV-2 [16, 17].

Sjogren's disease is characterized by the production of autoantibodies such as anti-SS-A/Ro, anti-SS-B/La and polyclonal activation of B lymphocytes. Autoantibodies associated with Sjögren's syndrome have been reported in the sera of patients with COVID-19 infection. Early reports include a study of 102 patients post-COVID-19 that identified antibodies to U1-snRNP and anti-SS-B/La in some patients. Both autoantibodies were positively associated with persistent symptoms of fatigue and dyspnoea [18]. Most of these patients had at least two known autoantibodies in their sera. The percentage of patients who had autoantibodies decreased from 79% at 3 months post-infection to 41% at 12 months. At 3 months post-COVID, 30% had anti-SS-B/La, declining to 21% at 12 months. At 3 months post-COVID, 23% had anti-SS-A/Ro60, and this percentage fell to 12% at 12 months.

Other evidence that SARS-CoV-2 infection is associated with the development of new autoimmune diseases, including Sjögren's disease, is provided by electronic health record studies that utilised diagnostic codes and other electronic diagnostic information to document new diagnoses. These studies include a study using German routine healthcare data that compared 641,704 cases with polymerase chain reaction confirmed COVID-19 through December 31, 2020, that were matched 1:3 with a control cohort without COVID-19 [19] and followed until June 30, 2021. Patients who had COVID-19 had a 42.63% higher likelihood of being diagnosed with a new autoimmune disease. The most common incident autoimmune diseases in the COVID-19 group were Hashimoto thyroiditis (Incident Rates (IR) COVID-19 = 4.41, Incident Rate Ratio (IRR) = 1.42), Graves' disease (IR

COVID-19 = 3.52, IRR = 1.41), psoriasis (IR COVID-19 = 3.17, IRR = 1.17), rheumatoid arthritis (IR COVID-19 = 2.43, IRR = 1.42), and Sjögren syndrome (IR COVID-19 = 1.24, IRR = 1.44). Patients with a more severe course of COVID-19 were at a greater risk for incident autoimmune disease.

Another large study of RECOVER, which contained EHR data from three large, national healthcare networks in the United States [20]. The goal was to estimate the frequency of new autoimmune disease diagnoses reported after SARS-CoV-2 infection and to determine if the risk of a new autoimmune diagnosis was related to the severity of COVID-19. Patients (n = 2,031,457) with SARS-CoV-2 infection between April 1, 2020, and April 1, 2021, were identified and classified according to the World Health Organisation's COVID-19 severity category for adults. Baseline health data were available for the year before the infection date, and identified patients were followed for 2 years for the development of a new autoimmune disease. Inflammatory arthritis was the most common new-onset autoimmune disease among adults, with an IR of 1.41 per 1000 person-years in the NC3 network and 0.79 per 1000 person-years in the PCORnet network. Sjögren's disease also had a high incidence of new onset, with an IR of 0.61 per 1000 person-years in the NC3 network and 0.72 per 1000 person-years in the PCORnet network. Severe acute COVID-19 was strongly associated with the risk of development of new autoimmune diseases.

Similar findings were reported in an earlier study by those examining EHR data in the Clinical Practice Research Datalink Aurum database in the United Kingdom [21]. Data from 458,147 adults aged ≥18 years with a confirmed SARS-CoV-2 infection and no prior diagnosis of immune-mediated inflammatory diseases (IMIDs) were matched to 1,818,929 adults with no diagnosis of confirmed or suspected SARS-CoV-2 infection. The primary outcome was a composite of any of the following: autoimmune thyroiditis, coeliac disease, inflammatory bowel disease (IBD), myasthenia gravis, pernicious anaemia, psoriasis, rheumatoid arthritis (RA), Sjögren's disease, systemic lupus erythematosus (SLE), type 1 diabetes mellitus (T1DM), and vitiligo. Patients exposed to SARS-CoV-2 had a 22% increased risk of developing an IMID compared to those without exposure. An increased incidence of type 1 diabetes mellitus, inflammatory bowel disease, and psoriasis was found in the exposed cohort, but the incidence of Sjögren's disease was low and was not increased in the SARS-CoV-2 group.

28.4 Treatment Recommendations for Dry Mouth After SARS-CoV-2 Infection

Supportive therapy for COVID-19 patients with significant dry mouth should address xerostomia by providing artificial saliva, prescribing sialagogues to stimulate salivary gland secretions, and following available guidelines to prevent dental caries in those with Sjögren's disease [22, 23]. These include using topical fluorides and non-fluoride remineralisation agents to reduce the incidence, arrest, or reverse coronal or root caries. Other possible complications include oral candidiasis, especially in those using inhaled corticosteroids frequently. This infection should be treated with topical or systemic antifungal agents.

Patients with dry mouth should be counselled to drink plenty of water throughout the day and to limit sugar intake. More frequent recall appointments could be considered for those who present with new carious lesions to manage incipient caries with agents that arrest progression. Application of in-office topical fluoride varnishes is also recommended.

28.5 Conclusions

In conclusion, possible direct glandular tissue and neurotoxic damage to the salivary glands and a significant autoimmune response resulting in the induction of Sjogren's like disease may be responsible for significant dry mouth in the different phases of SARS-CoV-2 infection.

Future longitudinal studies are needed to ascertain the natural history and severity of post-COVID-19 new-onset Sjögren's disease and other autoimmune diseases, such as rheumatoid arthritis, that often have associated Sjögren's disease. Does the disease persist, increase in severity, or resolve with time? Does it develop in genetically susceptible individuals, or is susceptibility universal? Are the features of new-onset Sjögren's disease after acute COVID-19 similar to those in well-characterised cohorts of Sjögren's disease patients [24, 25].

References

1. Qu B, Liu H, Zhu W, Wei M, Yin W, Liu Q, Zhu Z. Oral complications during the two waves of COVID-19 pandemic in China: a prospective cross-sectional analysis of 510 cases using questionnaire. BMC Oral Health. 2024;24(1):1265.
2. Patel D, Louca C, Machuca VC. Oral manifestations of long COVID and the views of healthcare professionals. Br Dent J. 2024;236(2):111–6.
3. Fernandes TJ, Ogrzewalska M, Martins EB, de Siqueira MAMT, Brasil P, Calvet GA. Oral manifestations of COVID-19 in unvaccinated patients: a cross-sectional study. BMC Oral Health. 2023;23(1):696.
4. Paszynska E, Gawriolek M, Hernik A, Otulakowska-Skrzynska J, Winiarska H, Springer D, Roszak M, Slebioda Z, Krahel A, Cofta S. Prevalence of oral complications in the course of severe SARS-CoV-2 infection under mechanical non-invasive ventilation. Eur J Med Res. 2023;28(1):293.
5. Saleem MKM, Lal A, Ahmed N, Abbasi MS, Vohra F, Abduljabbar T. Oral health related quality of life and the prevalence of ageusia and xerostomia in active and recovered COVID-19 patients. PeerJ. 2023;11:e14860.
6. Katz J. Prevalence of dry mouth in COVID-19 patients with and without Sicca syndrome in a large hospital center. Ir J Med Sci. 2021;190(4):1639–41.
7. Sawa Y, Ibaragi S, Okui T, Yamashita J, Ikebe T, Harada H. Expression of SARS-CoV-2 entry factors in human oral tissue. J Anat. 2021;238(6):1341–54.

8. Okada Y, Yoshimura K, Toya S, Tsuchimochi M. Pathogenesis of taste impairment and salivary dysfunction in COVID-19 patients. Jpn Dent Sci Rev. 2021;57:111–22.
9. Chang R, Yen-Ting Chen T, Wang SI, Hung YM, Chen HY, Wei CJ. Risk of autoimmune diseases in patients with COVID-19: a retrospective cohort study. EClinicalMedicine. 2023;56:101783.
10. Ely EW, Brown LM, Fineberg HV, National academies of sciences, engineering, and medicine committee on examining the working definition for long Covid. Long Covid Defined. N Engl J Med. 2024;391(18):1746–53.
11. Tonutti A, Motta F, Isailovic N, Selmi C, Timilsina S, Eric Gershwin M, De Santis M. Mechanistic considerations linking SARS-CoV-2 infection, inflammation, and the loss of immune tolerance. Curr Opin Immunol. 2025;95:102567.
12. Unger ER. Long COVID as an infection-associated chronic condition: implications. Am J Health Promot. 2025;39(6):960–5.
13. Silva MJA, Ribeiro LR, Gouveia MIM, Marcelino BDR, Santos CSD, Lima KVB, Lima LNGC. Hyperinflammatory response in COVID-19: a systematic review. Viruses. 2023;15(2):553.
14. Dobrowolska K, Zarębska-Michaluk D, Poniedziałek B, Jaroszewicz J, Flisiak R, Rzymski P. Overview of autoantibodies in COVID-19 convalescents. J Med Virol. 2023;95(6):e28864.
15. Notarte KI, Carandang THDC, Velasco JV, Pastrana A, Ver AT, Manalo GN, Ng JA, Grecia S, Lippi G, Henry BM, Fernandez-de-las-Peñas C. Autoantibodies in COVID-19 survivors with post-COVID symptoms: a systematic review. Front Immunol. 2024;15:1428645.
16. Jiang W, Johnson D, Adekunle R, Heather H, Xu W, Cong X, Wu X, Fan H, Andersson LM, Robertson J, Gisslén M. COVID-19 is associated with bystander polyclonal autoreactive B cell activation as reflected by a broad autoantibody production, but none is linked to disease severity. J Med Virol. 2023;95(1):e28134.
17. Son K, Jamil R, Chowdhury A, Mukherjee M, Venegas C, Miyasaki K, Zhang K, Patel Z, Salter B, Yuen ACY, Lau KS, Cowbrough B, Radford K, Huang C, Kjarsgaard M, Dvorkin-Gheva A, Smith J, Li QZ, Waserman S, Ryerson CJ, Nair P, Ho T, Balakrishnan N, Nazy I, Bowdish DME, Svenningsen S, Carlsten C, Mukherjee M. Circulating anti-nuclear autoantibodies in COVID-19 survivors predict long COVID symptoms. Eur Respir J. 2023;61(1):2200970.
18. Su Y, Yuan D, Chen DG, Ng RH, Wang K, Choi J, Li S, Hong S, Zhang R, Xie J, Kornilov SA, Scherler K, Pavlovitch-Bedzyk AJ, Dong S, Lausted C, Lee I, Fallen S, Dai CL, Baloni P, Smith B, Duvvuri VR, Anderson KG, Li J, Yang F, Duncombe CJ, McCulloch DJ, Rostomily C, Troisch P, Zhou J, Mackay S, DeGottardi Q, May DH, Taniguchi R, Gittelman RM, Klinger M, Snyder TM, Roper R, Wojciechowska G, Murray K, Edmark R, Evans S, Jones L, Zhou Y, Rowen L, Liu R, Chour W, Algren HA, Berrington WR, Wallick JA, Cochran RA, Micikas ME, ISB-Swedish COVID-19 Biobanking Unit, Wrin T, Petropoulos CJ, Cole HR, Fischer TD, Wei W, Hoon DSB, Price ND, Subramanian N, Hill JA, Hadlock J, Magis AT, Ribas A, Lanier LL, Boyd SD, Bluestone JA, Chu H, Hood L, Gottardo R, Greenberg PD, Davis MM, Goldman JD, Heath JR. Multiple early factors anticipate post-acute COVID-19 sequelae. Cell. 2022;185(5):881–95.
19. Tesch F, Ehm F, Vivirito A, Wende D, Batram M, Loser F, Menzer S, Jacob J, Roessler M, Seifert M, Kind B, König C, Schulte C, Buschmann T, Hertle D, Ballesteros P, Baßler S, Bertele B, Bitterer T, Riederer C, Sobik F, Reitzle L, Scheidt-Nave C, Schmitt J. Incident autoimmune diseases in association with SARS-CoV-2 infection: a matched cohort study. Clin Rheumatol. 2023;42(10):2905–14. https://doi.org/10.1007/s10067-023-06670-0. Epub 2023 Jun 19. Erratum in: Clin Rheumatol. 2023;42(10):2919–20.
20. Wuller S, Singer NG, Lewis C, Karlson EW, Schulert GS, Goldman JD, Hadlock J, Arnold J, Hirabayashi K, Stiles LE, Kleinman LC, Cowell LG, Hornig M, Hall MA, Weiner MG, Koropsak M, Lamendola-Essel MF, Kenney R, Moffitt RA, Abedian S, Esquenazi-Karonika S, Johnson SG, Stroebel S, Wallace ZS, Costenbader KH, RECOVER Initiative, RECOVER PCORnet EHR Cohort, and the N3C RECOVER EHR Cohort. Severity of acute SARS-CoV-2

infection and risk of new-onset autoimmune disease: A RECOVER initiative study in nationwide U.S. cohorts. PLoS One. 2025;20(6):e0324513.
21. Syed U, Subramanian A, Wraith DC, Lord JM, McGee K, Ghokale K, Nirantharakumar K, Haroon S. Incidence of immune-mediated inflammatory diseases following COVID-19: a matched cohort study in UK primary care. BMC Med. 2023;21(1):363.
22. Vivino FB, Carsons SE, Foulks G, Daniels TE, Parke A, Brennan MT, Forstot SL, Scofield RH, Hammitt KM. New treatment guidelines for Sjögren's disease. Rheum Dis Clin N Am. 2016;42(3):531–51.
23. Zero DT, Brennan MT, Daniels TE, Papas A, Stewart C, Pinto A, Al-Hashimi I, Navazesh M, Rhodus N, Sciubba J, Singh M, Wu AJ, Frantsve-Hawley J, Tracy S, Fox PC, Ford TL, Cohen S, Vivino FB, Hammitt KM, Sjögren's Syndrome Foundation Clinical Practice Guidelines Committee. Clinical practice guidelines for oral management of Sjögren disease: dental caries prevention. J Am Dent Assoc. 2016;147(4):295–305.
24. Shiboski SC, Shiboski CH, Criswell L, Baer A, Challacombe S, Lanfranchi H, Schiødt M, Umehara H, Vivino F, Zhao Y, Dong Y, Greenspan D, Heidenreich AM, Helin P, Kirkham B, Kitagawa K, Larkin G, Li M, Lietman T, Lindegaard J, McNamara N, Sack K, Shirlaw P, Sugai S, Vollenweider C, Whitcher J, Wu A, Zhang S, Zhang W, Greenspan J, Daniels T, Sjögren's International Collaborative Clinical Alliance (SICCA) Research Groups. American College of Rheumatology classification criteria for Sjögren's syndrome: a data-driven, expert consensus approach in the Sjögren's International Collaborative Clinical Alliance cohort. Arthritis Care Res (Hoboken). 2012;64(4):475–87.
25. Ng WF, Bowman SJ, Griffiths B, UKPSSR study group. United Kingdom Primary Sjogren's Syndrome Registry--a united effort to tackle an orphan rheumatic disease. Rheumatology (Oxford). 2011;50(1):32–9.

COVID-19 and Maxillofacial Surgery

29

S. M. Balaji

29.1 Introduction

The COVID-19 pandemic was a global challenge for healthcare systems. It forced surgical disciplines to adapt and change rapidly. Oral and maxillofacial surgery (OMFS), which combines both medical and dental practices, faced considerable difficulties during this period. The nature of many of its procedures, which can easily transmit aerosol infections, its vital role in managing airway compromise, and its involvement in treating a broad range of conditions, from infections to malignancies, have made it one of the specialities most impacted by the crisis.

This chapter describes the ongoing development of OMFS through five stages: beginning with addressing initial limitations in emergency care, then cautiously restructuring management systems in response to evolving disease patterns, prioritising and managing patients awaiting surgery, handling long-term consequences, and integrating acquired experience into a framework for future preparedness. The pandemic changed working methods within the speciality, prompting innovations in patient prioritisation, operator safety measures, and interdisciplinary collaboration that continue to influence current OMFS practice.

29.2 The Initial Phase: Service Contraction and Need-Based Patient Prioritisation

The initial global response to the SARS-CoV-2 outbreak resulted in the immediate suspension of OMFS services. Healthcare authorities directed a complete withdrawal from all but emergency and urgent care, prompting departments to swiftly adopt an emergency-based patient prioritisation system. This approach was expanded to include time-sensitive oncological resections, reconstructive surgeries

S. M. Balaji (✉)
Balaji Dental, Craniofacial Hospital & Research Institute, Chennai, Tamil Nadu, India

S. R. Prabhu et al. (eds.), *COVID-19 in Dental Practice*,
https://doi.org/10.1007/978-3-032-26000-0_29

for traumatic defects, and the management of progressively enlarging benign lesions [1]. The factors influencing this decision involved the uncertain risk of viral transmission, weighed against the well-understood disease process for which surgery was necessary and would otherwise be postponed during such a pandemic. In this context, the surgeon assumed a significant ethical responsibility [2].

In this context, the responsibilities of the OMF surgeon focused on airway management and infection control. Emergency dentoalveolar surgery proceeded despite critical shortages of personal protective equipment (PPE) and widespread concerns about aerosol-generating procedures (AGPs) [3], as shown in Fig. 29.1. This led to several technical innovations, including a shift to external drainage of abscesses, since intraoral drainage could potentially produce aerosols, increased use of local anaesthesia rather than general anaesthesia, and a notable reduction in high-speed drilling. A particular challenge was managing severe odontogenic infections in patients with a “Do Not Intubate” order, with some undergoing radical extraoral drainage under local anaesthesia as a definitive, life-saving measure.

The closure of general dental practices led to hospital-based OMFS services becoming the sole providers of emergency dental care in many areas, leaving many patients who would otherwise have been treated in the clinic setting without care. This further emphasised the existing ‘dental vs. surgical’ divide. In the interim, OMFS surgeons became vital members of surgical teams by performing surgical tracheostomies in critically ill COVID-19 patients. This was due to modifications in team structures and operative techniques aimed at safeguarding against viral exposure during surgery [4]. This period was marked by considerable stress for practitioners, with OMF surgeons performing only a limited range of interventions because of safety concerns, which led to frustration and worry over their inability to manage untreated dental diseases.

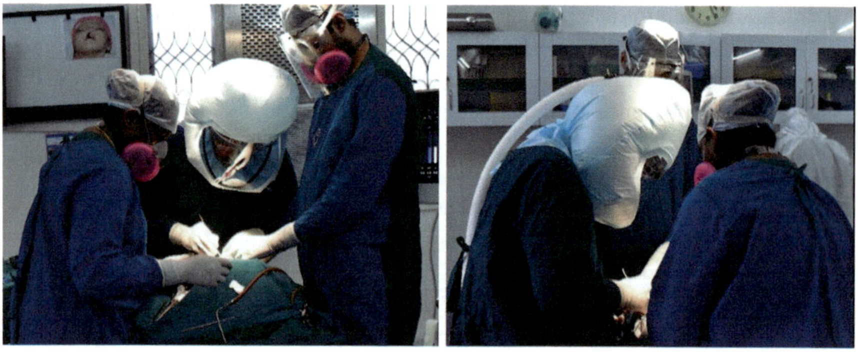

Fig. 29.1 Adaptations of modified PPE in oral and maxillofacial surgery during the COVID-19 pandemic. (Author performing emergency procedures and cleft cases using a powered air-purifying respirator (PAPR), with assistants supported by HEPA-filtered air supply units—measures implemented to ensure surgical team safety during the pandemic)

29.3 The Slow Reopening: Reinventing Treatment Processes and the Emergence of Pandemic-Related Diseases

The gradual resumption of services signified a fundamental restructuring of treatment processes rather than a return to complete normalcy. Altering the theatre infrastructure to lower the risk of viral transmission became essential. This involved upgrading the theatre's ventilation systems with high-efficiency particulate air (HEPA) filters and, where feasible, creating negative-pressure environments. These changes were vital to the resumption of procedures involving drills or nasal endoscopy, while also significantly reducing the risk of transmission of infection [5].

Necessary presurgical safety measures required that all patients undergo preoperative SARS-CoV-2 RT-PCR testing. Although important, these tests were performed with certain limitations. They were consistently associated with anxiety arising from the possibility of potential false negatives in elective surgery lists, and the insistence that a patient self-isolate not only impacted patient compliance but also compromised the optimal administration of service [6]. As a practical example, the introduction of PPE led to one of the most significant challenges: lens fogging, which invariably compromises vision during delicate procedures and affects surgical efficiency and ergonomics [7].

Clinically, during this period in India, the emergence of COVID-19-associated mucormycosis (CAM) infections was observed (Fig. 29.2). The pathogenesis was linked to three distinct factors: systemic steroid use worsening diabetic control, virus-induced endothelial injury, and impaired immunity [8]. The convergence of these factors enabled the disease to affect immunocompromised hosts, in whom omnipresent fungal spores caused severely destructive rhino-orbital-cerebral disease. OMFS surgeons found themselves on the frontline of this epidemic in countries like India, performing radical tissue debridement that was often disfiguring. Atypical oral manifestations beyond CAM were also observed, including an increase in necrotising periodontal diseases, which may be related to the virus causing injury to the cells lining the microvascular blood vessels [9]. This phase posed a dual challenge: adapting infrastructure to the new normal of sustained viral outbreaks while simultaneously safeguarding against a tragic opportunistic fungal complication. Figure 29.3a–l illustrates the management of a CAM case, demonstrating the step-by-step approach from resection to reconstruction.

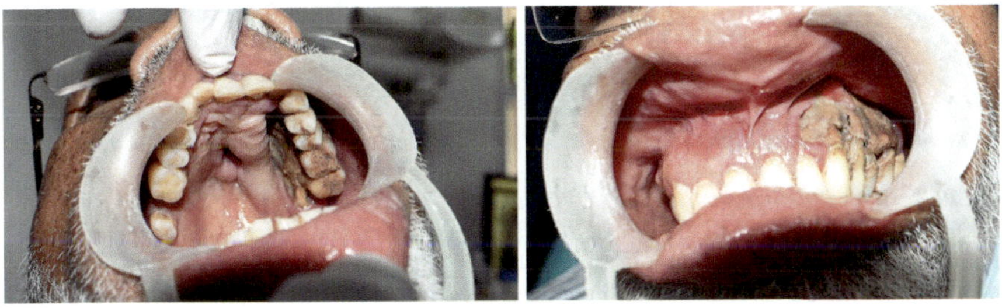

Fig. 29.2 COVID-19-associated mucormycosis involving the maxilla and palate—showing necrotic involvement of the maxilla and palate

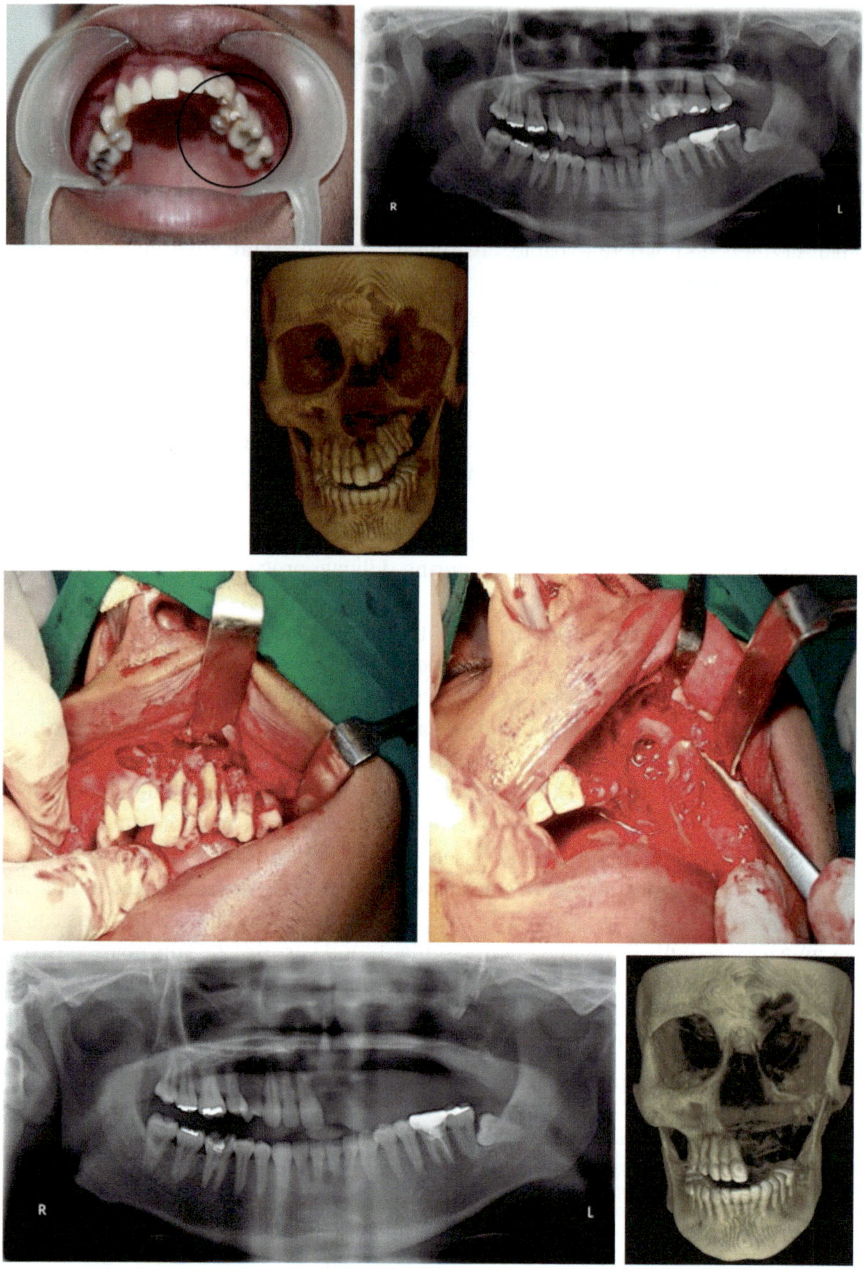

Fig. 29.3 (**a**–**c**) *Pre-operative, clinical, OPG, and 3D CT* views showing CAM involving the right maxilla. (**d**–**g**) *Intraoperative, OPG, and 3D CT views* showing complete debridement and resection of the right maxilla via intraoral approach. (**h**–**i**) *Reconstruction phase*—total left maxilla reconstructed using a costochondral rib graft and fixed with titanium miniplates and screws. (**j**–**l**) *Post-operative view* showing implant-supported prosthesis demonstrating restoration of aesthetic form and functional rehabilitation

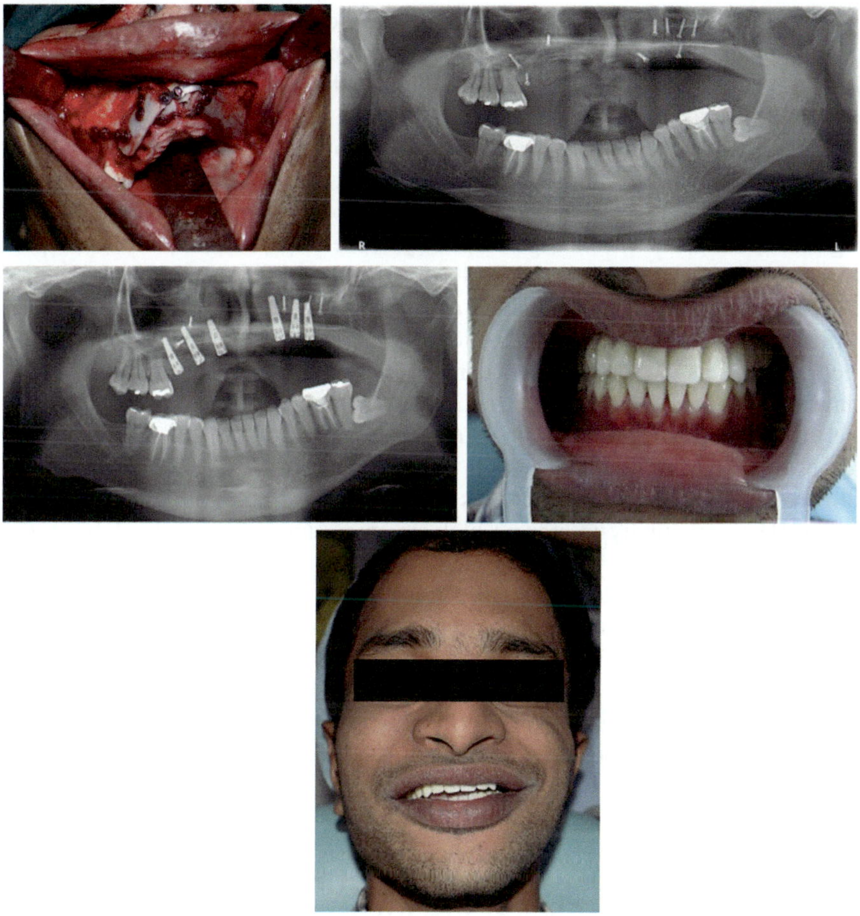

Fig. 29.3 (continued)

29.4 Backlog Clearance and Systemic Strain: A Multifaceted Challenge

The "recovery" phase underscored the significant difficulty of clearing the accumulated surgical backlog, which was far more than simply increasing operational output. The severity of this challenge differed across various healthcare systems, depending on pre-existing resource disparities. Initial efforts to extend theatre hours quickly reached the limits of available human resources, leading to exhaustion and burnout among the workforces. More accurate patient selection systems were developed and implemented to balance clinical urgency, disease progression, quality-of-life impairment, and resource availability [10].

There was universal agreement on prioritising cancer surgery and high-impact trauma surgery. However, this raised ethical dilemmas regarding the allocation of care for patients with benign but debilitating conditions. "Waiting list morbidity" was believed to compromise the delivery of care to patients presenting to the surgical service with conditions like progressive odontogenic cysts, orthognathic deformities contributing to obstructive sleep apnoea, or awaiting more complex pre-prosthetic surgery; all such patients experienced worsened function, psychological suffering, and increasing complexity of the surgical intervention with progressively delayed treatment [11]. Following the onset of the "lockdown," patients with acute trauma presented for care at an equally rapid rate, also adding unforeseen difficulties to the post-lockdown system, further straining the surgical care and recovery systems. The management burden for patients with delayed presentation to surgical services became evident when patients presented with malignancies, which were now more advanced, requiring more radical resections and more complex reconstructions.

Postoperative critical care facilities also remained under strain for an extended period. The opportunity to resume high-risk procedures depended solely on the availability of the ICU. In the months that followed, hospitals experienced multiple waves of the pandemic, leading to the redeployment of ICU resources. Each wave caused a cyclical pause in complex elective surgeries, illustrating how the speciality was at the mercy of the public health situation [12]. At the same time, the economic impact of halting elective surgeries placed significant pressure on the healthcare system. Addressing the backlog, while providing essential value to an expanding clinical backlog, has become a long-term endeavour that continues to expose systemic flaws.

29.5 Long COVID and Its Maxillofacial Implications: A Broadening Clinical Spectrum

A form of chronic debilitation in some SARS-CoV-2 patients, known as Long COVID, has emerged. Its complex symptoms have further expanded the scope of oral medicine and maxillofacial practice. Major musculoskeletal manifestations, such as temporomandibular joint (TMJ) disorders and myofascial pain, are often linked to virus-induced neuroinflammation and pandemic-related stress, necessitating multidisciplinary pain management [13]. Oral issues resulting from nerve damage, especially Burning Mouth Syndrome, were also common. Chronic loss of taste (ageusia) and smell (anosmia) due to chemosensory dysfunction significantly affected nutrition and overall quality of life [14]. Additionally, dry mouth (xerostomia) was a widespread symptom associated with an increased risk of dental caries and oral candida infection.

Reports also documented salivary gland dysfunction, with sialadenitis attributed to SARS-CoV-2's tropism for glandular tissue, leading to swelling and inflammation. A serious sequelae documented on a large scale in India, but reported worldwide, consisted of massive palatal and midfacial defects resulting from aggressive surgical management of CAM. These surgeries resulted in radical maxillectomies or palatectomies, creating large oronasal communications for the patient.

Reconstructing these large post-surgical structural defects was often a significant challenge. A high burden of fungal infection typically made immediate free tissue transfer unfeasible. Staged strategies were adopted: stabilising the defect, managing the infection immediately with obturators, and then undertaking definitive reconstruction after stabilisation. The submental artery flap is effective for managing small defects as a local flap. It is suitable for small to moderate defects, whereas the free anterolateral thigh (ALT) flap [15] remains the gold standard for reconstructing total or subtotal maxillectomy defects.

Emergency trauma management in cases such as maxillo-orbital fractures, along with airway complications, vision-threatening issues, and panfacial fractures, still requires immediate surgical intervention under strict infection-control protocols. Cleft cases with airway compromise sometimes need emergency tracheostomy. These situations demonstrate the ongoing commitment of OMFS teams to provide essential, life saving care even during the challenges of the pandemic.

This widespread experience in palatal reconstruction, developed from unfortunate necessity, has enhanced the technical skills in reconstructing major craniofacial defects and maintained the principles of staged, definitive reconstruction of significant post-infective defects.

29.6 Lessons Learnt and Future Pandemic Preparedness: A Strategic Blueprint

COVID-19 demonstrated the importance of a structured approach in oral and maxillofacial surgery, preparing us for both teaching and clinical practice in the future. First, curriculum reform should incorporate pandemic preparedness as more than just ad-hoc learning; it must be established as a core professional competence. Considering the clear link between PPE levels and moral distress during pandemics, residents need to be trained in high-risk AGP protocols (i.e., donning/doffing) and advanced emergency airway management, such as percutaneous tracheostomy. They should also receive training in disaster medicine, including careful resource allocation. This crystallisation of essential expertise should be a key element of residency training accreditation [16], with extensive simulation-based training to uphold excellence during periods of reduced operating exposure.

Secondly, the permanent biosafety enhancements, including HEPA-filtered, negative-pressure operating theatres and protected 'cold' surgical centres, should be upheld. This is essential to guarantee continuous elective and oncological surgeries. Although it required planning and investment at a national level, it functions as a lasting safeguard [17].

Operationally, the rapid adoption of technology driven by the crisis must now be firmly integrated into routine practice. Although studies highlight the shortcomings of virtual consultations compared to physical examinations in clinical practice, telemedicine should not be discarded. It functions as a valuable method for efficient patient selection, standard follow-up, and multidisciplinary meetings by creating opportunities for patient management if "Plan A" capabilities are diminished [18]. Simultaneously, digital workflows and 3D printing for pre-surgical planning and cutting guide fabrication should be fully incorporated into standard clinical practice, mainly for complex reconstructions, to reduce theatre time and enhance precision.

Moreover, the successful interdisciplinary cooperation with fields such as ENT, anaesthesiology, and critical care must be maintained at the organisational level. It required a certain degree of joint simulation-based training, and establishing integrated crisis protocols was vital, with these protocols being routinely practised. Most importantly, future preparedness and planning must specifically address the significant psychological impact on the healthcare workforce. Burnout was high due to moral injury from complex patient selection decisions and the ongoing stress of working in high-risk environments. To build a disaster-ready, resilient system, organisations must prioritise evidence-based support programmes to ensure that non-stigmatising mental health resources are easily accessible. The well-being of healthcare workers is crucial for an effective response to pandemics.

29.7 Conclusion/Summary

The COVID-19 pandemic has permanently transformed the field of OMFS, requiring a paradigm shift. It challenged the clinical skills, operational flexibility, and ethical standards of the specialty. The journey through service reductions, emerging pathologies, and system-wide backlogs has been quite challenging. The insights gained from the COVID-19 crisis highlight the importance of infrastructure, formal disaster preparedness, strategic integration of digital systems, and workforce well-being. Together, these elements create a practical and actionable framework for managing future crises. By integrating these lessons, the OMFS speciality not only endures but also becomes stronger and more resilient.

References

1. COVIDSurg Collaborative. Elective surgery cancellations due to the COVID-19 pandemic: global predictive modelling to inform surgical recovery plans. Br J Surg. 2020;107(11):1440–9.
2. Givi B, Schiff BA, Chinn SB, et al. Safety recommendations for evaluation and surgery of the head and neck during the COVID-19 pandemic. JAMA Otolaryngol Head Neck Surg. 2020;146(6):579–84.
3. Chawla G, Abrol N, Kakkar K. Personal protective equipment: a Pandora's box. Indian J Crit Care Med. 2020;24(5):371.
4. Takhar A, Walker A, Tricklebank S, Wyncoll D, Hart N, Jacob T, Arora A, Skilbeck C, Simo R, Surda P. Recommendation of a practical guideline for safe tracheostomy during the COVID-19 pandemic. Eur Arch Otorhinolaryngol. 2020;277(8):2173–84.
5. Workman AD, Jafari A, Welling DB, Varvares MA, Gray ST, Holbrook EH, Scangas GA, Xiao R, Carter BS, Curry WT, Bleier BS. Airborne aerosol generation during endonasal

procedures in the era of COVID-19: risks and recommendations. Otolaryngol Head Neck Surg. 2020;163(3):465–70.
6. Woloshin S, Patel N, Kesselheim AS. False negative tests for SARS-CoV-2 infection — challenges and implications. N Engl J Med. 2020;383(6):e38.
7. Kumar A, Qureshi OA, Arora R, Kumar S, Jameel J, Khan R. Comparison of three low-cost techniques to control fogging of sealed eyewear in a simulated operating room environment: a preliminary analysis. J Clin Orthop Trauma. 2020;11:S696–9.
8. Dravid A, Kashiva R, Khan Z, Bande B, Memon D, Kodre A, Mane M, Pawar V, Patil D, Kalyani S, Raut P. Epidemiology, clinical presentation and management of COVID-19 associated mucormycosis: a single centre experience from Pune, Western India. Mycoses. 2022;65(5):526–40.
9. Patel J, Woolley J. Necrotizing periodontal disease: oral manifestation of COVID-19. Oral Dis. 2021;27(Suppl 3):768–9.
10. Samson B. The difficult clearance of the elective surgical backlog caused by the cancellation of cases due to the COVID-19 pandemic. Can J Anesth. 2021;68(6):932–3.
11. Kaufman HW, Chen Z, Niles J, Fesko Y. Changes in the number of US patients with newly identified cancer before and during the coronavirus disease 2019 (COVID-19) pandemic. JAMA Network Open. 2020;3(8):e2017267.
12. Nepogodiev D, Abbott TE, Ademuyiwa AO, AlAmeer E, Bankhead-Kendall BK, Biccard BM, Chakrabortee S, Chaudhry D, Edwards JG, El-Boghdadly K, Ghosh D. Projecting COVID-19 disruption to elective surgery. Lancet. 2022;399(10321):233–4.
13. Tate W, Walker M, Sweetman E, Helliwell A, Peppercorn K, Edgar C, Blair A, Chatterjee A. Molecular mechanisms of neuroinflammation in ME/CFS and long COVID to sustain disease and promote relapses. Front Neurol. 2022;13:877772.
14. Coelho DH, Reiter ER, French E, Costanzo RM. Decreasing incidence of chemosensory changes by COVID-19 variant. Otolaryngol Head Neck Surg. 2023;168(4):704–6.
15. Mohebbi S, Zabihidan M, Omidvari A, Abrishami M. Post-COVID-19 maxillary bony sequestration: a case report on mucormycosis challenges. Clin Case Rep. 2025;13(10):e71080.
16. Klein M, Weksler N, Kaplan DM, Weksler D, Chorny I, Gurman GM. Emergency percutaneous tracheostomy is feasable in experienced hands. Eur J Emer Med. 2004;11(2):108–12.
17. Williams BA, Jones CH, Welch V, True JM. Outlook of pandemic preparedness in a post-COVID-19 world. npj Vaccines. 2023;8(1):178.
18. Aashima, Nanda M, Sharma R. A review of patient satisfaction and experience with telemedicine: a virtual solution during and beyond COVID-19 pandemic. Telemed e-Health. 2021;27(12):1325–31.

Protective Measures Against COVID-19 and Infection Control in Dental Practice

30

T. S. Roberts

30.1 Introduction

The COVID-19 pandemic has led to a global reassessment of infection control protocols. Oral health professionals face an increased risk of contracting or spreading SARS-CoV-2 because of their exposure to saliva, blood, respiratory secretions, and routine aerosol-generating procedures (AGPs). This chapter discusses how infection control practices in dentistry have evolved during the COVID-19 pandemic. It also highlights the lessons learned from COVID-19, supported by a stronger evidence-based approach for managing future public health emergencies.

30.2 Tiered PPE System

The COVID-19 pandemic prompted a paradigm shift in the management of dental infections, transitioning from standard measures to a risk-based PPE approach. Before the pandemic, control efforts primarily focused on blood-borne pathogens, with standard precautions such as surgical masks, gloves, and basic clothing [1]. The SARS-Cov-2 pandemic has prompted a re-evaluation of established infection control protocols and the implementation of more advanced measures, including the use of N95 respirators, face shields, liquid-tight clothing, and enhanced ventilation systems. The upgraded system, known as the PPE-tiered system, aligns the level of protection with the risk associated with each clinical procedure [2], reflecting a move towards evidence-based infection control practices.

T. S. Roberts (✉)
Faculty of Dentistry, Maxillofacial Pathology, University of the Western Cape, Cape Town, South Africa
e-mail: trobert@uwc.ac.za

S. R. Prabhu et al. (eds.), *COVID-19 in Dental Practice*,
https://doi.org/10.1007/978-3-032-26000-0_30

30.2.1 Masks and Respirators

One aspect of personal protective equipment that was reviewed during the COVID-19 pandemic was mask use. Both N95 respirators and surgical masks were widely employed during this period. Although both played a vital role in infection control, the type of mask used in a dental setting depended on the risk level of the procedure, with higher-filtration (N95) masks required for procedures that generated aerosols [3].

Surgical masks prevent particulate droplets from infecting healthcare practitioners while they breathe, talk, and sneeze. They serve as filters to avoid contamination of the surgical environment and must therefore be fluid-resistant. A high-quality surgical mask can filter particles with an average size of 2.7 μm [4].

Respirators, on the other hand, create effective facial seals around the nose and mouth, preventing inhalation of airborne particles, gases, and vapours. Respirators offer varying degrees of filtration. Three key criteria are required for a respirator to be effective [5]:

1. The filter materials should be effective at capturing hazardous particles.
2. The respirator needs to fit snugly around the face to create and maintain an effective facial seal.
3. The respirator needs to be put on (donned) and removed (doffed) correctly.

While filtration capacity is an important factor in infection control, the clinical effectiveness of masks and respirators is primarily influenced by proper fit and consistent use [6]. demonstrated that, regardless of filtration rating, consistent use of surgical masks and N95 respirators was associated with a lower risk of infection transmission. Furthermore, although N95 respirators are designed to provide superior filtration, their protective benefit is realised only when a tight facial seal is achieved. Ill-fitting N95 respirators leak air and significantly reduce their effectiveness.

Despite their lower theoretical filtration, well-fitting surgical masks can still provide meaningful protection when worn correctly and consistently. Table 30.1 summarises the comparative evidence and appropriate indications for the use of N95 respirators and surgical masks in dental practice, including their filtration efficiency, fit requirements, and real-world effectiveness.

Universal masking is more effective in clinical settings than selectively using high-performance respirators, which ignores the broader risk of airborne contagion in shared spaces. Universal masking provides two layers of protection by reducing the release of infectious particles from unknowingly infected individuals and preventing healthy individuals from inhaling them. This two-fold effect significantly decreases the overall airborne viral concentration. De Araujo et al. (2021) support this argument. The authors found that the risk of transmission was reduced if all subjects wore masks in the clinical setting [12].

Table 30.1 Comparison of N95 respirators and surgical masks in dental settings: Indications, filtration performance, and evidence base

Criteria	N95 respirators	Surgical masks
Recommended use	Aerosol-generating procedures High-risk clinical settings with airborne transmission concerns Source control in highly infectious environments	Routine patient care without AGPs General droplet precautions When N95s are unavailable
Filtration performance	98–99% filtration efficiency Reduces aerosol emissions by 90% (speaking) and 74% (coughing)	54–88% filtration efficiency Less effective in aerosol-rich environments
Real-world clinical effectiveness	High filtration efficiency only when properly fitted No definitive superiority over surgical masks for routine care	Effective for droplet control when used consistently Still protective in non-AGP situations
Fit requirements	Requires proper fit-testing ensures seal and protection	Looser fit, no seal Less dependent on fit
Resource considerations	Preferred in high-risk scenarios More costly and less widely available	Cost-effective Widely available Acceptable for lower-risk settings

Adapted from Refs. [7–11]

30.2.2 Eye Protection and Face Shields

Eye injuries are common in dental settings. In a study involving 54 dentists preparing and performing anterior tooth preparations, Skibitskyi and Ryzhova (2025) found that 20.4% of participants experienced eye injuries or infections. The injuries mainly resulted from foreign bodies (e.g., hard tissue or tooth particles), aerosols, biologically active fluids, and soft dental deposits. In the context of SARS-CoV-2, the eyes can serve as entry points for viral particles, and physical hazards encountered during routine dental procedures can increase the risk of infection. The authors also noted that dentists who wore regular glasses experienced more eye injuries than those who wore either side-shield or face-shield glasses [13]. Manzar et al. (2022) agreed with Skibitskyi and Ryzhova (2025) that side-shield safety glasses offer a practical balance between adequate coverage and clear visibility, which is especially critical during high-precision procedures [14]. These findings suggest that equipment covering more of the eye area reduces the risk of ocular injury and viral infection, providing a basis for recommending eye protection during AGPs [15]. Table 30.2 outlines the main clinical and ergonomic factors influencing the selection of eye protection, including the impact of different AGPs and procedural visibility challenges.

30.2.3 Gowns

Although traditionally considered secondary to masks and gloves in infection control protocols, gowns have played an essential role in preventing contamination in

Table 30.2 Challenges impacting the selection and efficacy of eye protection during dental aerosol-generating procedures (AGPs)

Clinical challenge	Key findings
1. Aerosol production from instruments	High-speed rotating instruments produce the most aerosol at the operator, assistant, and patient sites Air polishing causes more aerosol than ultrasound scaling The contamination decreases with distance from the source Eye protection required for all AGPs
2. Visibility and ergonomic barriers	Full-face shields can impair visibility during fine procedures Safety glasses performed equally to goggles when paired with surgical masks Side-shield glasses with loupes provided the best balance of protection and visibility
3. High-power laser dentistry	Laser procedures produce both aerosols and surgical smoke Face shields must accommodate laser safety glasses underneath Proper fit and spacing between the shield and the eyes is essential Laser eyewear must be decontaminated after each use

Adapted from Refs. [13, 16–19]

Table 30.3 Functions and limitations of medical gowns

Aspect	Functions	Limitations
Contact transmission	Prevent microbial transfer from the patient to the provider by acting as a physical barrier against saliva, blood, and other contaminated fluids	Gowns alone do not prevent microbial transfer via hands or surfaces if proper glove use, hand hygiene, and environmental cleaning are not followed
Droplet spread	Block large droplets that may carry viral particles Part of a layered PPE strategy that includes masks, gloves, and face shields	Do not filter airborne particles Do not protect against aerosolised *viruses* without complementary respiratory PPE (e.g., N95 masks)
Standards-based barrier performance	Regulatory standards (e.g., AAMI PB70, EN 14126) assess gowns for fluid resistance and biological protection. Proper gown use has been shown to reduce the risk of infection in clinical settings.	Gowns that are damaged, improperly worn, or reused beyond manufacturer guidelines can fail to provide adequate protection Poor laundering practices with reusable gowns may increase the risk of infection

Adapted from Refs. [20–22]

dental settings. Their effectiveness as barriers to microbial transmission was highlighted during the COVID-19 pandemic, which emphasised the need to reassess PPE priorities in clinical dentistry. Table 30.3 summarises the functions and limitations of medical gowns.

After confirming that saliva and the upper respiratory tract were reservoirs for SARS-CoV, it became clear that oral health workers faced a high risk of viral exposure. Researchers and regulatory authorities revisited gown protocols and updated evidence-based guidance on gown choice, performance, and sustainability [2, 23].

The World Health Organisation (WHO) advised that healthcare workers should consistently wear gowns when caring for patients with suspected or confirmed COVID-19, especially when there is a risk of exposure to bodily fluids. The guidelines stress that the entire body must be covered [24].

During the pandemic, either disposable or reusable gowns were worn in dental and clinical settings. The suitability of these gowns depended on their barrier effectiveness, the nature of the clinical procedure, the number of patients, and access to laundry facilities. Table 30.4 summarises the considerations that influenced the clinical relevance of each type, along with their economic and environmental impacts.

Table 30.4 Comparative overview of the clinical, economic, and environmental considerations of disposable and reusable gowns in dental infection control during COVID-19

Feature	Disposable gowns	Reusable gowns
Material composition	Non-woven polypropylene (SMS: Spunbond-Meltblown-Spunbond)	Polyester or polyester-cotton blends
Intended use	Single-use only; ideal for high-risk, aerosol-generating procedures	Reused after laundering; suitable for routine or moderate-risk procedures
Regulatory standards	Must meet ANSI/AAMI PB70 Level 2+ or EN 14126/ISO 16604 for biological risk	Must meet ANSI/AAMI PB70 initially Performance may decline over repeated washes
Barrier performance	High fluid resistance when new	Maintains fluid resistance over 75–100 washes Some decline in tear strength
Infection control evidence	Reuse is associated with 2× higher infection rates	When properly maintained, offer comparable protection
Donning & doffing	Faster donning/doffing; disposable after each use	Requires proper laundering protocols; doffing protocols are still essential
Cost implications	High cost during pandemic; price spike up to 2000% [25]	Long-term cost savings; up to 50% reduction in gown expenditure
Environmental impact	High medical waste contribution	Lower environmental footprint; reduced waste, energy, and water usage
Feasibility in resource-limited areas	Limited use due to recurring procurement costs and disposal needs	Feasible and acceptable in low-resource settings

Adapted from Refs. [25–27]

30.3 Procedural Innovations: Aerosol Minimisation and Equipment Use

30.3.1 Rubber Dams

Rubber dams have re-emerged as a method to reduce aerosolised contaminants generated by AGPs, including high-speed drills and ultrasonic scalers. Table 30.5 summarises key findings from studies assessing the effectiveness of rubber dams in limiting aerosol spread and bacterial contamination in dental settings.

Rubber dams are cost-effective, simple to implement, and efficient at isolating aerosols and particles, making them ideally suited for resource-constrained environments.

Although evidence linking rubber dams to reduced SARS-CoV-2 transmission is limited, changes in bacterial and particulate contamination can act as surrogate indicators. When combined with HVE and proper PPE, rubber dams are a cost-effective strategy to improve safety in dental practice.

30.3.2 High-Volume Evacuators (HVE)

HVEs, intraoral suction systems, are designed to remove aerosols and have become vital in decreasing airborne contamination. When positioned correctly, HVEs can eliminate up to 90% of aerosols. Their effectiveness is significantly boosted when used together with extraoral vacuum aspirators (EOVA) [31]. Together, they capture residual splatter and droplet spread in the clinical environment. Table 30.6 summarises the evidence supporting suction systems used for aerosol reduction in dental practice.

Table 30.5 Effectiveness of rubber dams

Study	Intervention	Key findings	Clinical implications
Samaranayake et al. (1989) [28]	Rubber dam use during dental procedures	Approximately 70% decrease in contaminated aerosol concentrations within a 3-meter radius	Significant decrease in aerosol spread in clinical areas
Scott et al. (2020) [29]	Rubber dam use	Between 80 and 99% decrease in bacterial contamination on surrounding surfaces 33% decrease in aerosol/droplet spread within 1 meter of the patient	Effective in limiting bacterial aerosol and droplet dispersion
Nasiri (2020) [30]	Rubber dam + high-volume evacuation (HVE)	Significant reduction in ultrafine aerosol particles generated during AGPs	Supports a layered infection control

Adapted from Refs. [28–30]

Table 30.6 Evidence supporting intraoral and extraoral suction for aerosol reduction in dentistry

Study	Methodology	Intervention	Key findings	Implications
Suwandi et al. (2022) [32]	Simulation study	HVE alone and HVE + EOVA	Significantly reduced contamination among clinicians Combination HVE + EOVA is more effective	A combination of suction devices enhances protection for dental staff
Kim et al. (2023) [33].	Laser light-sheet analysis	Intraoral HVE	Minimised lateral and vertical aerosol dispersion	Controls aerosol spread during procedures
Wang et al. (2025) [31]	Experimental particle measurement	HVE + EOVA	98% reduction in aerosol particles (0.3–10 μm)	Validates the combined suction approach for mitigating airborne viral transmission

Adapted from Refs. [31–33]

These findings support current infection control guidelines, which advocate a layered strategy integrating intraoral and extraoral suction, adequate ventilation, and consistent PPE use.

30.3.3 Mouth Rinses

The COVID-19 pandemic prompted an interest in the use of antiseptic mouthwashes as a preventive strategy to reduce viral load in the oral cavity.

Evidence supports the effectiveness of certain formulations in temporarily reducing the SARS-CoV-2 load in saliva, thereby decreasing the risk of transmission. However, this effect is brief and should be seen as an additional measure, not a replacement, for standard personal protective equipment (PPE) and established infection control protocols [34, 35].

A Bayesian network meta-analysis conducted by Seijas-Otero et al. (2025) evaluated the effectiveness of 16 oral and nasal antiseptics across 26 studies. Among these, the most active were povidone-iodine (PVP-I), hydrogen peroxide (H_2O_2), and chlorhexidine (CHX). PVP-I emerged as the most effective (SUCRA = 0.85), followed by cetylpyridinium chloride (CPC) and CHX (SUCRA = 0.72), with H_2O_2 (SUCRA = 0.70). Compared to control groups, only PVP-I achieved statistical significance, showing a 34% reduction in viral load [36]. These findings were supported by Espejo-Carrera et al. (2025), who carried out a systematic review and meta-analysis of 16 clinical trials evaluating PVP-I, PVP-V, CHX, and CPC. PVP-I demonstrated a statistically significant reduction in SARS-CoV-2 viral load, whereas CPC and CHX showed contrasting results [37].

Current findings suggest that PVP-I is the most promising agent available for reducing salivary viral load.

30.4 Clinic Design and Environmental Controls

30.4.1 Air Purification Systems

The COVID-19 pandemic accelerated the rapid deployment and testing of air purification systems. Research shows that combining multiple technologies is more effective than using single methods. Table 30.7 summarises the effectiveness and limitations of both combined and individual air purification systems.

30.4.2 Operatory Ventilation Spacing and Follow Time Between Patients

During the COVID-19 pandemic, dental and medical facilities implemented specific protocols, including a follow-up interval. This is the time period needed between patients to allow aerosols to settle, clear, and minimise viral transmission during aerosol-generating procedures [44].

Implementing extraoral high-volume air evacuation devices (HVAED) offers a solution to the prolonged fallow time required between patients during aerosol-generating procedures (AGPs). Haseeb et al. (2023) found that without HVAED, the fallow time after AGPs was approximately 1 h. This significant interval between patients limited clinical throughput and reduced access to care. However, with the HVAED, fallow time was decreased to 15 min [43].

These devices therefore enhance safety by reducing airborne contamination and improve operational efficiency. Apart from improving general appointment throughput and other procedures such as examinations, restorations, and extractions, the most important gains were observed in AGPs. As ultrasonic scaling was the focus of the study, the procedure served as a practical benchmark for assessing aerosol control using these devices.

30.4.3 Ventilation

Building on this, adequate ventilation was consistently recognised as another vital element of infection control in dental and clinical environments. Deery [44] emphasised the importance of good airflow and suggested that these could be enhanced with the use of air cleaners and disinfection fogging systems.

Table 30.7 Comparative effectiveness of air purification technologies for reducing airborne viral particles and improving indoor air quality during COVID-19

Effectiveness category	Combined HEPA + UV-C + Ionizer)	Combined UV-C + filtration (portable air cleaner)	UV-C radiation alone	HEPA filtration alone	Negative pressure systems
Virus inactivation	>4-log reduction of aerosolised SARS-CoV-2 in 36 s	99.8% reduction of coronavirus model in 20 mins	Inactivated SARS-CoV-2 by RNA disruption	No direct inactivation (traps only)	Indirect—prevents airborne virus spread
Particulate matter removal (PM2.5)	Not directly reported	Likely improved due to the filtration component	97% (with 3D media + filtration)	39.9% lower PM2.5 in classrooms vs. standard filters	Achieved via a ventilation system (6–12 ACH)
Time to effect	36 s	20 min	Varies (requires direct exposure)	Continuous passive capture	Continuous with system in place
Limitations	Lab-based; real-world variability	May vary with virus type & room design	Poor penetration in dense filters; exposure angle limits	Traps but does not kill microbes	High infrastructure cost; not suitable for all settings
Best use case	Rapid viral load reduction in closed spaces	Mobile settings, clinics, classrooms	Supplemental disinfection in air ducts/surfaces	Classrooms, offices, general indoor air quality	Hospitals, isolation rooms

Adapted from Refs [38–42]

30.4.4 Contactless Workflow in Dentistry During COVID-19

During the COVID-19 pandemic, dental practices swiftly adopted contactless workflows and digital technologies to minimise physical contact and decrease disease transmission (Table 30.8).

Despite the efficiency of the contactless workflow, there were certain challenges, including concerns about diagnostic accuracy, technical reliability, privacy issues, and the need for adequate internet infrastructure and digital literacy [47].

Table 30.8 Examples of digital dental technologies used during the COVID-19 pandemic

Category	Description & tools used	Primary benefits
Teledentistry & virtual consultations	Telecommunications (video conferencing, mobile phone cameras) to conduct remote consultations, diagnosis, and treatment planning	Enabled remote patient management Assisted with COVID-19 screening and triage of dental emergencies
Digital check-in & communication	Online forms and instant messaging platforms replaced paper-based intake processes	Reduced in-person contact Improved real-time communication between patients and providers
Remote monitoring systems	Patients captured self-taken intraoral images (SELFIE models) from home, shared for professional review	Enabled treatment triage and self-monitoring Reduced unnecessary clinic visits

Adapted from Refs. [45–48]

30.5 Patient-Centred Protocols

During the COVID-19 pandemic, dental practices adopted comprehensive pre-appointment screening protocols to identify potentially infected patients before they entered the clinic (Table 30.9).

Table 30.9 Triage and screening methods implemented in dental settings during COVID-19

Screening approach	Description	Key strengths	Limitations/ considerations
Temperature & questionnaire screening	Pre-appointment temperature checks and symptom/exposure questionnaires are used to triage patients	Simple and rapid implementation Standardised across many practices	Unable to identify asymptomatic SARS-CoV-2
Multilayered screening processes	Combined symptom questionnaires, exposure history, and organisational eligibility criteria for in-person visits	Improved risk stratification Supported appointment decision-making	Relies on patient self-reporting
Teledentistry	Remote triage via virtual consultations prior to scheduling in-person care	Reduced unnecessary clinic visits Minimized exposure risk for staff and patients	Depends on patient access to technology
Standard operating procedures (SOPs)	Workplace-specific SOPs covered screening, hand hygiene, waiting room modifications, universal precautions, and vaccination checks	Ensured consistency and compliance Supported organisational infection control strategies	Required regular updating as guidance evolved
Testing protocols	RT-PCR or rapid antigen testing for patients and staff prior to appointments	Higher diagnostic accuracy Enhanced infection detection	Costly and logistically impractical in many settings
Best practice frameworks (3 Ps model)	Systematic approach based on *preparation, protection, and prevention* for patients and healthcare workers	Evidence-based framework Supported monitoring and communication of protocols	Required organisational commitment and oversight

Adapted from Refs. [49–52]

30.6 Conclusion

The COVID-19 pandemic has reshaped infection control protocols in dentistry. They highlight the need for a continually changing, risk-based approach. These have been clearly evident in the shift from standard precautions to the tiered PPE system, which strategically adapts to procedural risk. The comparative analysis of surgical masks and N95 respirators underscores that effective infection control relies not only on equipment but also on proper use and universal compliance. Universal masking, fit-tested respirators, and improved awareness of aerosol risks have become cornerstones of safer dental practice. As the sector adapts to a post-pandemic reality, these lessons provide a blueprint for future resilience and preparedness in dental infection control.

References

1. Harrel SK, Molinari J. Aerosols and splatter in dentistry: a brief review of the literature and infection control implications. J Am Dent Assoc [Internet]. 2004 [cited 2025 Dec 27];135(4):429–37. Available from: https://jada.ada.org/action/showFullText?pii=S0002817714612277
2. Ge ZY, Yang LM, Xia JJ, Fu XH, Zhang YZ. Possible aerosol transmission of COVID-19 and special precautions in dentistry. J Zhejiang University-SCI B [Internet]. 2020 [cited 2025 Dec 27];21(5):361–8. Available from: https://link.springer.com/article/10.1631/jzus.B2010010
3. Diaz KT, Smaldone GC. Quantifying exposure risk: surgical masks and respirators. Am J Infect Control. 2010;38(7):501–8.
4. Mulder R, Layloo N, van Staden SM. COVID-19: focus on masks and respirators - implications for oral health-care workers. South African Dent J. 2020;75(4)
5. D'Alessandro A, MM. Proper N95 respirator use for respiratory protection preparedness [Internet]. 2020 [cited 2026 Jan 14]. Available from: https://blogs.cdc.gov/niosh-science-blog/2020/03/16/n95-preparedness/
6. Andrejko KL, Pry JM, Myers JF, Fukui N, DeGuzman JL, Openshaw J, et al. Effectiveness of face mask or respirator use in indoor public settings for prevention of SARS-CoV-2 infection — California, February–December 2021. MMWR Morb Mortal Wkly Rep [Internet]. 2025 [cited 2026 Jan 14];71(6):212–6. Available from: https://www.cdc.gov/mmwr/volumes/71/wr/mm7106e1.htm
7. Smith JD, MacDougall CC, Johnstone J, Copes RA, Schwartz B, Garber GE. Effectiveness of N95 respirators versus surgical masks in protecting health care workers from acute respiratory infection: a systematic review and meta-analysis. CMAJ [Internet]. 2016 [cited 2026 Jan 11];188(8):567–74. Available from: https://www.cmaj.ca/content/188/8/567.
8. Rengasamy S, Shaffer R, Williams B, Smit S. A comparison of facemask and respirator filtration test methods. J Occup Environ Hyg [Internet]. 2017 [cited 2026 Jan 11];14(2):92–103. Available from: https://www.tandfonline.com/doi/pdf/10.1080/15459624.2016.1225157
9. Asadi S, Cappa CD, Barreda S, Wexler AS, Bouvier NM, Ristenpart WD. Efficacy of masks and face coverings in controlling outward aerosol particle emission from expiratory activities. Sci Rep. 2020;10:1 [Internet]. 2020 [cited 2026 Jan 11];10(1):15665-. Available from: https://www.nature.com/articles/s41598-020-72798-7
10. Chou R, Dana T, Jungbauer R, Weeks C. Update alert 4: masks for prevention of respiratory virus infections, including SARS-CoV-2, in health care and community settings. [Internet]. 2020 [cited 2026 Jan 11];174(2):W24. Available from: https://doi.org/10.7326/L20-1429.

11. Howard J, Huang A, Li Z, Tufekci Z, Zdimal V, van der Westhuizen HM, et al. An evidence review of face masks against COVID-19. Proc Natl Acad Sci U S A [Internet]. 2021 [cited 2026 Jan 11];118(4):e2014564118. Available from: https://doi.org/10.1073/pnas.2014564118.
12. de Araujo CM, Guariza-Filho O, Gonçalves FM, Basso IB, Schroder AGD, Cavalcante-Leão BL, et al. Front lines of the COVID-19 pandemic: what is the effectiveness of using personal protective equipment in health service environments?—a systematic review. Int Arch Occup Environ Health. 2021 95:1 [Internet]. 2021 [cited 2025 Dec 28];95(1):7–24. Available from: https://link.springer.com/article/10.1007/s00420-021-01775-y
13. Skibitskyi VS, Ryzhova IP. Prevalence of eye injuries in the professional practice of a dentist and their prevention. Part 1. Act Dent [Internet]. 2025 [cited 2025 Dec 28];124(1):55–9. Available from: https://dentalexpert.com.ua/index.php/stomatology/article/view/685
14. Manzar S, Kazmi F, Shahzad H Bin, Qureshi FA, Shahbaz M, Rashid S. Estimation of the risk of COVID-19 transmission through aerosol-generating procedures. Dent Med Probl [Internet]. 2022 [cited 2025 Dec 28];59(3):351–6. Available from: https://pubmed.ncbi.nlm.nih.gov/36128802/
15. Brunello G, Gurzawska-Comis K, Becker K, Becker J, Sivolella S, Schwarz F, et al. Dental care during COVID-19 pandemic: follow-up survey of experts' opinion. Clin Oral Implants Res [Internet]. 2021 [cited 2025 Dec 28];32(S21):342–52. Available from: https://doi.org/10.1111/clr.13783.
16. Matys J, Grzech-Leśniak K. Dental aerosol as a hazard risk for dental workers. Materials. 2020 [Internet]. 2020 [cited 2025 Dec 28];13(22):5109. Available from: https://www.mdpi.com/1996-1944/13/22/5109/htm
17. Kaufmann M, Solderer A, Gubler A, Wegehaupt FJ, Attin T, Schmidlin PR. Quantitative measurements of aerosols from air-polishing and ultrasonic devices: (How) can we protect ourselves? PLoS One [Internet]. 2020 [cited 2025 Dec 28];15(12):e0244020. Available from: https://journals.plos.org/plosone/article?id=10.1371/journal.pone.0244020
18. Ng JH, Daniel D, Sadovoy A, Teo CEH. Eye protection in ENT practice during the COVID-19 pandemic. OTO Open [Internet]. 2021 [cited 2025 Dec 28];5(2):2473974X211010408. Available from: https://doi.org/10.1177/2473974X211010408.
19. Ferreira MVL, de Souza LN. High power laser use in the COVID-19 pandemic era in dentistry: tips for the readers. Lasers Dent Sci. 2020;4:3 [Internet]. 2020 Aug 9 [cited 2025 Dec 28];4(3):165–6. Available from: https://link.springer.com/article/10.1007/s41547-020-00102-x
20. Caggiano M, Acerra A, Martina S, Galdi M, D'Ambrosio F. Infection control in dental practice during the COVID-19 Pandemic: what is changed? Int J Environ Res Public Health. 2023;20:3903 [Internet]. 2023 [cited 2026 Jan 13];20(5):3903. Available from: https://www.mdpi.com/1660-4601/20/5/3903/htm
21. Coronavirus Disease 2019 (COVID-19) | COVID-19 | CDC [Internet]. [cited 2025 Dec 27]. Available from: https://www.cdc.gov/covid/?CDC_AAref_Val=https://www.cdc.gov/coronavirus/2019-ncov/hcp/dental-settings.html
22. U.S. Food and Drug Administration (FDA). Medical gowns. [online] U.S. Department of Health & Human Services [Internet]; 2024 [cited 2026 Jan 13]. Available from: https://www.fda.gov/medical-devices/personal-protective-equipment-infection-control/medical-gowns?utm_source=chatgpt.com
23. Meng L, Hua F, Bian Z. Coronavirus disease 2019 (COVID-19): emerging and future challenges for dental and oral medicine. J Dent Res [Internet]. 2020 [cited 2025 Dec 27];99(5):481–7. Available from: https://pubmed.ncbi.nlm.nih.gov/32162995/
24. World Health Organization (WHO). Rational use of personal protective equipment for coronavirus disease (COVID-19) and considerations during severe shortages. [pdf] [Internet]; 2020 [cited 2026 Jan 13]. Available from: https://iris.who.int/bitstream/handle/10665/331695/WHO-2019-nCov-IPC_PPE_use-2020.3-eng.pdf. Accessed 13 Jan 2026.
25. Baker N, Bromley-Dulfano R, Chan J, Gupta A, Herman L, Jain N, et al. COVID-19 solutions are climate solutions: lessons from reusable gowns. Front Public Health [Internet]. 2020 [cited 2025 Dec 28];8:590275. Available from: www.frontiersin.org

26. Limani F, Garley D, Cocker D, Patel P, Patel P, Gordon S, et al. Lessons learnt from the rapid implementation of reusable personal protective equipment for COVID-19 in Malawi. BMJ Glob Health [Internet]. 2021 [cited 2025 Dec 28];6(9):6498. Available from: https://gh.bmj.com/content/6/9/e006498
27. Easter E, Dabbain S. An evaluation of the barrier and durability performance of reusable level 2 isolation gowns over their promoted service life. AATCC J Res [Internet]. 2024 [cited 2025 Dec 28];11(1):58–70. Available from: https://scholar.google.com/scholar_url?url=https://journals.sagepub.com/doi/pdf/10.1177/24723444231212950&hl=en&sa=T&oi=ucasa&ct=ufr&ei=-U5RacTjGNrJieoPiYyysAk&scisig=ALhkC2QqgPb_Zv5AD3qvXxy0amq2
28. Samaranayake LP, Reid J, Evans D. The efficacy of rubber dam isolation in reducing atmospheric bacterial contamination. ASDC J Dent Child. 1989;56(6):442–4.
29. Scott D, Hogan T, John J. Rubber dam evidence. Br Dent J [Internet]. 2020 [cited 2025 Dec 28];229(3):150. Available from: https://www.nature.com/articles/s41415-020-2011-y
30. Nasiri K. The role of rubber dam in preventing coronavirus diseases 2019 (Covid-19) in dentistry. Interv Pediatric Dent Open Access J. 2020;4(4).
31. Wang CT, Yang G, Chao CYH, Fu SC. Effective control of dental aerosols and splatters via commercial extraoral suction and an innovative design with an annular air curtain. Indoor Built Environ [Internet]. 2025 [cited 2025 Dec 29];34(7):1305–21. Available from: https://scholar.google.com/scholar_url?url=https://journals.sagepub.com/doi/pdf/10.1177/1420326X251331390%3Fcasa_token%3DXIvs5ZpkjYYAAAAA:_vBLiLN2pJn9mgjih034qef5lCY-fJiKc9gkwnxnOaYLz3Ti0H28rE2pfYnUGGWiE6-x1Y0_TeQju&hl=en&sa=T&oi=ucasa&ct=ucasa&ei=yapRaaDjEa-nieoPz8HDqAc&scisig=ALhkC2TkwKNgI7EhgmjUEGyQfQr3
32. Suwandi T, Nursolihati V, Sundjojo M, Widyarman AS. The efficacy of high-volume evacuators and extraoral vacuum aspirators in reducing aerosol and droplet in ultrasonic scaling procedures during the COVID-19 pandemic. Eur J Dent [Internet]. 2022 [cited 2025 Dec 28];16(04):803–8. Available from: http://www.thieme-connect.de/products/ejournals/html/10.1055/s-0041-1739448
33. Kim MJ, Kuroda M, Kobayashi Y, Yamamoto T, Aizawa T, Satoh K. Visualization of airborne droplets generated with dental handpieces and verification of the efficacy of high-volume evacuators: an in vitro study. BMC Oral Health 2023;23:1 [Internet]. 2023 Dec 7 [cited 2025 Dec 29];23(1):976. Available from: https://link.springer.com/article/10.1186/s12903-023-03725-1
34. Ebrahimi T, Shamshiri AR, Alebouyeh M, Mohebbi SZ. Effectiveness of mouthwashes on reducing SARS-CoV-2 viral load in oral cavity: a systematic review and meta-analysis. BMC Oral Health [Internet]. 2023 [cited 2026 Jan 14];23(1):443. Available from: https://pmc.ncbi.nlm.nih.gov/articles/PMC10318743/
35. Sánchez Barrueco Á, Mateos-Moreno MV, Martínez-Beneyto Y, García-Vázquez E, Campos González A, Zapardiel Ferrero J, et al. Effect of oral antiseptics in reducing SARS-CoV-2 infectivity: evidence from a randomized double-blind clinical trial. Emerg Microbes Infect [Internet]. 2022 [cited 2026 Jan 14];11(1):1833. Available from: https://pmc.ncbi.nlm.nih.gov/articles/PMC9336498/
36. Seijas-Otero N, Blanco-Pintos T, Regueira-Iglesias A, Suárez-Rodríguez B, Sánchez-Barco A, Balsa-Castro C, et al. Antiseptics as effective virucidal agents against SARS-CoV-2: systematic review and Bayesian network meta-analysis. Jpn Dent Sci Rev [Internet]. 2025 [cited 2025 Dec 28];61:138–54. Available from: https://www.sciencedirect.com/science/article/pii/S1882761625000092
37. Espejo-Carrera RE, Asmat-Abanto AS, Carruitero-Honores MJ, Caballero-Alvarado JA. Effectiveness of mouthwashes to reduce the SARS-COV-2 load in saliva of adults with diagnosis of COVID-19: systematic review and meta-analysis. J Clin Exp Dent [Internet]. 2025 [cited 2025 Dec 28];17(1):e96. Available from: https://pmc.ncbi.nlm.nih.gov/articles/PMC11829719/
38. Liu J, Liu J, Fan Y, Wang P. Combination of UV radiation with 3D structure media filter for indoor air disinfection. E3S Web Conf [Internet]. 2022 [cited 2026 Jan 11];356:05054. Available from: https://www.e3s-conferences.org/articles/e3sconf/abs/2022/23/e3sconf_roomvent2022_05054/e3sconf_roomvent2022_05054.html

39. Li P, Koziel JA, Macedo N, Zimmerman JJ, Wrzesinski D, Sobotka E, et al. Evaluation of an air cleaning device equipped with filtration and UV: comparison of removal efficiency on particulate matter and viable airborne bacteria in the inlet and treated air. Int J Environ Res Public Health [Internet]. 2022 [cited 2026 Jan 11];19(23):16135. Available from: https://www.mdpi.com/1660-4601/19/23/16135/htm
40. Reissner J, Reichelt B, Siller P, Brockmann G, Kriegel M, Roesler U, et al. Evaluation of the decontamination efficacy of a portable air cleaner using 275-nm UVC-LED radiation against airborne Coronavirus and Influenza virus. GMS Hyg Infect Control [Internet]. 2025 [cited 2026 Jan 11];20:Doc44. Available from: https://pubmed.ncbi.nlm.nih.gov/40979864/
41. Law CK, Lai JHK, Sze-To RGN, Tuttle RS, Solocinski K, Wilkinson JE, et al. Efficacy of flow-through air purification device in removing aerosolized SARS-CoV-2. Indoor Air [Internet]. 2025 [cited 2026 Jan 10];2025(1):6684377. Available from: https://doi.org/10.1155/ina/6684377.
42. Simona SC, Bartell SM, Vieira VM. Classroom air quality in a randomized crossover trial with portable HEPA air cleaners. J Expo Sci Environ Epidemiol. 2025;35:4 [Internet]. 2025 [cited 2026 Jan 11];35(4):644–8. Available from: https://www.nature.com/articles/s41370-025-00743-9
43. Haseeb M, Khalid N, Syed AUY, Khan ZA, Qureshi F, Ahsen I. The standard operating procedures in COVID-19 Pandemic for periodontal aerosol-generating procedures: a process audit. Eur J Dent [Internet]. 2023 [cited 2026 Jan 11];17(4):1084–8. Available from: http://www.thieme-connect.de/products/ejournals/html/10.1055/s-0042-1758067
44. Deery C. The legal position of delivering dental care in a time of COVID-19. Evid Based Dent [Internet]. 2021 [cited 2026 Jan 11];22(2):84. Available from: https://www.nature.com/articles/s41432-021-0180-4
45. Deshpande S, Patil D, Dhokar A, Bhanushali P, Katge F. Teledentistry: a boon amidst COVID-19 lockdown—a narrative review. Int J Telemed Appl [Internet]. 2021 [cited 2026 Jan 11];2021:8859746. Available from: https://pmc.ncbi.nlm.nih.gov/articles/PMC7894051/
46. Singhal S, Mohapatra S, Quiñonez C. Reviewing teledentistry usage in Canada during COVID-19 to determine possible future opportunities. Int J Environ Res Public Health. 2022;19:31 [Internet]. 2021 [cited 2026 Jan 11];19(1):31. Available from: https://www.mdpi.com/1660-4601/19/1/31/htm
47. Bhuyan L, Mahapatra N, Dhull KS, Doddawad VG, Sahoo N, Panda A. Tele dentistry - its practical applicability, hurdles and future prospects. Bangladesh J Med Sci [Internet]. 2023 [cited 2026 Jan 11];22(Special Issue):52–7. Available from: https://www.banglajol.info/index.php/BJMS/article/view/66307
48. Xiao J, Kopycka-Kedzierawski D, Ragusa P, Mendez Chagoya LA, Funkhouser K, Lischka T, et al. Acceptance and usability of an innovative mDentistry eHygiene model amid the COVID-19 pandemic within the US National Dental Practice-Based Research Network: mixed methods study. JMIR Hum Factors [Internet]. 2023 [cited 2026 Jan 11];10(1):e45418. Available from: http://www.ncbi.nlm.nih.gov/pubmed/37594795.
49. Nathwani S, Rahman N. The 3 P's model enhancing patient safety during the COVID-19 pandemic. Oral Surg [Internet]. 2021 [cited 2026 Jan 11];14(3):246–54. Available from: https://doi.org/10.1111/ors.12607.
50. Pittayapat P, Ampornaramveth R, Jirachoksopon C, Suvarnbriksha K, Kattapong S, Pethprasert T, et al. Procedures used in managing SARS-CoV-2 infected dental personnel or patients: a case study from a Thai dental hospital. Front Oral Health [Internet]. 2021 [cited 2026 Jan 11];2:750394. Available from: www.frontiersin.org
51. Hung M, Lipsky MS, Phuatrakoon TN, Nguyen M, Licari FW, Unni EJ. Teledentistry implementation during the COVID-19 pandemic: scoping review. Interact J Med Res [Internet]. 2022 [cited 2026 Jan 11];11(2):e39955. Available from: https://www.i-jmr.org/2022/2/e39955
52. Kajal K, Mohammadnezhad M. Organizational preventative strategies undertaken by dental clinics in Fiji during COVID-19 pandemic: a qualitative study. Open Dent J. 2022;17(1)

Recommended COVID-19 Guidelines for Dental Service

31

Sue-Ching Yeoh

Objective

To present a concise, evidence-based set of guidelines that enable dental professionals to deliver safe and effective care while minimising the risk of COVID-19 transmission.

Scope and Relevance

These recommendations extend beyond emergency response. They offer a framework for preparedness, ongoing audit, and continuous refinement of clinical protocols. The chapter demonstrates a commitment to safety, adaptability, and the enduring importance of oral health care in public health systems.

31.1 Introduction and Rationale

The COVID-19 pandemic significantly changed healthcare delivery worldwide. Dental services were particularly affected due to the inherent risk of aerosol generation and close patient contact [1]. Although the worst phase of the pandemic has now passed, the ongoing presence of SARS-CoV-2 and other respiratory pathogens requires ongoing vigilance and strict adherence to infection prevention and control (IPC) guidelines.

S.-C. Yeoh (✉)
Sydney Dental School, Faculty of Medicine and Health, The University of Sydney, Sydney, Australia
e-mail: sue-ching.yeoh@sydney.edu.au

S. R. Prabhu et al. (eds.), *COVID-19 in Dental Practice*,
https://doi.org/10.1007/978-3-032-26000-0_31

The protocols enhanced during the pandemic have become integral to universal precautions, serving as a critical defence against a broad spectrum of infectious agents [1]. This represents a fundamental shift from a reactive to a proactive approach to managing communicable diseases in the dental setting.

Many dental procedures produce fine mists of aerosols and droplets from high-speed handpieces, ultrasonic scalers, and air-water syringes [2, 3]. These airborne particles, containing saliva, blood, and other bodily fluids, can carry various micro-organisms, including viruses and bacteria. The fundamental challenge is inherent in dental work itself: it occurs in the most pathogen-rich environment of the human body—the mouth. The mechanical action of dental instruments, especially those operating at high speeds, propels this bio-rich fluid into the surrounding air, forming an invisible cloud of potential contagions [4]. Therefore, maintaining the highest IPC standards is essential, regardless of the current COVID-19 alert level. The lessons learned have cemented IPC as an integral and vital part of quality dental care [1]. This chapter offers comprehensive guidance based on recommendations from authoritative sources, including the World Health Organisation (WHO), the Centres for Disease Control and Prevention (CDC), and national dental associations [5–9].

31.2 Infection Prevention and Control (IPC)

A successful IPC strategy for dental services relies on several core principles. These principles are not separate steps but form an integrated framework aimed at providing multiple layers of protection.

31.2.1 Standard Precautions and Enhanced PPE Use

Use of appropriate personal protective equipment (PPE) by all healthcare staff is mandatory. The level of PPE required will correlate with the assessed risk of exposure to infectious agents and the nature of the necessary procedure. PPE acts as a physical barrier between the healthcare worker and potential pathogens [10].

For routine non-aerosol-generating procedures (non-AGPs):

- Disposable clean gloves are changed between patients and after touching any contaminated surface
- Level 2 or 3 surgical masks changed if wet/soiled, and between every patient [10]
- Full face shield or safety glasses with side shields for protection against splatter and splashes

For all aerosol-generating procedures (AGPs):

- N95 or P2 respirators that are fit tested to ensure a proper seal, providing superior filtration [11]
- Fluid-resistant gowns with long sleeves and cuffed wrists
- Full face shield in addition to the respirator
- Disposable gloves

31.2.2 Hand Hygiene Protocols

Hand hygiene is the most effective method for preventing the spread of infection and is a fundamental part of IPC protocols [12]. Proper hand hygiene must be performed at key points during patient care. Hands must be washed:

- Before and after direct contact with any patient
- Before performing any aseptic procedure
- After removing gloves or any PPE
- After touching a patient's immediate environment
- Before handling clean equipment

Hand hygiene can be achieved through handwashing with soap and water for at least 20 s, or by using an alcohol-based hand rub with at least 60% alcohol content [12, 13]. Alcohol-based hand rubs are effective when hands are not visibly soiled and are preferred in most clinical situations due to their superior antimicrobial activity.

31.2.3 Aerosol-Generating Procedures: Risk Stratification and Mitigation

The most significant potential risk of transmission is associated with Aerosol-Generating Procedures (AGPs), which generate airborne particulate matter. AGPs include the use of high-speed handpieces, ultrasonic scalers, air polishing devices, and air-water syringes [2, 3, 8]. Whenever possible, the use of non-AGPs should be prioritised as a primary risk-reduction measure.

When AGPs are necessary, risk mitigation protocols include:

- Mandatory use of appropriate enhanced PPE (N95/P2 respirator, fluid-resistant gown, face shield) [10, 11]
- Environmental engineering controls, including HEPA filtration systems that capture at least 99.97% of airborne particles 0.3 micrometres in size [14]

- Optimised clinical teamwork using four-handed dentistry practices and high-volume suction (HVS) [15]
- Consistent and effective use of rubber dam isolation of the operative site [4]
- Administration of antiseptic pre-procedural mouth rinse (1% hydrogen peroxide or 0.2% povidone-iodine) for 30–60 s [16]

31.2.4 Surface Disinfection and Sterilisation Protocols

All clinical surfaces must be cleaned and disinfected with hospital-grade disinfectants effective against SARS-CoV-2 and other pathogens [5, 17]. Surfaces should be cleaned between each patient. All reusable dental instruments and devices must be sterilised in accordance with established protocols. Single-use items must be appropriately disposed of and never reused.

31.2.5 Ventilation and Air Filtration Recommendations

Advanced ventilation and air-purification systems are vital environmental-engineering controls. Installing HEPA filters that can capture at least 99.97% of airborne particles 0.3 micrometres in size is essential [14, 18]. These systems operate by continuously purifying the air in a room, thereby decreasing the concentration of airborne viral particles. Adequate ventilation with increased air changes per hour and proper directional airflow patterns should be maintained.

31.3 Patient Management and Scheduling

31.3.1 Pre-appointment Screening

Effective patient screening forms the first line of defence against the introduction and transmission of infection in the dental setting [19, 20]. Screening should commence before the patient's appointment by using online forms or phone calls to inquire about:

- Current respiratory symptoms
- Recent travel history
- Recent high-risk exposure to COVID-19
- Vaccination status

This pre-screening process facilitates early detection of potential risks and supports making informed decisions regarding scheduling and treatment protocols.

31.3.2 Tele-Triage and Remote Consultations

Consideration of teledentistry in select circumstances may be a valuable tool in reducing the risk of viral transmission while balancing the need for ongoing patient support [21]. Recent advances in secure videoconferencing platforms enable remote consultations, non-emergency assessments, follow-up appointments, patient education, and pre-treatment discussions, thereby reducing the need for in-person appointments and minimising potential exposure risks.

31.3.3 Appointment Spacing and Staggered Scheduling

Appointments should be spaced adequately to allow sufficient time for proper room turnover, cleaning, and disinfection between patients. Staggered scheduling helps minimise the number of people in the waiting area and reduces the risk of cross-contamination [22]. Consideration should be given to adequate air exchange time between appointments, particularly following AGPs.

31.3.4 Entry Protocols

The clinic entrance should display signage instructing patients with current respiratory symptoms not to enter [20]. Hand sanitiser or an alcohol-based hand rub should be available at the doorway to emphasise the importance of hand hygiene upon entry. Temperature checks may be introduced as an extra screening measure when community transmission rates are high.

31.3.5 Consent Updates and COVID-Specific Disclosures

Informed consent procedures should be revised to include COVID-19-specific information, such as acknowledgement of potential exposure risks, the introduction of enhanced infection control measures, and any alterations to standard treatment protocols [9]. Patients should be educated about their role in infection prevention, including the importance of disclosing symptoms and rescheduling if unwell.

31.4 Clinic Layout and Workflow Modifications

31.4.1 Waiting Room Redesign

Waiting areas should be rearranged to ensure physical distancing with at least 1.5 metres between seats [22]. Clear signage should be displayed to inform about respiratory hygiene, hand hygiene, and physical distancing measures. Physical barriers, such as plexiglass screens at reception desks, offer extra protection. The number of seats should be decreased to avoid crowding, and patients should be advised to wait outside or in their vehicles whenever possible until their appointment.

31.4.2 Clinical Zoning

Clinical zoning involves creating 'clean' and 'contaminated' zones within the practice to minimise cross-contamination [23]. This includes:

- Dedicated areas for donning and doffing PPE, separate from the clinical space
- Clear separation between patient treatment areas and staff break areas
- Designated pathways for the movement of contaminated materials
- Isolation rooms for patients with suspected or confirmed respiratory infections requiring emergency dental care

31.4.3 Staff Rotation and Cohorting Strategies

Staff rotation and cohorting strategies can help reduce exposure and ensure workforce continuity. This involves organising staff into consistent teams that work together, which decreases the number of contacts within the practice. In the event of an outbreak, this method helps limit the number of staff needing to isolate.

31.4.4 Digital Documentation and Contactless Payment Systems

Digital documentation systems should be adopted to lessen the use of paper forms and reduce contact points. Contactless payment options ought to be provided to decrease physical handling of payment cards and cash. Electronic communication methods should be employed for appointment reminders, consent forms, and post-treatment instructions.

31.5 Prioritisation of Dental Care

31.5.1 Classification of Urgent, Emergent, and Elective Procedures

Dental procedures should be classified according to urgency [6, 9]:

Emergency procedures (life-threatening conditions requiring immediate treatment): uncontrolled bleeding, cellulitis or soft tissue infection with systemic involvement, trauma involving facial bones with potential airway compromise.

Urgent procedures (requiring prompt treatment to relieve severe pain or infection risk): severe dental pain, pericoronitis, dental abscess, and post-operative complications.

Elective Procedures (non-urgent routine care): routine cleanings, preventive care, cosmetic procedures, and non-symptomatic restorative work.

31.5.2 Deferral Criteria for Non-essential Treatments

Non-urgent dental treatment should be postponed for patients with confirmed or suspected respiratory infections, including COVID-19 [5, 24]. This is an essential measure to safeguard staff and other patients. The decision to postpone treatment should be based on:

- Current community transmission rates
- Patient's health status and risk factors
- Urgency of the dental condition
- Availability of appropriate PPE and infection control measures

31.5.3 Management of Dental Emergencies

Emergency dental care for patients with confirmed or suspected respiratory infections should be performed in dedicated isolation rooms using full AGP-level PPE (N95/P2 respirator, fluid-resistant gown, and face shield) [5, 11]. The room should be thoroughly cleaned and disinfected after the appointment, with re-occupancy only allowed once sufficient air changes have occurred to remove any remaining airborne particles.

31.6 Staff Health and Vaccination

31.6.1 Staff Vaccination Policies

All staff should be strongly encouraged to receive vaccinated against COVID-19, influenza, and other relevant communicable diseases [25]. This safeguards both staff and patients and ensures workforce continuity. Vaccination policies should be clearly communicated and documented, with booster doses administered in accordance with current public health guidelines.

31.6.2 Monitoring and Reporting of Symptoms

Staff should be educated and encouraged to monitor themselves for symptoms of illness. Clear policies for sick leave and guidelines for return-to-work should be established that align with current public health advice [24]. If unwell, staff members must stay home to prevent the transmission of illness to colleagues and patients. A precise reporting mechanism should be in place for staff to notify management of potential exposures or symptoms.

31.6.3 Mental Health and Burnout Support

The health and resilience of the dental team are essential to providing safe and effective services. The considerable stress and psychological burden faced by healthcare workers during and after the COVID-19 pandemic must be recognised [26]. Practices should offer access to mental health support and promote a supportive work environment. Regular check-ins, peer support programmes, and access to professional counselling should be available to all staff members.

31.7 Ethical and Legal Considerations

31.7.1 Duty of Care vs. Risk to Providers

Dental professionals have a duty of care to their patients, but this must be balanced with their own right to a safe working environment [7]. Providing appropriate PPE, engineering controls, and administrative measures is essential to fulfilling this dual responsibility. Dental professionals are not expected to deliver care when proper safety measures are unavailable.

31.7.2 Informed Consent and Patient Autonomy

Patients must be fully informed about the risks of dental treatment during a pandemic, including the possibility of exposure to infectious diseases despite all precautions [9]. They have the right to make autonomous decisions about their care, including the right to postpone non-urgent treatment. The consent process should ensure patients understand both the risks of proceeding with treatment and the risks of delaying it.

31.7.3 Compliance with Public Health Mandates

Dental practices must stay compliant with changing public health mandates and guidelines from local health authorities [5, 8]. Regularly reviewing current regulations and guidance documents is crucial to maintaining compliance. This includes following requirements related to vaccination, testing, isolation protocols, and case reporting.

31.7.4 Documentation for Medico-Legal Protection

Comprehensive documentation of infection control measures, risk assessments, patient screening, consent discussions, and any incidents is vital for medico-legal protection [19, 23]. Clear protocols and procedures for handling and disposing of clinical waste, including sharps and contaminated PPE, should be documented in accordance with local environmental regulations. Records should demonstrate that all reasonable precautions were taken to reduce the risk of transmission.

31.8 Post-Pandemic Transition and Legacy Practices

31.8.1 Phased Relaxation of Restrictions

As pandemic conditions evolve, restrictions may be gradually eased in phases. This process should be guided by local public health authorities and based on factors such as community transmission rates, healthcare capacity, and vaccination coverage [5, 8]. Nevertheless, core IPC principles should be maintained regardless of the pandemic stage.

31.8.2 Retention of Effective IPC Measures

Many of the enhanced IPC measures introduced during COVID-19 should be kept as standard practice [1, 27]. These include better hand hygiene, routine use of appropriate PPE for AGPs, improved environmental cleaning protocols, and upgraded ventilation systems. The lessons learned have shown that these measures protect not only against COVID-19 but also a wide range of infectious agents.

31.8.3 Integration of Telehealth and Digital Tools

The expanded use of teledentistry and digital tools during the pandemic has demonstrated their value in enhancing access to care and simplifying practice operations [21]. These tools should be incorporated into routine care where suitable, including for initial consultations, follow-up appointments, patient education, and some aspects of treatment planning.

31.8.4 Lessons Learned: Resilience, Adaptability, and Preparedness

The COVID-19 pandemic vividly demonstrated the dynamic and evolving nature of public health challenges. Dental practices must foster a culture of continuous learning and adaptability. It is essential to stay up-to-date with the latest recommendations from authoritative sources such as the World Health Organisation (WHO) and local health authorities [8]. Regular training and updates on IPC protocols for all staff should be provided, alongside ongoing review of current protocols and guidelines to ensure they remain current and reflect emerging research and experience. The commitment to a proactive, robust, and continuously evolving IPC framework is not merely a response to a past pandemic but a fundamental obligation in safeguarding public health and safety amid ongoing and future infectious disease threats.

31.9 Summary

By consistently applying these comprehensive, evidence-based guidelines, dental services can continue to offer essential oral healthcare safely and effectively. The protocols outlined in this chapter and summarised in the Table 31.1 represent a synthesis of current best practices for infection prevention and control in dental settings [1–27]. Although developed in response to COVID-19, these measures provide a framework for managing present and future infectious disease challenges. The commitment to upholding high standards of infection prevention and control ensures the safety of both patients and the dedicated professionals who serve them while supporting the ongoing delivery of quality dental care.

Table 31.1 Practical guidance summary

Area	Key actions
Personal protective equipment	Use N95/P2 respirators for all AGPs Ensure proper fit-testing of respirators Wear fluid-resistant gowns and full-face shields for AGPs Change gloves between patients and after contact with contaminated surfaces
Hand hygiene	Wash hands before and after patient contact Use alcohol-based hand rub (≥60% alcohol) when hands not visibly soiled Wash for at least 20 s with soap and water Perform hand hygiene after removing PPE
Patient screening	Screen patients before appointment via phone or online forms Ask about respiratory symptoms, exposure history, and vaccination status Defer non-urgent treatment for symptomatic patients Display signage instructing symptomatic patients not to enter
Aerosol mitigation	Use high-volume suction during all AGPs Apply rubber dam isolation when feasible Administer pre-procedural antiseptic mouth rinse (1% H_2O_2 or 0.2% povidone-iodine) Consider non-AGP alternatives when clinically appropriate

(continued)

Table 31.1 (continued)

Area	Key actions
Environmental controls	Install HEPA filtration systems (99.97% efficiency for 0.3 μm particles) Ensure adequate ventilation with increased air changes per hour Clean and disinfect all surfaces between patients Allow sufficient air change time after AGPs before room re-occupancy
Clinic workflow	Space appointments to allow adequate turnover time Create clinical zoning (clean and contaminated areas) Implement contactless payment and digital documentation Minimize waiting room occupancy through staggered scheduling
Staff health	Encourage vaccination against COVID-19 and influenza Establish clear sick leave policies aligned with public health advice Provide access to mental health support resources Conduct regular training on IPC protocols
Emergency care	Treat symptomatic patients requiring emergency care in dedicated isolation rooms Use full AGP-level PPE for emergency treatment of suspected cases Thoroughly clean and disinfect room after treatment Follow triage protocols to prioritize truly urgent cases
Documentation	Document all infection control measures and risk assessments Record patient screening results and consent discussions Maintain protocols for clinical waste disposal Keep records demonstrating compliance with current guidelines

References

1. Caggiano M, Acerra A, Martina S, Galdi M, D'Ambrosio F. Infection control in dental practice during the COVID-19 pandemic: what is changed? Int J Environ Res Public Health. 2023;20(5):3903.
2. Al-Yaseen W, Al-Yaseen W, Jones R, et al. Aerosol and splatter generation with rotary handpieces used in restorative and orthodontic dentistry: a systematic review. BDJ Open. 2022;8(1):26.
3. Lahdentausta L, Sanmark E, Lauretsalo S, et al. Aerosol concentrations and size distributions during clinical dental procedures. Heliyon. 2022;8(10):e11074.
4. Rathore K, Rathore HS, Singh P, Kumar P. Redefining aerosol in dentistry during COVID-19 pandemic. Dent Res J (Isfahan). 2022;19:53.
5. Centers for Disease Control and Prevention. Interim infection prevention and control recommendations for dental settings during the COVID-19 pandemic. Atlanta: CDC; 2023.
6. American Dental Association. ADA interim guidance for minimizing risk of COVID-19 transmission. Chicago: ADA; 2020.
7. The British Dental Association. COVID-19: a guide to risk assessment and management in dental practice. London: BDA; 2020.
8. World Health Organization. Interim guidance for dental services during the COVID-19 outbreak. Geneva: WHO; 2020.

9. Australian Dental Association. COVID-19: managing dental patients. Sydney: ADA; 2022.
10. World Health Organization. Rational use of personal protective equipment for coronavirus disease 2019 (COVID-19) and considerations during severe shortages. Geneva: WHO; 2020.
11. National Institute for Occupational Safety and Health. N95 respirators and surgical masks. Atlanta: NIOSH; 2023.
12. World Health Organization. WHO guidelines on hand hygiene in health care. Geneva: WHO; 2009.
13. Australian Commission on Safety and Quality in Health Care. National hand hygiene initiative. Sydney: ACSQHC; 2022.
14. American Society of Heating, Refrigerating and Air-Conditioning Engineers. ASHRAE guidance for building operations during the COVID-19 pandemic. Atlanta: ASHRAE; 2020.
15. Finkbeiner BL. Four-handed dentistry revisited. J Contemp Dent Pract. 2000;1(4):74–86.
16. Garcia-Sanchez A, Peña-Cardelles JF, Ordonez-Fernandez E, et al. Povidone-iodine as a preprocedural mouthwash to reduce the salivary viral load of SARS-CoV-2: a systematic review of randomized controlled trials. Int J Environ Res Public Health. 2022;19(5):2877.
17. Therapeutic Goods Administration. Australian regulatory guidelines for medical devices. Canberra: TGA; 2023.
18. Morawska L, Tang JW, Bahnfleth W, et al. How can airborne transmission of COVID-19 indoors be minimised? Environ Int. 2020;142:105832.
19. Australian Dental Association. ADA guidelines for dental practice. Sydney: ADA; 2021.
20. Public Health England. COVID-19: infection prevention and control dental appendix. London: PHE; 2021.
21. Lee J, Park JS, Feng B, Wang KN. The utilisation of teledentistry in Australia: a systematic review and meta-analysis. J Dent. 2024;149:105265.
22. Australian Government Department of Health. Physical distancing for COVID-19. Canberra: Australian Government; 2022.
23. The Dental Council of New Zealand. COVID-19: infection prevention and control practice. Wellington: DCNZ; 2021.
24. Australian Government Department of Health. Isolation and testing for COVID-19. Canberra: Australian Government; 2023.
25. World Health Organization. WHO SAGE roadmap for prioritizing uses of COVID-19 vaccines in the context of limited supply. Geneva: WHO; 2020.
26. American Dental Association. COVID-19 mental health resources. Chicago: ADA; 2022.
27. Kathree BA, Khan SB, Ahmed R, et al. COVID-19 and its impact in the dental setting: a scoping review. PLoS One. 2020;15(12):e0244352.

GPSR Compliance

The European Union's (EU) General Product Safety Regulation (GPSR) is a set of rules that requires consumer products to be safe and our obligations to ensure this.

If you have any concerns about our products, you can contact us on ProductSafety@springernature.com

In case Publisher is established outside the EU, the EU authorized representative is:

Springer Nature Customer Service Center GmbH
Europaplatz 3
69115 Heidelberg, Germany

Batch number: 10577050

Printed by Printforce, the Netherlands